Deconstructing Scandinavia's "Achievement Generation"

Ole Jacob Madsen

Deconstructing Scandinavia's "Achievement Generation"

A Youth Mental Health Crisis?

Translated by Diane Oatley

palgrave
macmillan

Ole Jacob Madsen
Department of Psychology
University of Oslo
Oslo, Oslo, Norway

Translated by
Diane Oatley
Oslo, Norway

ISBN 978-3-030-72554-9 ISBN 978-3-030-72555-6 (eBook)
https://doi.org/10.1007/978-3-030-72555-6

This Palgrave Macmillan imprint is published by the registered company Springer Nature Switzerland AG.
The registered company address is: Gewerbestrasse 11, 6330 Cham, Switzerland

Contents

1 Introduction 1
What's New? 6
How Are We, Really? 8
The Circle and the Line 12
Left and Right 14
A Diagnosis for Us—A Diagnosis for You 16
The Organization of This Book 17

2 The Pathologies of Modernity 19
Nietzsche's Last Human 21
Marx's Alienation 22
Durkheim's Anomie 24
Weber's Iron Cage 25
Freud's Discontentment Within Culture 27
Adorno and Horkheimer's Enlightenment 29
Fromm's Contentment in Culture 31
Rieff's Therapeutic Turn 33
Erikson's Identity Crisis 34
Mitscherlich's Fatherlessness 35
Conclusion: The Tragic View of Life 37

3 The Pathologies of Late Modernity 41
Ziehe's Society of Choices 43
Beck's Individualization 44
Bauman's Liquid Modernity 45
Rosa's Social Acceleration 46
We Are Not Thriving in Late Capitalism 48
Dufour's Anthropological Mutation 50
The Market as a New "God" 53
Between the Guilt and the Shame 54
Failure to Thrive in the New Millennium 56
Conclusion 64

4 Young, Privileged and Sick 67
Illness Experiences from Life in Late Modernity 71
Norway: "I Get So Afraid of Missing Out on Myself" 71
The Road to Depression 73
Self-Realization's Exhausting Downside 78
Optimization of the Self 80
Sweden: "You Should Really Make the Most of What You've Received" 83
Denmark: "You Bloody Well Better Perform Well in This Society, Right?" 85
Where Are We Now? 87
Somewhere Over the Rainbow 90
Conclusion 92

5 Youth Under Pressure 95
Suicide in Norway 97
Suicide Among Young People 98
Suicide Internationally 99
Suicide and Psychological Disorders 100
Psychological Disorders and Complaints 101
Psychological Complaints in Young People 104
Why the Increase in the Reporting of Psychological Complaints? 107
Which Group of Young People Is Hardest Hit? 110

Use of Medication 111
Self-Harm 112
Externalizing Behaviours 114
The New Digital Existence 118
Generational Differences 122
Conclusion 127

6 **Social Representations** 129
The Achievement Society 131
The Achievement Generation 140
Good Girl 148
The Good Girl: A Media History 150
The Good Girl Syndrome 154
Conclusion 167

7 **Self-Fulfilling Prophecies** 169
The Problem Without a Name 173
When the Meritocracy Came to Norway 177
Finally Somebody Who Understands Us 182
Students Provide a Causal Explanation 186
Identifying with the Research 188
Talking About It 189
Conclusion 191

8 **The Paradox of Health** 193
Cultural Oblivion 196
Scientific Myths 197
British Resistance 199
How Does Infection Occur? 201
The Illness Epidemic in Sweden 207
Reaping as We Sow 208
Professional Whistleblowing Systems 214
Double Reflexivity 218
Conclusion 222

9 Conclusion 225
Summing Up the Book 227
The Answer Is Served 229
The Unbearable Distortion of the Media Society 231
Media Templates 232
Media Favouritism 234
Skewed Reporting 235
The Reality 2.0 237
The Generation Label 238
Wanted: "The Stagnation Generation" 239
Left-Wing Media? 241
What Must Be Done? 243
A Good Enough Society 243
Different Medicine 244
The Disadvantaged Among Us 245
We Need to Talk About It 246
Life Sucks 248
Existentialism, Where Did You Go in the Midst of All the Chaos? 249
To the Root of the Problem 251
Silence Is Golden 252
Nothing New Under the Sun: The Youth of the Past 254
Don't Speak: The Young People of Today 257
Generation Screwed: The Young People of the Future 260
Conclusion: Overloading "Young People" 262

References 267

Index 297

1

Introduction

"LATE MODERN HUMANKIND is to be pitied" wrote Swedish journalist Kristofer Ahlström a few years ago,[1] echoing August Strindberg famous line from *A Dream Play*.[2] Yes, you have to pity the human race, but is this particularly true for the human population of our times? If we are to take seriously the widespread, universal concern for today's youth, this would appear to be the case. From a historical perspective, on the other hand, there is every reason to maintain that no generation ever before has had better conditions for self-realization. This antimony is the underlying theme of this book.

New Year's Eve 2016. In keeping with tradition, His Majesty King Harald of Norway gives a speech to the Norwegian people. On the last day of the year, he speaks about a special tree that was planted in the Palace Park the summer before: The Wishing Tree. On the branches of this tree, visitors could hang their hopes and wishes for Norway and the world. One of the wishes, written by a child, had read: "I wish that everyone would be kinder to themselves", which His Majesty selected as

[1] Kristofer Ahlström, "Jag är inte narcissist, men", *Dagens Nyheter*, 16 April 2017, 15.

[2] August Strindberg, *The dream play*, (1902), https://www.gutenberg.org/files/45375/45375-h/45375-h.htm

O. J. Madsen, *Deconstructing Scandinavia's "Achievement Generation"*,
https://doi.org/10.1007/978-3-030-72555-6_1

a particularly meaningful wish, the implication being that this is the right medicine for the particular challenges faced by the coming generation of young people:

> Many teenagers become psychologically and physically worn out by what they experience as the pressure of enormous requirements. But my impression is that we impose many of these requirements on ourselves. We quite simply wear ourselves out with thoughts of our own inadequacy.[3]

A bit later, His Majesty King Harald acknowledges the universal nature of this theme, but simultaneously expresses his agreement with the far more widespread perception that the problem is more serious today than ever before:

> Being a teenager has always been a challenge. But I feel sincere compassion for the young people of today who are faced with so many more choices and influences, so much more external pressure than was the case for the past two generations.[4]

Even readers in Norway who have paid only scant attention to newspaper headlines, research reports and other unanimous expressions of concern for the coming generation of recent years will be familiar with the ideas behind His Majesty's comments, because of the prevalence in the Norwegian media of labels such as *the achievement society, generation Y or Z, pathological perfection, a pathologically serious generation of youth and the good girl syndrome.* The basis for a number of these headlines is the Norwegian nationwide Ungdata study, which gathered the responses of half a million Norwegian thirteen- to nineteen-year-olds. Since 2010, surveys commissioned by the public authorities have been carried out on a regular basis to determine how adolescents in Norway are *really* doing. In the 2017 report, the main findings were summarized as follows:

---

[3] His Majesty King Harald V of Norway, "Nyttårstalen 2016. Det norske kongehus", (2016), http://www.kongehuset.no/nyhet.html?tid=139780&sek=26939, paragraph 7–8.

[4] Ibid., paragraph 22.

> The young people who are growing up today can to a large extent be described as a well-adjusted, active and home-loving generation of youth. Although the majority are thriving and content, there are many who experience worries in daily life. In particular, many girls experience school as stressful. An important finding from this year's survey is that the scope of mental health complaints continues to expand. There is a marked increase for both girls and boys.[5]

The percentage of girls who report symptoms of depression has gradually increased since 2010 by 0.2–0.3 percent annually until 2015, while the findings for 2016 and 2017 show an increase of 2.8 percent for girls in lower secondary school and 3.6 percent for upper secondary school girls.[6] Because the increase is so dramatic compared to previous years, there is some cause for concern, although one should exercise caution so as not to place exaggerated emphasis on isolated findings. The findings of recent years have shown a slight downturn among boys in the number reporting a high level of depressive symptoms, but we have seen, in more recent years, an increase in reported mental health complaints for this group as well, although it is not as pronounced.[7] Since the findings show an increase in depressive symptoms for both boys and girls, it is appropriate to try to ascertain the cause, at least if one takes into account not only the number of young people who also report recurring physical symptoms such as headaches and stomach pains and the fact that one out of every four girls in their mid-teens self-medicates using under-the-counter pain relievers—a substantial increase since the early 2000s.[8] The Ungdata report highlights a conflict-ridden home environment, an inadequate social support system and bullying as factors increasing the risk of poor mental health. Other possible causes mentioned are the growth of individualism and greater pressure to perform well at school, which can lead to an increase in stress levels and because of which many now state that "everything is hard work" and that they "worry too much about

[5] Anders Bakken, "Ungdata. Nasjonale resultater 2017, NOVA Rapport 10/17", (Oslo: NOVA, 2017), 2.

[6] "Ungdata. Nasjonale resultater 2018, NOVA Rapport 8/18", (Oslo: NOVA, 2018).

[7] Ibid.

[8] Ibid.

things".[9] As I will illustrate clearly throughout this book, particularly the latter social factors appear to be emphasized all the more in the explanations for young people's psychological disabilities, as psychiatrist Anne Kristine Bergem illustrates here in her comments from the online newspaper *VG+*: "It is disturbing that so many young people experience anxiety. This can be related to the so-called achievement generation syndrome. They live with an experience of stress and pressure over their appearance, schoolwork and other performance areas."[10]

If one remains unconvinced by mathematical research data or expert opinions, there is no shortage of more personal accounts about how demanding growing up today can be. One such example is found in an account from the newspaper *Adresseavisen* and is typical of the times. The anonymous source who refers to herself as "Good Girl" describes how she experiences her daily life:

> I am one of many girls who suffer from the good girl syndrome. For me, receiving a B on a test is not acceptable. For me, coming in second in sports competitions is not good enough. No matter how many hours I spend in front of the mirror before school, I never feel 'pretty' enough. No matter how many hours I spend at the gym, I never feel 'fit' enough. No matter how many hours I spend on social media, I never feel that I am visible enough. I know there are incredibly many girls out there who can identify with these statements. We impose unrealistic requirements on ourselves that we must live up to. We must basically be perfect in all areas. The word perfect, which was formerly associated with something inhuman and that nobody could live up to, has become the ideal. The ideal of today's society is to be perfect.[11]

The life of "Good Girl" sounds undeniably exhausting: the writer feels that she must achieve excellence in all areas of life. And apparently none of these areas offers any relief from the imagined or real requirements imposed. On the contrary. A term such as "down time" seems passé,

[9] Ibid.

[10] Marie Moen Kingsrød-Olsen and Kaja Storrøsten, "Slik tok Therese og Jannicke kontroll over panikkangsten", *VG+* (2018), http://pluss.vg.no/2018/01/15/3027/3027_24232719, paragraph 13.

[11] "Flink pike", "'Flink pike'-syndromet", *Adresseavisen*, 20 January 2014, 15.

given the anonymous writer's total absorption with herself and her self-realization project twenty-four hours a day. Norwegian philosopher Arne Johan Vetlesen has used the term "the open 24/7 human being" to depict this development in which even our sleep is threatened by a mentality of "round-the-clock availability".[12] The average American now sleeps an average of 6.5 hours a night, while just one generation ago, the average was 8 hours and at the start of the twentieth century, 10 hours.[13] *Psychology Today* posed the question "Have we lost our ability to dream?".[14] Studies on the use of time show that Norwegians still sleep around eight hours a night, which is about the same as in 1980,[15] but sleep problems are on the rise in Norway too, especially in the 18–30 years age group.[16]

Simultaneously, the "Good Girl" also relates the experience of growing up in a country and time period offering many opportunities. The anonymous contributor would appear to have opportunities for education, recreational activities and friends easily within reach. Having these factors intact is what makes it possible for her to have great ambitions for herself in the first place. Perhaps her plans are overly ambitious, but nonetheless they indicate that the writer is living in an era when real opportunities exist that permit young people to pursue countless educational, career and life paths. Indeed, the many options are in themselves a part of the problem. His Majesty King Harald mentioned this as well in his New Year's Eve speech. But the alternative, that is, *not* having these choices, which has been the state of affairs for most generations up until the present day and remains so in countries less privileged than Norway, would certainly have been worse. For as the main character in Lasse Hallström's film *My Life as a Dog*—twelve-year-old Ingemar—thoughtfully states, "You have to compare."[17] Ingemar

[12] Arne Johan Vetlesen, "Det døgnåpne mennesket", *Morgenbladet*, 4 September 2014.

[13] Jonathan Crary, *24/7: late capitalism and the ends of sleep* (London: Verso, 2014).

[14] Michelle Carr, "Dream deprived: a modern epidemic?", *Psychology Today* (2017). https://www.psychologytoday.com/blog/dream-factory/201708/dream-deprived-modern-epidemic#_=_

[15] Statistics Norway, "Tidene skifter: tidsbruk 1971–2010", (Oslo: Statistisk sentralbyrå, 2012).

[16] Ståle Pallesen et al., "A 10-year trend of insomnia prevalence in the adult Norwegian population", *Sleep Medicine* 15, no. 2 (2014); NTB, "Unge voksne sliter mer med søvnen", *Aftenposten* (2016), https://www.aftenposten.no/norge/i/PAnOR/Unge-voksne-sliter-mer-med-sovnen

[17] Lasse Hallström, "Mitt liv som hund", (Stockholm: AB Svensk Filmindustri, 1985).

tackles life's challenges by putting things in perspective, for example, by thinking of the dog Laika that was sent into outer space and died.

Nonetheless, everyone who has been met with the "think about the children in Africa" response has felt frustration at having one's own complaints dismissed on the grounds that somebody else's situation, somewhere else in the world, is worse. Sometimes such problems are called *first world problems,* but first world problems are also problems worthy of attention, even though somebody else may be worse off. From such a perspective, we can perhaps conceive of the current generation's challenges as characteristic of our own times and as worthy of our attention, just as the problems of former generations have merited analysis and discussion.

What's New?

What's new here, and what does the problem consist of? As early as in 1990, Zygmunt Bauman described a defining feature of the shift from *modernity* to *postmodernity*: while previously we sacrificed freedom for security, the tendency in postmodern-day culture is to sacrifice security for freedom.[18] The individual freedom which formerly was restricted to ensure the construction of an orderly society has now been liberated and become the yardstick against which everything is gauged. The old world's encumbrances were about the dissatisfaction that arose when men and women's freedom and possibilities for development were curtailed in the name of security. The dream of breaking free is still very much alive and well. Countless examples can be found in the real-life stories found in magazine articles about men or women who quit their day jobs and dared to follow their dreams. And many still believe that more of us should follow suit: "Far too few dare to follow their dreams" career counsellor Eivind Bøe declared in the national daily *Dagens Næringsliv*.[19] Realizing one's dreams is a recent invention that can be found in a number of

[18] Zygmunt Bauman, *Postmodernity and its discontents* (London: Polity, 1997).

[19] Line Kaspersen, "Altfor få tør å følge drømmene sine", *Dagens Næringsliv* (2016), https://www.dn.no/jobbledelse/2016/02/07/1201/Karriere/-altfor-f-tr%2D%2Dflge-drmmene-sine

literary depictions, mainly of women breaking out of unfulfilling marriages such as Emma, in Gustave Flaubert's nineteenth-century novel *Madame Bovary*,[20] or in Elisabeth Gilbert's more current globetrotter bestseller *Eat, Pray, Love*.[21] In fact, the appeal to seek self-realization appears to have become so all-encompassing today that the librarian of the Norwegian National Library Aslak Sira Myhre found himself compelled to come forward and offer his own recommendation for the hopeful souls of the nation: "Don't follow your dream."[22]

The new world's encumbrances demonstrate that in the struggle to do away with all encumbrances, new ones will inevitably arise. When you are told that all manner of opportunities are lying at your feet, insecurity, uncertainty and the feeling of being overwhelmed by what to choose and subsequently about whether you have made the right decision will quickly sneak in. The price of freedom has been called "*to suffer from indecision*".[23] A couple of years ago one of the therapists at the Student Mental Health Service in Bergen told me that when she started working there in the 1990s, her typical client was a student struggling with anxiety about exams, while today the anxiety is more free-floating. The students are not merely anxious about how they will perform on their exams. They are also anxious about most of life's many choices and whether they are managing themselves in the best possible way. In response to this, Bauman remarks: "There's no such thing as a free lunch"—we both win something and lose something else. And as is the case for all kinds of social changes, they will favour some and disfavour others. Or as stated about progress in the television series *The Handmaid's Tale*: "Better never means better for everyone. It always means worse, for some."[24]

[20] Gustave Flaubert, *Madame Bovary* (London: Penguin, 2003).

[21] Elisabeth Gilbert, *Eat, pray, love* (Riverhead Books: New York, 2006).

[22] Aslak Sira Myhre, "Ikke følg drømmen din", *Dagsavisen* (2016), http://www.dagsavisen.no/nyemeninger/ikke-f%C3%B8lg-dr%C3 %B8mmen-din-1.773216.

[23] Jonas Jakobsen, "Å lide av ubestemthet. Axel Honneths hegelianske samtidsdiagnose", *Agora – Journal for metafysisk spekulasjon* 27, no. 4 (2009).

[24] Mike Barker, "The Handmaid's Tale: Faithful Episode 5", (Los Angeles: Hulu, 2017), 32:40.

How Are We, Really?

A paradoxical but striking feature of our freedom-obsessed society pertains to whether the young people of today have the backbone to take it. The question is whether we are sicker now than before, or are we simply better at talking about it? Overall, collective concerns, especially about young people, seem to be rampant in the modern age. Someone has commented that discussion pertaining to young people often encompasses more universal questions about society's challenges: the questions about young people are actually about all of us.[25] Perhaps we lack a satisfactory, acceptable answer since the concerns persist and resurface constantly. Perhaps there is something unique to our contemporary culture that unceasingly compels us to brood over this. In this book, my ambition is to present what I consider to be some credible, potential answers.

As stated, the question of whether we are sicker now than before contains an apparent paradox. Objectively speaking, we have never been better off—measured in terms of material prosperity or average life expectancy—while subjectively speaking, more and more people would appear to be feeling worse[26] and are struggling with a range of different mental health problems of varying degrees of severity. This pertains especially to young people. This riddle is therefore referred to as "one of the greatest paradoxes of our time"[27] and is revisited again and again, such as in this podcast from the Norwegian radio station P1 entitled *"The Psychologist"*:

> We live in a peaceful country. A rich country in so many ways. Most of us have jobs. We have at least a roof over our heads. And we have families or

[25] Thomas Ziehe, "Ungdom och modernitet", in *Kulturanalyser. Ungdom, utbilding, modernitet*, Johan Fornäs and Joachim Retzlaff, eds. (Stockholm: Brutus Östlings Bokförlag Symposion, 1994), 50.

[26] Anthony J. Barsky, "The paradox of health" *New England Journal of Medicine* 318 (1988).

[27] Per Anders Nordengen, "Pjusk eller syk?", *Tidsskriftet Den Norske Legeforeningen* 137, no. 1 (2017).

> friends. For the most part healthy. And nonetheless, we become depressed. [...] Is our own prosperity so intolerable?[28]

The description of the problem is typical: we are dealing with an apparent contradiction between how we are doing, objectively speaking, and how we feel, subjectively speaking. A question that some people have begun to ask is therefore whether it is the very knowledge of all the unprecedented opportunities that is causing mental health complaints and disorders on such a large scale? French sociologist Alain Ehrenberg defines depression as the shame of tolerating the knowledge that *everything is possible* while simultaneously failing in its achievement.[29]

And perhaps Norwegians are especially concerned about such questions, given that they are living in such a privileged country. In 2017, Norway was ranked as the happiest country in the world, ahead of its Nordic neighbours Denmark and Iceland.[30] However, from 2018 to 2021, Finland has taken over the throne as the happiest country in the world. Although Norway is relegated down to fifth place, the so-called Nordic exceptionalism continues to prevail. The concern about the state of the nation's mental health can perhaps also explain the prevalent myth about Norway being the world leader in the number of suicides, a claim that is repeated constantly. In the newspaper *Moss Avis,* the otherwise well-read columnist Kai Holtan offered the following observation:

> There is little doubt that we live in one of the world's safest, most equality-based, and well-organized societies, even though comment threads and parliamentary debates do not attest to this. And most of us have quite ample financial resources. [...] But if we are so damned happy, why is the consumption of anti-depressants (also called la-la pills) on the increase, particularly among young people? Why is the Norwegian suicide rate said to be among the highest in the world?[31]

---

[28] NRK P1, *Deprimert og ulykkelig i lykkelandet*, podcast audio 2016, http://podtail.com/podcast/nrk-psykologen/deprimert-og-ulykkelig-i-lykkelandet/, 0:02.

[29] Alain Ehrenberg, *The weariness of the self: diagnosing the history of depression in the contemporary age* (Montreal: McGill-Queen's University Press, 2010).

[30] Kjersti Strømmen, "Norge kåret til verdens lykkeligste land. NRK", (2017), https://www.nrk.no/norge/norge-karet-til-verdens-lykkeligste-land-1.13435868

[31] Kai Holtan, "La-la land", *Moss Avis*, 25 March 2017, 31.

The latter claim is demonstrably incorrect. The little-coveted first place is currently held by the poor South American country of Guyana with around 30 suicides per 100,000 inhabitants, while Norway comes in 73rd place with around 10 suicides.[32] In other words, there is little evidence to suggest that Norway is distinctive in a negative sense. The statistics are also based on the assumption that the individual nations in question have a sufficiently developed infrastructure in place to enable the keeping of records on suicides, not to mention a political or religious will to recognize fatalities as suicides. It is highly probable that such factors have contributed to the Caribbean island kingdoms of Antigua and Barbuda and Barbados taking the two last places and reportedly having close to zero registered suicides. The equally resilient myth about *the suicidal nation of Norway* can be viewed as an indication of a recurring sense of guilt on the part of many Norwegians over not feeling particularly happy, when objectively speaking they should. The culmination of this paradox is reached when it is combined with the historically unprecedented, privileged situation of today's young people in *the happy nation of Norway*. In the perhaps most canonized Norwegian film of the 2010s, Joachim Trier's portrait of a generation *Oslo, August 31st*, this is the basic premise and onerous insight embodied by the main character Anders, who commits suicide in the end.[33] *Feeling no hunger*, unlike Knut Hamsun's aspiring author self at the beginning of the twentieth century, is paradoxically a situation late modern human beings can't seem to escape from unscathed.[34] The literary critic Marta Norheim highlights this in particular as a defining feature of Norwegian contemporary literature:

> With the knowledge I have acquired about the characters in Norwegian novels, I know with reasonable certainty that such reports will have a directly disheartening impact on them: when you fail to be happy in the happiest country in the world, yes, then you are a loser.[35]

---

[32] WHO, "Suicide rates, age-standardized", (2017), http://apps.who.int/gho/data/node.main.MHSUICIDEASDR?lang=en

[33] Joachim Trier, "Oslo, August 31st", (Oslo: Motlys, 2011).

[34] Knut Hamsun, *Sult* (Copenhagen: P. G. Philipsens forlag, 1890).

[35] Marta Norheim, *Oppdateringar frå lykkelandet. Røff guide til samtidslitteraturen* (Oslo: Samlaget, 2017), 16.

This paradox has also been staged in the theatres of Norway. In the production *Det går bra* ("All is Well"), the theatre company Antiteateret put seven young, privileged characters on stage, all dressed up for Norway's Constitution Day, to speak about how they actually feel. The other side of the coin was thereby revealed. The critic from the national daily newspaper *Aftenposten*, Per Christian Selmer-Anderssen, expresses his approval of this paradox: "What they have in common is that they are almost as depressed as they are privileged. In a country where the consumption of anti-depressants is increasing in step with the oil fund, Antiteateret is without a doubt onto something."[36] Not unlike the perception of Norway as the suicidal nation, a cunning point is made here about depression in Norway being underpinned by privilege, a point supported by an increase in the consumption of antidepressants on a par with the growth of the oil fund. However thought-provoking this may be, does this paradoxical description of the contemporary age necessarily fit most young people?

The recurring discussion about the coming generation's wealth and well-being can also be viewed as the preliminary culmination of an uneasiness that has long saddled the modern era, specifically, the idea that the entire development of modernity is veiled in a latent, long-heralded spiritual crisis. This is perhaps only now becoming evident in a serious fashion in the form of a grave defect in the mental fitness of young people.

The idea of modernity, however, has always been marked by an element of ambivalence. On the one hand, there is the uplifting vision of a step-by-step departure from the wars between civilizations, superstition and premature death of "the dark Middle Ages", as expressed by Immanuel Kant: "Enlightenment is man's exit from his self-inflicted incapacity",[37] and the entrance into a perfectly and completely rationalized society founded on science, technology and democracy, where happiness lies easily within reach for everyone. On the other hand, there is modernity as a feeling of doom, anxiety and despair, as captured by Edvard Munch's iconic painting *The Scream*. Political scientist Steven Smith stresses that

---

[36] Per Christian Selmer-Anderssen, "Generasjon Depresjon speiler seg selv", *Aftenposten*, 2 April 2017, 5.

[37] Immanuel Kant, "Svar på spørsmålet: Hva er opplysning?", in *Store pedagoger i egne skrifter. III. Opplysningstiden*, ed. Reidar Myhre (Oslo: Fabritius & Sønners forlag, 1969), 14.

modernity must be viewed as a form of governance dedicated to happiness but surrounded by discontent.[38]

Nonetheless, it can appear that modernity's promise of a unilaterally happier life is irresistible and the absence of happiness correspondingly offensive. French philosopher Pascal Bruckner has pointed out how the Enlightenment and the French Revolution in 1789 did not merely do away with original sin—the sin that every human is born into, according to the doctrines of the Christian Church, but was also a harbinger of a historical development based on a promise of happiness for all.[39] Happiness was no longer to be considered a metaphysical figment of the imagination, an improbable goal like the singular salvation, but something obtainable here and now—in spite of the fact that happiness always seems to slip away at the very moment it is within one's grasp, just like salvation and the Promised Land. A consequence of this shift was a nascent aversion to suffering at a time when it was no longer possible to turn to God for consolation. When the goal of existence is no longer doing one's duty, but enjoying it, even the smallest discomfort will be experienced as offensive. The foundation is thereby in place for a cultural climate in which *not* having achieved this stage of happiness produces a sensation of something scandalous. And if even young people with all the opportunities offered them are unable to be happy, who then is able to be happy? The teenager is the twenty-first century's seismometer, and everyone around them is intently observing the tiniest quiver in the needle recording the tremors.

The Circle and the Line

The Norwegian author Jan Kjærstad claims that in the intellectual history of the Western world you can find two fundamental views of human life based on the geometric figures of the circle and the line, respectively. The circle view maintains that people essentially do not change and that human beings' dreams and burdens are essentially the same today as they

---

[38] Steven B. Smith, *Modernity and its discontents: making and unmaking the bourgeois from Machiavelli to Bellow* (New Haven: Yale University Press, 2016).

[39] Pascal Bruckner, *Perpetual euphoria: on the duty to be happy* (Princeton, NJ: Princeton University Press, 2000).

were thousands of years ago. The line view, on the other hand, holds that human beings undergo constant change, so human nature, during Antiquity, for example, was fundamentally different than it is today:

> For a long time, I have believed there to be an opposition in literature, a kind of competition between the circle and the line, between something repetitive and something that seeks to transcend former limitations. I could illustrate this through reference to two important Norwegian authors. On the one hand we have Sigrid Undset, who concludes her rendition of the King Arthur legends with the pronouncement: 'But human hearts have not changed whatsoever throughout all of time.' It's as if Undset wants to say there is no difference between the human being of the Middle Ages and the human being of today; for that reason, every novel from the Middle Ages will also be contemporary literature. There is nothing new under the sun. On the other hand, we have Henrik Wergeland and his equally famous words from the poem 'Follow the Call': 'But our world must still be young, Saga of each race must be still merely its cradlesong and its childhood fairy tale.' Wergeland is also responsible for the title in the form of the impatient question: 'Why does humanity progress so slowly?'[40]

It can be useful to include these two perspectives on human nature in a discussion about being human. Why? Well, because they represent two fundamentally different views and it can be constructive to confront the one with the other, so we do not lose sight of either of them. An exaggeration of the aspect of changeability can lead to losing our sense of history. Then it is easy to believe that all the challenges of today are new and consequently make them more serious than they actually are. To exaggerate un-changeability can lead to an apolitical stance with respect to how external historical events affect our opportunities as human beings. If everything remains unchanged regardless, the external framework conditions for human life are of no importance. I would hold that in addressing contemporary culture, we need these perspectives to both fully grasp the essence of the culture and avoid exaggerations of what is new or old in the situation.

[40] Jan Kjærstad, *Menneskets vidde* (Oslo: Aschehoug, 2013), 15–16.

Left and Right

Further, it is possible to discern at least two main views in the understanding of present-day psychological disorders. One of these views emphasizes that the idea that young people of today experience more stress and pressure than previous generations is very real. Here reference is typically made to developmental features associated with *late capitalism, neoliberalism* or *the new individualism,* which have in turn spawned diagnoses of the contemporary era such as *the competition state, the achievement society* and *the achievement generation.* According to this school of thought, late modernity is permeated with a collective pathologizing and a lapse in subjectivation, producing a breakdown of identity and disorders on a grand scale. This is, for example, how the sociologists Anthony Elliott and Charles Lemert open their co-authored work *The New Individualism: The Emotional Costs of Globalization*:

> Corporate networking, short-term project work, organizational downsizing, self-help manuals, compulsive consumerism, cybersex, instant identity makeovers and therapy cultures: These are just some of the core features of global individualist culture, and throughout this book we developed the argument that immersion in such a world carries profound emotional consequences for people's private and public lives.[41]

According to the two social scientists, life in late modernity has profound emotional costs for human existence. Such a view is often coupled with a Leftist radical criticism of the status quo that seeks an upheaval of the existing social conditions and where the problem is *political.*

In the other main school of thought, however, the idea that it is particularly difficult to be a human being today is considered to be greatly exaggerated and that it is instead a matter of human beings' inherent shortcomings. In seeking an explanation for the impression that many people nonetheless believe this to be the case, it makes more sense to explore the misleading role models that instil unrealistic expectations in

[41] Anthony Elliott and Charles Lemert, *The new individualism: the emotional costs of globalization (revised edition)* (New York: Routledge, 2009), xi.

young people about how much social change can increase the feeling of happiness in the population and how happy one can be at any given time. It is highly probable that it has always been difficult to be young, presumably more difficult than today in many areas, but there were no Ungdata questionnaires, no "Speak Up" commentary pages for young people hosted by national media organizations and no social media channels where one could share frustrations or answer questions along the lines of "Do you sometimes think that everything is hopeless?" A term such as the *paradox of health* also highlights the idea that the public authorities' health policy and campaigns, however much they undoubtedly contribute, objectively speaking, to improved public health, in many cases will lead to people feeling worse, subjectively speaking. The reason being that they cause people to become more attentive to internal bodily states, more inclined to apply illness categories to themselves and to remain bedridden longer when suffering from transitory illnesses.[42] Accordingly, the right medicine here is to improve individuals' awareness about how well-off they actually are, to remind the young people of today that failure, pain and suffering are not necessarily evidence of something wrong with them or with society, but a natural part of life, and then motivate them to assume more personal responsibility. Canadian psychologist Jordan Peterson does something along these lines with his popular twelve rules for life: "If you are suffering–well, that's the norm. People are limited and life is tragic", he reminds the reader and then instructs them to put their house and life in order before they "blame capitalism".[43] This view is often coupled with a conservative analysis intent on preserving the status quo, with primary importance placed on *morality*.

These two main views of modern-day pathologies correspond with well-known political distinctions of the Left and Right. From a moderate vantage point, irrespective of political views, I hope to show throughout the book that both perspectives may have some merit in explaining how the world and the people inhabiting it are connected.

---

[42] Barsky, "The paradox of health".

[43] Jordan B. Peterson, *12 rules for life: an antidote to chaos* (London: Allen Lane 2018), 157–58.

A Diagnosis for Us—A Diagnosis for You

Educator Arne Klyve has asked rhetorically: "Why are we coming up with so many diagnoses for people and not for our times?"[44] The scope of psychiatric diagnoses has increased dramatically in number since the first edition of DSM—the diagnostic manual of the American Psychiatric Association—from somewhere around 60 in 1952 to more than 400 diagnoses in the DSM-5 edition from 2013. The likelihood of receiving a psychiatric diagnosis in the course of one's lifetime has increased in keeping with the increase in types of diagnoses with each successive generation since the post-war period.[45]

But given the accelerating incidence of the pseudo-diagnoses typical of recent years, particularly for young people, such as "the achievement generation" and "a pathologically serious adolescent generation", it can appear that there has been a full-scale endeavour to diagnose our times based on the model of individual psychiatric diagnoses, along with the generation coming of age within these times. The question is merely whether these social diagnoses are the correct ones and if the prescribed treatment is expedient when it comes to the considerable challenges faced by society. A somatic or mental health diagnosis is justified only if it proves to be a useful tool for the physician or psychologist seeking to provide the most adequate treatment.

The premise of this book is that regardless of whether one believes that the young people of today face uniquely difficult challenges and deserve even more help and support or that they are unprecedentedly privileged cry-babies who first and foremost should pull themselves together, our understanding of how we have reached this point is relatively underdeveloped. Explanations with an emphasis on the *realities* of the unique challenges young people must overcome to live the best possible life in late modernity and accounts of the *imaginary* nature of the notion that it is supposed to be especially difficult for them today both merit a more thorough investigation.

---

[44] Arne Klyve, "Samtidsdiagnose", *Tidsskrift for Psykisk Helsearbeid* 14, no. 1 (2017), 73.

[45] Myrna M. Weissmann, "The changing rate of major depression", *Journal of the American Medical Association* 268 (1992).

In the research field comprising diagnoses of contemporary Western society, it is well known that self-fulfilling prophecies are an ongoing risk—in other words, by labelling a tendency of the current day, such as "the therapeutic culture", there is always a danger of this well-meaning manoeuvre having the effect of solidifying and strengthening the very phenomenon one intended to warn about in the first place.[46] To an even larger extent, this applies to presumably inflammatory concepts pertaining to today's youth such as "the achievement generation" or "the good girl syndrome"—and for that reason I have also included chapters about social representations and self-fulfilling prophecies that are intended to illuminate this risk. This exercise need not exhaust the relevance of what has been called the traditional Leftist critique of culture, in which "the capitalistic competitive society makes us overly preoccupied with self-realization and places undue pressure on the individual".[47] However, by also exercising greater resistance to these ideas, a more thorough examination is enabled than is usually the case to ascertain the relation between language and reality, concept and phenomenon.

The Organization of This Book

In Chap. 2, "The Pathologies of Modernity", and Chap. 3, "The Pathologies of Late Modernity", I present a review from the perspective of intellectual history of central social philosophical, sociological and socio-psychological interpretations of the development of modernity and late modernity. A key question is, "What is it about the current era?" In other words, does modern-day Western culture give the individual the tools required to become a whole human being or is the trajectory of modernity leading up to the contemporary society of the twenty-first century in reality a story of faulty subjectivation? In Chap. 4, "Young, Privileged and Sick", I present qualitative interviews of young adults from Norway, Sweden and Denmark on the subject of how these individuals

[46] Torben Hviid Nielsen, "De 'frisatte'. Om individualisering og identitet i nyere samtidsdiagnoser", in *Klassebilder: Ulikheter og sosial mobilitet i Norge*, Kenneth Dahlgren and Jørn Ljunggren, eds. (Oslo: Universitetsforlaget, 2010).

[47] Arne Borge, "–Kierkegaard var ingen selvhjelpsguru!" *Vårt Land*, 13 May 2017, 34.

experience being young today, with a particular focus on the consequences of performance requirements and the danger of becoming exhausted, stressed and depressed by the latter. In Chap. 5, "Youth Under Pressure", I give a summary of statistics and reports that can tell us how young people growing up in Norway today are faring. Here I will address suicide, mental health complaints and psychological disorders, use of medication, self-harm, acting-out behaviour, digital media and generational differences. In Chap. 6, "Social Representations", I conduct a psycholinguistic investigation of some wholly key images that are disseminated through the media. Here I provide a historical review of the concepts "achievement society", "the achievement generation" and "the good girl syndrome". In Chap. 7, "Self-Fulfilling Prophecies", I address the issue of how the terms we use in reference to young people and the contemporary age may instigate the very phenomena they describe. In Chap. 8, "The Paradox of Health", I illustrate how humans always interact with scientific classifications, but when it comes to psychological disorders, we don't seem willing to acknowledge the interactive nature of the illnesses, for fear of their being defined as culture. In Chap. 9, "Conclusion", I present a comparative evaluation of the different perspectives and conclude with the classical, utopian challenge "What must be done?"

2

The Pathologies of Modernity

Idleness is the beginning of all psychology.[1] (Friedrich Nietzsche)

ANYONE WHO HAS READ A MINIMUM of intellectual history, philosophy or sociology about the distinctive features of modernity and late modernity as time periods will have almost inevitably picked up on the warnings about the peculiar pathologies to which the development of society gives rise. The idea of *The Modern* extends all the way back to the fifth century as a division between the Christian and pagan eras. In more recent history, the term purportedly stems from a discussion at the French Academy in Paris in the early 1690s about whether modern culture is artistically superior to the Classical Greek-Roman culture. The use of the expression *modernity* appears for the first time in the nineteenth century as an epoch-defining concept in reference to our own times as the new and modern era. German idealists such as Hegel and Schelling used the term "modernity" as a secular affirmation that the future had begun, in contrast to the historical past, as if the world now found itself in a state in which it was wholly open to all that was new about the future. The break with

[1] Friedrich Nietzsche, *Twilight of the idols/The anti-Christ* (London: Penguin, 1990), 33.

O. J. Madsen, *Deconstructing Scandinavia's "Achievement Generation"*,
https://doi.org/10.1007/978-3-030-72555-6_2

the continuum of the past entailed that: "Modernity cannot and will no longer use the criteria by which it takes its orientation from the models supplied by another epoch: it has to create its normativity out of itself."[2] Modernity was thereby experienced as something fundamentally different from and more immediately present than the traditional existence that had predictably unfolded in the past. The present day became more present. "By 'modernity' I mean the ephemeral, the fugitive, the contingent", the French poet Charles Baudelaire wrote in 1864,[3] capturing the essence of the Modern: a self that transcended fixed roles and institutions, where the subjective dimensions of life could blossom, independent of the duty-bound necessities of daily life.

The optimism that was attached to modernity rested on the masses' expectation of becoming modern and thereby realizing their inner essence, which shone like a promise for the twentieth century. But as always, new opportunities brought new social problems, and modernity gave rise to the establishment of several of the social sciences dedicated to these problems. This was the case for sociology at the end of the nineteenth century and the beginning of the twentieth century, when pioneers such as Auguste Comte, Karl Marx, Émile Durkheim and Max Weber attempted to provide scientific answers for the many challenges accompanying modernity, such as industrialization, urbanization, secularization and rationalization. A leading figure in sociology, Georg Simmel, depicted modernity's pitfalls as follows: "The deepest problems of modern life derive from the claim of the individual to preserve the autonomy and individuality of his existence in the face of overwhelming social forces."[4] The psychological burden of living under modernity's law of gravitation would become the defining focus of the continental philosophy and social sciences. As I will show in this chapter, most Western philosophers with any self-respect have their own diagnoses of present-day society, intended to capture the essence of living in modernity. The thesis about what is called *individuation*—the development of a

[2] Jürgen Habermas, *The philosophical discourse of modernity: twelve lectures* (Cambridge: Polity Press, 2007), 7.

[3] Charles-Pierre Baudelaire, *The painter of modern life* (London: Penguin Classics, 2010), 13.

[4] Georg Simmel, "The metropolis and mental life", in *Simmel: on individuality and social forms*, ed. Donald Levine (Chicago: Chicago University Press, 1971), 324.

unique self, *socialization* and *subjectivation*, whereby the individual is honoured with an identity extraneous to his or her own will—has with time acquired an extensive history in fields such as psychoanalysis, social and community psychology, social philosophy and sociology. And equally extensive, at least, is the history of theories about faulty individuation, socialization or subjectivation. In other words, culture either produces individuals who are neurotic or gives rise to psychotic character formation. Psychological disorders cannot thereby merely be considered an exception but are instead the rule for the modern human being, according to the most pessimistic interpretations. This perception appears to have arisen in the aftermath of the emergence of modernity, at which time a series of psychologists, sociologists and philosophers asked themselves whether modern man can manage without "God" and if the science-based Enlightenment's promise of secular happiness would hold water.

Nietzsche's Last Human

The most fabled social diagnostician of them all, the German philosopher Friedrich Nietzsche (1844–1900), is famous for his declaration that "God is dead" and correspondingly renowned for his alter-ego Zarathustra's prophecy of the *Übermensch*, to a large degree attributed to Adolf Hitler's twisted aspirations for a pure Arian race. Nietzsche's *Übermensch* was the intended remedy for the decline of Christianity, whereby humans would be obliged to learn the meaning of the world instead of addressing life on the basis of a celestial hope of eternal life for the soul. But the *Übermensch* remained an ideal, the stewardship of which proved to exceed the abilities of contemporary human beings. The hearts of the people in *Thus Spoke Zarathustra* do not comprehend Zarathustra's prophetic teachings: "They do not understand me; I am not the mouth for these ears."[5] Nietzsche therefore urges us to prepare for the diminutive alternative to the *Übermensch*: the last man who is no longer able to "give birth to any star", in other words, unable to create a new "God" and instead lives on earth where everything has become small. The device

[5] Friedrich Nietzsche, *Thus spoke Zarathustra* (London: Penguin, 1969), 45.

invented to replace the gods is happiness and good health: "One has one's little pleasure for the day and one's little pleasure for the night: but one has a regard for health 'We have invented happiness,' say the last men and blink."[6] Nietzsche anticipates here in many ways what one hundred years later would be held up as the present day's final, surviving value. In the modern-day concept of *healthism,* it is precisely health that is held up as the sole remaining effective ideology in Western contemporary culture; optimized healthiness has become a super-value into which all other values must be subsumed.[7] Why the last man then? In Zarathustra's prophecy lies a warning that the cultural development of the modern age can be irreversible if the insight throughout history about "God" being a human construction is in the process of being forgotten and thereby also the motivation to become an *Übermensch* capable of instilling the world with meaning through the creation of new gods. The creative, enthusiastic human is on his deathbed. When the last man populates the earth, he will no longer be able to create, and despair itself will cease to exist: "Alas, the time is coming when man will no longer give birth to a star. Alas, the time of the most despicable man is coming, he that is no longer able to despise himself."[8] According to Nietzsche's prediction then, it is not anxiety which will be the quintessential emotion of the modern era, but rather satiety and apathy. Modern man is condemned to become a passive spectator in an ever more trammelled existence.

Marx's Alienation

The giants of the sociology also have their own present-day diagnoses of society: perhaps the best known of them all—Karl Marx (1818–1883)—is associated more than any other with the term *alienation*. Alienation is one of three components in Marx's critique of capitalism, along with inefficiency and exploitation. Alienation can be defined as "the absence of

[6] Ibid.

[7] Robert Crawford, "Healthism and the medicalization of everyday life", *International Journal of Health Services* 10, no. 3 (1980).

[8] Nietzsche, *Thus spoke Zarathustra*, 46.

a sense of meaning".[9] The lack of self-realization is commonly considered to be one of the most important forms of alienation. Marx held that the good life implies a life of active self-realization. He understood self-realization as "the full and free development of the powers and abilities of the individual".[10] The dream of the communist society was also a dream of everyone having the opportunity to live a life dedicated to self-realization. But the capitalism of that time ensured that only a select few were permitted to be a part of this, while the greater majority were excluded.

Alienation also arose as a consequence of the emergence of modern working life, which did not begin to resemble Marx's idea of work as a creative activity.[11] Modern work was instead characterized by the production of alien objects which did not develop the inner life of the workers or belong to them. The methods of production implied that work became something external to human nature. For most men and women, work as such engendered an inability to find satisfaction in it. They had no opportunity to develop their creativity and were instead exhausted and debased. Only in their free time could the majority feel that they were present, while the individual during working hours was homeless. Neither did the work provide any direct satisfaction of needs, but instead became a means of satisfying other needs. As such, alienation occurs, since for a better part of the day human beings are occupied with an activity that is only a means of continued survival. For many people, working life under capitalism also entails alienation from others, according to Marx. People are now assessed according to their profit value as workers. Social relations are no longer between individuals, but rather between workers and the capitalist, or farmers and landowners. As we will see below, this is also a central critique in the warnings about the achievement society.

---

[9] Jon Elster, *Making sense of Marx* (Cambridge: Cambridge University Press, 1985), 41.

[10] Ibid., 56.

[11] Karl Marx and Friedrich Engels, *Økonomisk-filosofiske manuskripter og andre ungdomsverker* (Oslo: Falken, 1991).

Durkheim's Anomie

In the writings of yet another of the founders of sociology, Émile Durkheim (1858–1917), we find the term *anomie*, which comes from the Greek word *anomia* meaning lawlessness. In his doctoral thesis *The Division of Labour in Society*, Durkheim uses the term anomie to characterize the pathological economy that is free from all regulations and where everyone's war against everyone else has become a natural state.[12] In the sequel, *On Suicide*, anomie is used as a description of the pathological, mental state of a person who is not sufficiently regulated by society and suffers from infinite aspirations. A distinguishing feature of *the anomic suicide* is a situation in which society is not sufficiently present in the individual's emotional life, so that the people of that society become completely dissolute. These conditions had purportedly become so common at the end of the nineteenth century that people virtually began to view them as normal:

> People constantly say that it is part of human nature to be constantly discontented, to keep pressing forward without pause or rest towards an indeterminate goal. A passion for the infinite is daily presented as a sign of moral distinction, when in fact it can only occur in disturbed minds which accord the status of a norm to the very disturbance from which they are suffering.[13]

Durkheim connects the development of the anomic suicide to the doctrine of progress, which he maintains has become a creed in its own right and where the greatest human cost and incidence of suicide are to be found in the pecuniary fields, such as trade and industry, since the chaotic circumstances are most prominent in the economic sector. In Durkheim's work, we find the apparent source of what with time came to be the defining understanding of a modernity implicitly critical of capitalism, in which economic competition considerations profit from

[12] Émile Durkheim, *The division of labor in society* (New York: Free Press, 1997).

[13] Émile Durkheim, *On suicide* (London: Penguin Books, 2006), 282.

human dissatisfaction and restlessness in the constant striving towards unknown goals.

The American sociologist Robert Merton was inspired by Durkheim and later developed an influential theory about deviance in which anomie denotes an acute state of normlessness that can arise when there is a discrepancy between cultural ideals and the opportunities available for members of society to achieve these.[14] Merton viewed the American dream of the 1930s of becoming rich as a goal of financial success, in the absence of sufficient opportunities for the majority to achieve the same goal. Merton therefore claims that the capitalistic system's inherent logic would result in a greater incidence of deviant behaviour.

In addition to the anomic suicide, Durkheim operated with three other suicide motifs: *the egoistic, altruistic* and *fatalistic* suicide. The first in particular is interesting in this context, in that Durkheim here explains a higher suicide rate in Protestant than in Catholic European nations by the fact that Protestantism to a greater extent allows free thought, while collective forces have a stronger presence in the lives of devout Catholics. Here Durkheim anticipates the idea that if individualism is developed excessively, the suicide rate in the population will increase, since many will experience the loss of something larger than themselves, which gave life meaning and provided a buffer against life's challenges.

Weber's Iron Cage

Another related feature of the development of modernity was that human behaviour was controlled more by a goal-oriented rationality as opposed to traditions and values. The German sociologist Max Weber (1864–1920) explains this situation in his well-known work *The Protestant Ethic and the Spirit of Capitalism*:

> The Puritan wanted to work in a calling; we are forced to do so. For when asceticism was carried out of monastic cells into everyday life, and began to dominate worldly morality, it did its part in building the tremendous

[14] Robert K. Merton, "Social structure and anomie", *American Sociological Review* 3, no. 5 (1938).

> cosmos of the modern economic order. This order is now bound to the technical and economic conditions of machine production which to-day determine the lives of all the individuals who are born into this mechanism, not only those directly concerned with economic acquisition, with irresistible force. Perhaps it will so determine them until the last ton of fossilized coal is burnt. In Baxter's view the care for external goods should only lie on the shoulders of the 'saint like a light cloak, which can be thrown aside at any moment'. But fate decreed that the cloak should become an iron cage.[15]

Weber describes how the ascetic set out to reconstruct the world, but in the process the world's external goods acquired increasing power over humans. Weber's "iron cage" has since prevailed as one of sociology's ultimate metaphors for the fate of modern man, imprisoned behind bars he himself has created. But as several people have since pointed out, the true author of the "iron cage" is not Weber, but one of his first English translators, the not unknown American sociologist Talcott Parsons.[16] Parsons concedes in a letter that the "iron cage" was a relatively free translation, inspired by Parsons' own Puritan background and extensive knowledge of John Bunyan's edifying novel of piety *The Pilgrim's Progress*. In this work, a man sits in an iron cage after having rejected God, and a bird symbolizing his soul flies out of the cage. In short: Man has now been left alone with his own misery. But Weber's original phrasing "*stahlhartes Gehäuse*" has a somewhat different meaning.[17] A more precise translation would have been "skull as hard as steel" which is after all more optimistic than the fatalistic iron cage metaphor, since Weber originally described how the spirit of capitalism enshrouds man like a cape, which he could ideally remove. Weber's staunch human being has not yet become like Gregor Samsa in Franz Kafka's novel *The Metamorphosis*, who one day finds himself transformed into a gigantic insect lying on a hard, armoured back and whose first thought is tellingly not concern

---

[15] Max Weber, *The protestant ethic and the spirit of capitalism*, (1920), https://pages.uoregon.edu/kimball/Wbr%20Protestant.Eth.ch5.htm

[16] Peter Baehr, "The 'iron cage' and the 'shell as hard as steel'", *History and Theory* 40, no. 2 (2001).

[17] Ibid.

about the altered state of his body, but about his job and schedule.[18] The story of the "iron cage" nonetheless illustrates how concepts are always dynamic and in their evolution can gain significance far afield from their original meanings.

Freud's Discontentment Within Culture

> That man should be 'happy' is not included in the scheme of 'Creation'. (Sigmund Freud)[19]

Besides Nietzsche and the sociologists Marx, Durkheim and Weber, the Austrian physician Sigmund Freud's (1856–1939) work *Civilization and Its Discontents,* written late in his life, probably reigns supreme as the most impressive diagnosis of civilization and would come to colour the future view of the individual's opportunities for development in Western society. In the original German, the work was entitled *Das Unbehagen in der Kultur*. The English title, *Civilization and Its Discontents*, underscores that the book is about modern culture and the discontent still to be found there, despite its many improvements. And according to Freud, this discontent will only increase in step with the development: "the price of progress in civilization is paid in forfeiting happiness through the heightening of the sense of guilt".[20] Freud's thesis is that the opposition between the individual and society can never find happy resolution. The reason for this is that society necessarily requires the individual to repress his or her natural drives. So-called normal people are able to bear this but not the neurotic and psychotic individuals among us.

Man's cultural advancement is essentially an abstraction of the individual's development, so one would expect the development of the individual and the community to reach a unified, positive conclusion. But as Freud points out, in the individual's developmental process finding happiness is of primary importance. In the struggle to achieve an expansive

[18] Ibid.

[19] Sigmund Freud, *Civilization and its discontents,* (1930), https://archive.org/details/in.ernet.dli.2015.221667/page/n7, 31.

[20] Ibid., 125.

human community, on the other hand, happiness is usually shoved into the background. Collective social forms are most easily implemented when the happiness of the individual is not considered. The individual and the community are like revolving planets, the meeting of which is the exception rather than the rule, Freud comments. It is only if absorption into the community is the foremost objective of the individual's developmental process that the latter will coincide with the cultural process.

Freud also asserts that the community forms its own super-ego. The cultural super-ego is eventually condensed into an ethics tied to the most vulnerable point of every culture, thereby concealing where *the culture's work* has been inadequate. Freud refers here to human beings' tendency towards aggression in relation to one another. The cultural super-ego's attempt to solve the problem of aggression in Western, Christian culture becomes the commandment: "Love thy neighbour as thyself." Here Freud draws a parallel to the treatment of neuroses in which the individual's super-ego cares little about the happiness of mankind and is wholly indifferent to the resistance that inevitably arises to compliance with external decrees. The goal of therapy becomes therefore to try and mitigate the requirements. The same problem appears with Christianity's commandment to love thy neighbour, whereby an inhuman requirement is imposed that not even so-called normal people will manage to satisfy without developing neuroses, rebelling and most certainly becoming unhappy. The cultural super-ego is essentially un-psychological in its conduct. The result is that young people in the West are released into the world equipped with the belief that everybody else is completely moral and fulfils society's ethical obligations. This thereby turns into a twofold strain—the young must both tolerate an aggression which has no outlet, out of consideration for the community, and live with the illusion that other people are living in happy, inner harmony with this troublesome imperative.

Having learned his lesson from the devastations of World War I and as an omen of what was to come, Freud concedes that anyone in the current culture who follows the rules will quickly find themselves helplessly confronted with those who choose to put themselves above them. Meanwhile, neither natural nor religious ethics have anything more to offer human beings here and now, beyond a narcissistic satisfaction in believing oneself to be better than others or a vague promise of relief in the afterlife.

Despite the dismal prospects, Freud nevertheless asks the promising question in conclusion: if the development of culture is the same as the development of the individual, can't one then also employ the same method to diagnose the times—have we all become neurotic under the pressure of cultural influence? And even more promising: Won't we subsequently be able to come up with suggestions for a therapeutic remedy? However, Freud quickly puts a damper on any hopeful expectations that might be bubbling up in his readers: a social diagnosis, unlike a diagnosis of a patient, will not have a normal state with which to compare itself and what purpose will even the most discerning analysis serve, if we don't have the power to impose therapy on society? Freud concludes the passage on sick society with words of encouragement for his followers: "In spite of all these difficulties, we may expect that one day someone will venture upon this research into the pathology of civilized communities."[21] His hopes would prove to be prophetic and it is no exaggeration to say that Freud's relatively intricate master work successfully laid the foundation for a unique cultural-philosophical genre about the nature of the connection between the individual and society and the disorders that must be expected to arise there.

Adorno and Horkheimer's Enlightenment

However, the discontent within culture appeared only to continue in the years following Freud's death. The German philosophers Max Horkheimer (1895–1973) and Theodor W. Adorno (1903–1969) open their illustrious work *Dialectic of Enlightenment* as follows: "Enlightenment, understood in the widest sense as the advance of thought, has always aimed at liberating human beings from fear and installing them as masters. Yet the

[21] Ibid., 142.

wholly enlightened earth is radiant with triumphant calamity."[22] Not unlike Freud's magnum opus, the two Frankfurt philosophers' co-authored work was a reaction to the Second World War's systematic barbarism and from their exile in the USA understandably full of pessimism on behalf of the human race. The formula they launch for the development of modernity is 'the more enlightenment, the more unhappiness'. Horkheimer and Adorno discuss the programme of enlightenment as the *disenchantment* of the former, myth-based world. The price of the road leading to modern science was that humans have been obliged to sacrifice meaning: "From now on matter was finally to be controlled without the illusion of immanent powers or hidden properties. For enlightenment, anything which does not conform to the standard of calculability and utility must be viewed with suspicion."[23] The myths slowly transition into enlightenment and nature becomes purely an objective matter. But this has a price, as Horkheimer and Adorno see it: the price for the human race is that the increase in power is proportionate to the alienation from what it has subjugated. This may sound like an echo of both Marx and Freud, although guilt has been replaced by alienation. Enlightenment's dominion becomes totalizing and makes no distinction between work and time off: "The rowers, unable to speak to one another, are all harnessed to the same rhythms, like modern workers in factories, cinemas, and the collective."[24] Of central importance for the Frankfurt school was also the claim, based on Marx's alienation thesis, that under capitalism man doesn't even discern that he is alienated. When modern human beings passively choose mass consumption rather than active self-realization, it is not because the opportunities for the latter are out of reach, but because they no longer desire anything else.[25]

[22] Theodor W. Adorno and Max Horkheimer, *Dialectic of enlightenment: philosophical fragments* (Stanford, CA: Stanford University Press, 2002), 1.

[23] Ibid., 3.

[24] Ibid., 29.

[25] Elster, *Making sense of Marx.*

Fromm's Contentment in Culture

The German psychoanalyst Erich Fromm (1900–1980), who early in his career was affiliated with precisely the Frankfurt school, later tried in *The Sane Society* to outline a positive alternative to the misery-inducing Viennese culture described by Freud.[26] Fromm opens the book by sowing seeds of doubt regarding some unquestioned truisms of the Western understanding of reality. There is a widespread assumption that man in the twentieth century is extremely normal. And although many people suffer from serious mental disorders, we have no doubts about the psychological health of the average human being. But can we be sure that we are not fooling ourselves? Fromm asks tellingly. Is the development of society *actually* healthy?

The analysis that Fromm expounds on a grand scale in *The Sane Society*, in close dialogue with Freud, is that Western cultural development in the modern era had the objective of creating a foundation for a complete experience of individuality.[27] By liberating the individual both politically and economically, by teaching humans to think for themselves and freeing them from authoritarian pressure, the aim was to put the subject in a central position, so that he or she could actively put their abilities to use and, as a result, feel their unique selves. But in reality, this is a project that has only proven successful for a minority. For the majority of the population, modern individualism is nothing more than a façade that conceals the failure experienced in the loss of a feeling of identity.

Fromm highlights a paradox that appears to be equally relevant today: humankind appears to have reached the beginning of a new, richer and happier era, but the existence of both the current and subsequent generations seems to be more threatened than ever before.[28] Man gained freedom from clerical and secular authorities and was left alone with common sense and the conscience as guides, but was simultaneously afraid of the newly won freedom. The freedom achieved is primarily a *freedom from*, whereas the *freedom to*—to be oneself, creative and fully

---

[26] Erich Fromm, *The sane society* (New York: Holt, Rinehart & Winston, 1976).

[27] Ibid.

[28] Ibid.

awake—was yet to come. As a result, human beings have sought to escape from the freedom—a theme of Fromm's book *Escape from Freedom.*[29] And man's great achievement, specifically, dominion over nature, made this escape possible. The establishment of new industrial machines became so all-engrossing that it became the foremost purpose of existence. Man's striving, once focused on a search for God or salvation, was now directed towards the domination of nature and a constant search for material well-being. Production is no longer merely a means to a better life; it has now become the end in its own right, taking precedence over life itself.[30]

Fromm describes a form of alienation from the growing consumer society during the phase of reconstruction in Western nations following World War II. Clearly inspired by Marx, Fromm maintains that man perceives himself as a commodity, a replaceable part of the machinery rather than its master. The objective is to achieve success and sell oneself at the highest possible price on the market. The esteem of every single human being is thereby reduced to his or her sales value, to the detriment of genuine, human qualities. Happiness too is now embedded in the commodity logic and synonymous with the consumption of ever new products or the consumption of entertainment, sex and intoxication, Fromm writes. His diagnosis of the contemporary era is correspondingly pitch-dark:

> He is alienated from himself, worships the products of his own hands, the leaders of his own making, as if they were above him rather than made by him. He is in a sense back where he was before the great human evolution began in the second millennium B.C.[31]

The creative human being Nietzsche tried to save appears lost. During the geopolitical period of the 1950s, Fromm sees the West evolve in the direction of Aldous Huxley's futuristic novel *Brave New World,* saturated with material prosperity and seamless efficiency by way of psychological

---

[29] Eric Fromm, *Escape from freedom* (New York: Farrar & Rinehart, 1941).

[30] Fromm, *The sane society.*

[31] Ibid., 122.

adaptation methods, mass hypnosis and pecuniary reward. In the East, there is also a more blatant exploitation and abuse of the population, reminiscent of George Orwell's reverse dystopia in *1984*. Alienation in both cases leads to an ever more widespread meaninglessness. In the end, life has no meaning, in that joy, faith and reality slip away from us. Everyone is indeed "happy", except for the fact that nobody feels, thinks intelligently or loves to any real extent any longer, Fromm claims to observe. The nineteenth century's big problem "God is dead" has its corollary in the twentieth century: "Human is dead". And where the consequence in the 1800s was inhuman cruelty, the consequence in the 1900s is a schizoid estrangement from the self, Fromm argues. Where our forefathers—the primitive people—helplessly faced the forces of nature, the modern human being is just as helpless in confrontation with the socio-economic forces we have created ourselves.

Fromm also describes the features of a utopian alternative—a healthy society in harmony with human beings' fundamental needs, in which love and brotherhood comprise a lowest common denominator, not blood and soil, and where everyone has the opportunity to achieve wholeness as a subject. But Fromm fears that if the current development continues, a more likely outcome will be a robotic power or a nuclear war that brings to an abrupt end civilization as we know it.

Rieff's Therapeutic Turn

One of Freud's most intelligent readers, the American religion sociologist Philip Rieff (1922–2006), in his doctoral work *Freud: The Mind of a Moralist* from 1959, threw a shadow of doubt on Freud's view of society and the spill-over effects it would have.[32] Rieff highlights how Freud expressed distrust in the radical political movements in the Europe of his day during the early decades of the twentieth century, "the frenzied revolutionaries", as Freud somewhat condescendingly referred to them.[33]

[32] Philip Rieff, *Freud, the mind of the moralist (3rd edition)* (Chicago: University of Chicago Press, 1979).

[33] Freud, *Civilization and its discontents*, 143.

The political struggle of the time over how to best organize society was understood by Freud to be an expression of an eternal battle between the individual and society's conflicting needs. And since society of necessity must be oppressive, there are no grounds for thinking that Freud would view the struggles after the revolution as anything but a refusal to abandon the illusion that a better world should be possible. Freud's sympathies will therefore always gravitate towards the status quo. Psychoanalysis' exaltation of the private individual and corresponding disillusionment with the community implies that each individual human being's inner, mental balance can just as easily be found in oppressive regimes as in the democratic, free society. Happiness will remain a subjective matter, Freud insists. The universal opposition between nature and culture acquires its alter ego in Freud's postulate regarding an eternal conflict between the individual and society. In contrast to Freud, Rieff is a fundamentally *communitarian* thinker, inspired by Durkheim, for whom only the community can ensure the good life. He therefore warns against the incipient softening of the super-ego and the moral conscience which Freud prescribed for Western culture, whereby instead of a pre-eminent morality the therapeutic question, "How does it feel?" becomes the guide. The result is a form of value nihilism in which psychoanalysis' incentive to reveal the self becomes a threadbare substitute for the moral superstructure of Western culture. As a political thinker, Freud can be viewed as an individualist of the liberalist school, for whom the social sphere is only highlighted when it interferes with individual adjustment. In this sense, Freud anticipated the widespread contemporary idea in the West that society is not primarily an arena in which the individual can realize him or herself, but rather a conformist hindrance from which the individual is urged to seek liberation.

Erikson's Identity Crisis

In 1950 the German American psychologist Erik Erikson (1902–1994) published his work *Childhood and Society*, in which he presented his well-known developmental theory on the eight stages of psychosocial development in human beings. The individual's personality will unavoidably be faced with unique challenges during all eight of the different life phases, encompassing both potential crises and opportunities,[34] from an infant's fundamental trust or distrust of his or her closest caregivers to old age's experience of integrity or despair. Erikson held that in adolescence the challenge is to establish a personal *identity* as a psychological connection between infancy and adult life, in which the outcome will be either identity affiliation or role confusion. The term *identity crisis* therefore comes from Erikson and refers to the insecurity that can arise in adolescence. The concept, however, would turn out to be characteristic of the entire modern era. Even a sober-minded organization such as the Language Council of Norway noted an increase beginning in the 1960s in a "preoccupation with who we are as human beings and where we belong. The Norwegian language has developed new words, such as identity crisis, loss of identity, identity problem."[35] At the time when Erikson conceived his theory in the 1940s, the identity-related challenges were probably not of such a nature as to extend beyond adolescence, but starting in the 1960s, a clear need arose for a term that captured the identity-related challenges that came to characterize not solely the challenges of puberty, but the overall lot of human beings in late modernity.

Mitscherlich's Fatherlessness

In traditional societies, children were ordinarily incorporated into the occupations of their parents, and familial relationships for this reason were consolidated throughout the course of the working day. During the industrial revolution, which involved the migration of labourers into the cities to work in factories, this changed and along with it also the nature of the dealings between the generations. In 1963 the German psychoanalyst Alexander Mitscherlich (1908–1982) published the book *Society without the Father*, in which he investigates the impact of the

[34] Erik H. Erikson, *Childhood and society* (New York: Pelican, 1950).

[35] Språkrådet, "Identitet", (2009), http://www.sprakradet.no/Vi-og-vart/hva-skjer/Aktuelt-ord/Identitet/

breakdown of Western society's traditional structures of authority, as the customary passing-down of traditions from parents to children was phased out.[36] Mitscherlich describes post-war Germany, in which the father figure in particular lost authority as a role model. Here the emphasis is on how a role model is an ideal which young people seek to live up to in the formation of the self and a positive identification with the father is a necessary condition for such role modelling.

Why precisely the father? For the psychoanalytic tradition of the inter- and post-war period, the father was an impetus driving the constitution of social authority structures such as the super-ego, ego idealism, guilt and the development of a social conscience. These terms were often connected to the child's experience with the father.[37] This was a narrative originally developed by Freud through his inroads into anthropology and group psychology in the 1920s. In *Totem and Taboo* Freud pondered over whether social psychology's fundamental problem could be solved on the basis of a single element—the individual's relationship to the father.[38] Mitscherlich identified the mass society of contemporary culture on the other hand as a *sibling society*, in which no specific person was the authority: "We grow up from the power relationships of childhood, which are tied to persons, into an incomprehensible system of power relationships, under which we spend our working life."[39]

Mitscherlich's thesis about the fatherless society pops up all the time in emphatically conservative cultural analyses of late modernity's anomic features. The American author Robert Bly, for example, writes words of warning in the preface to the English translation of the book: "In the fatherless society, the children – particularly the sons – have holes in their psyche that (they) fill with demons."[40] In Bly's own book *The Sibling Society*, he claims to see a pervasive crisis in men all around him, which

---

[36] Alexander Mitscherlich, *Society without the father: a contribution to social psychology* (New York: Harper Perennial, 1993).

[37] Matt Ffytche, "Psychoanalytic sociology and the traumas of history: Alexander Mitscherlich between the disciplines", *History of the Human Sciences* 30, no. 5 (2017), 8.

[38] Ibid.

[39] Mitscherlich, *Society without the father: a contribution to social psychology*, 277.

[40] Robert Bly, "Foreword: Mitscherlich and his uncomfortable thoughts", in *The society without the father* (New York: Harper Perennial, 1993), xvi.

he connects to the absence of traditional fatherhood in modern-day culture, so boys are now left more to their own devices, even in the transition from childhood to adulthood.[41] For that reason there are many who never leave childhood. In Denmark, the historian Henrik Jensen published the book *Det faderløse samfund* ("The Fatherless Society") in which, like Bly, he holds that the contemporary, horizontally designed Danish matriarchy finds reflection in a lack of direction and norms for young men.[42] Paradoxically, the Norwegian mass murderer Anders Behring Breivik, who lamented his fatherless upbringing, included a paragraph in his clip and paste manifesto *2083* that was entitled "The Fatherless Civilization". The chapter was written by Peder "Fjordman" Jensen, who claims that the father figure has been demonized and ridiculed in the West and that the Norwegian social democratic state sought to replace it with the kindergarten system, which he holds will give rise to social diseases in the future.[43]

Conclusion: The Tragic View of Life

Although Fromm tried to develop a positive alternative to the prior illness-generating Viennese culture, the question is raised as to whether his starting point in his progenitor Freud's inherently tragic view of life coloured his own and others' subsequent analyses. As shown, Freud was sceptical on the whole towards the idea of happiness as a realistic objective to strive for in life. He added laconically: "It is much less difficult to be unhappy."[44] Freud broke down the origins of suffering into three main categories that can be summarized as follows: (1) our body is a source of suffering in that it inexorably decays and breaks down, (2) the natural world descends upon us with its overpowering, destructive forces on a regular basis, and (3) relationships with other human beings inflict suffering. Most people will moderate their demand for happiness due to

---

41 Robert Bly, *The sibling society* (New York: Penguin, 1997).

42 Henrik Jensen, *Det faderløse samfund* (Copenhagen: People's Press, 2006).

43 Anders Behring Breivik, *2083 – A European declaration of independence* (London: Andrew Berwick, 2011).

44 Freud, *Civilization and its discontents*, 28.

the pressure suffering continually imposes upon them. The reality principle, whereby behaviour is controlled by the ego to meet the conditions imposed by the external world, will therefore replace the pleasure principle, according to which one makes do with being thankful for avoiding evil. When it comes to the sources of suffering, the reality is that we are obliged to accept the first two and resign ourselves to their inevitability, Freud writes. We will never be able to control nature completely. And the human body, also a part of nature, will always be an ephemeral organism with limited adaptive and performance abilities, even though we have succeeded to a certain extent in eliminating some natural illnesses and dangers. The third category of suffering, however, holds a privileged position. In confrontation with the social source of suffering, we are not as willing to accept resignation, because we expect this mechanism, which we have established ourselves, to provide us with protection and be a source of joy.[45] However, Freud is sceptical towards this idea: behind the source of social suffering, or that which we can simply call culture, the history of humankind indicates that the alleviation of suffering has not been particularly successful, precisely because, here too, an unbeatable nature lies behind it—the human psyche.

Freud stresses how in more recent times we have experienced progress within technology and the natural sciences of which previous generations could scarcely have dreamed. Simultaneously, these advances have not produced the anticipated results in terms of the feeling of happiness. It is thus perhaps not so strange that he has little faith in the development of culture as a strategy to improve the fundamental human condition. And vice versa: Freud's meagre expectations for the social sphere also make him distrustful of the idea promoted by many critics of modernity, the idea that modern culture is particularly illness-inducing. Freud's inherent scepticism entails that he also dismisses the idea that it is even possible to compare the feeling of happiness in the populations of different eras:

> Happiness, on the contrary, is something essentially subjective. However we may shrink in horror at the thought of certain situations, that of the

[45] Freud, *Civilization and its discontents*.

> galley-slaves in antiquity, of the peasants in the Thirty Years War, of the victims of the Inquisition, of the Jews awaiting a pogrom, it is still impossible for us to feel ourselves into the position of these people.[46]

It is not difficult to understand Freud's reservations against claiming certain knowledge about how our forefathers were *actually* feeling. At the same time, the question arises as to whether Freud nevertheless draws too extreme a conclusion. Although it is impossible to know with certainty how our forefathers experienced different historical, cultural and political eras, this does not necessarily imply that it's meaningless to try to pin down certain principles that can be presumed to be reasonably universal and which at the very least provide more or less tenable conditions for achieving a good life.

[46] Ibid. 49.

3

The Pathologies of Late Modernity

A NUMBER OF WORKS FROM THE SECOND HALF OF THE 1960s reflect how Marx's concept of alienation has actually advanced into another phase, moving from work and production into leisure time and consumption. The Italian film director Michelangelo Antonioni, known for his black and white "trilogy about modernity and its discontent"[1] *L'Avventura, La Notte* and *L'Eclisse* and the colourful sequel *Blow-Up*, captures this transition precisely as the protagonist Thomas in the latter film, together with workers who have ended their shift, leaves one of London's pipe factories.[2] The filmography of the art enthusiast Antonioni appears undeniably to have been inspired by Edvard Munch's painting *Workers Returning Home*, the motif of which was allegedly taken from the glassworks of Jeløya Island in Moss, Norway. The glassworks shut down the year before the new millennium and have since been levelled to the ground to make room for modern housing units where instead of manufacturing glass one can now enjoy the view of the Værlebukten Bay through imported glass windows. The existential drama of *Blow-Up*,

[1] Stephen Holden, "Antonioni's nothingness and beauty", *New York Times* (2006), https://www.nytimes.com/2006/06/04/movies/04hold.html, paragraph 10.

[2] Michelangelo Antonioni, "Blow-up", (Beverly Hills, CA: Metro-Goldwyn-Mayer, 1966).

O. J. Madsen, *Deconstructing Scandinavia's "Achievement Generation"*,
https://doi.org/10.1007/978-3-030-72555-6_3

narrated through the life of a successful, but passive fashion photographer who is only able to create representations of reality, foreshadows the era of post-production. The French Situationist Guy Debord's collection of aphorisms *Society of the Spectacle* from 1967 opens with the paradigmatic opening statement: "Everything that was directly lived has receded into a representation."[3] One year later, the Canadian philosopher Marshall McLuhan published *The Medium is the Massage*, about how the medium of our times—electronic technology—transforms everything that is familiar—yourself, your family, your neighbourhood, your job and your relationships with others—in a dramatic fashion.[4] The book was originally entitled *The Medium is the Message,* until a random typo purportedly led McLuhan to choose the alternative "massage", which intimates how the growing stream of images we have been fed with from as early as in the 1960s has produced a comfortable numbness. It was henceforth necessary to remind the revolutionary masses that "the revolution will not be televised", as the jazz poet Gil Scott-Heron from this period put it.[5] The entire idea of how the representation of reality is more real for us than the original was developed further by the French sociologist Jean Baudrillard, who, in *The Consumer Society,* provided an influential analysis of how consumerism capitalizes on human desire.[6] The consumer society's economic growth is contingent upon a steady flow of capital and therefore relies on the population's willingness to buy. Restless souls with a deficient inner spiritual life can be counted on to constantly hunt for something new to fill their emptiness. All human activities are reduced to the logic of consumption. Even political involvement finds expression at the mall where you can choose to purchase fair trade coffee or organic eggs to signal your support of the farmers in the global south, or free-range hens. The consumer society's universe of meaning is thereby levelled into: "A society with no myth other than itself."[7]

---

[3] Guy Debord, *The society of the spectacle*, (London: Zone Books), 2.

[4] Marshall McLuhan, *The medium is the massage* (London: Penguin, 1971).

[5] Gil Scott-Heron, "The revolution will not be televised" in *Small talk at 125th and Lenox* (1970).

[6] Jean Baudrillard, *The consumer society: myths and structures* (London: Sage, 2003).

[7] Ibid., ix.

Ziehe's Society of Choices

In the German pedagogue Thomas Ziehe's doctoral dissertation *Puberty and Narcissism*, he alleges that young people's personality patterns are currently evolving in the direction of increased narcissism. Ziehe is interested in the consequences of cultural modernization for human subjectivity and above all for our possibilities to address the challenges of modernity. The period around 1970 in the West was a watershed moment involving what Ziehe calls the phasing out of the *society of fates*, in which the life of the individual was predominantly tied to cultural traditions, followed by a transition to the *society of choices*, in which identity is no longer something that is passed down and the influence of previous generations on the next is diminished. The loss of traditions results in greater value-relativism, which in turn demands greater self-reflection and more choices. Performance must gradually give way to pleasure. Ziehe holds that the social changes are of such a scope that we must presume that the entire youth culture and the mentality of young people are undergoing change. In short, we are faced with a new form of socialization.[8] The new type of young person emerging is characterized by both greater emotional engagement and awareness of own worth, but also a greater inner emptiness, less psychological stability and an inadequately developed self. The emergent narcissistic character structure has less of an authority orientation and is more inclined to seek support from friends. Ziehe appears to be ambivalent about how this development will affect young people, insofar as their vulnerability and authenticity will become more pronounced. Young people in particular will be more receptive to cultural modernization processes such as reflexivity, plasticity and individualization because they are in the midst of a critical life phase during which they must forge an identity. They will therefore also to a larger degree be influenced by external societal changes than the members of the adult generation, who can still seek the support of old traditions and routines.

---

[8] Thomas Ziehe, *Pubertät und narzissmus: sind jugendliche entpolitisiert?* (Hamburg: Europäische Verlagsanstalt, 1984).

Beck's Individualization

The development described above appears to be continuing unimpeded in our times and the effects for young people appear to be a larger realm of opportunities than previously, but also greater vulnerability. In 1986, the German sociologist Ulrich Beck (1944–2015) published his book *Risk Society*, which made him world-famous, right after the Chernobyl accident.[9] The analyses of how new risks brought about by scientific and social changes have become humankind's new destiny, in contrast to the old dangers from the natural world such as plagues, earthquakes and starvation, were disturbingly topical. The new risks had a broader scope than before: "Poverty is hierarchic, smog is democratic."[10] While it was possible to ignore the necessities of former periods, nobody can now permit themselves to be indifferent about the threats of the nuclear age. A less obvious risk but an equally essential part of life in late modernity also involves social, biographical and cultural risks and uncertainties. A social transformation is underway within modernity through which the human being is freed from the social forms of the industrial society such as class, family and gender roles, just as the population was freed from the Church's rules for society during the Reformation. The individualization emerging in the aftermath of modernization is unlike that of former periods such as the Renaissance and the early industrial age, at which time it was a luxury usually reserved for the bourgeoisie. Beck gives a historical example from his own times, the unemployment in West Germany between 1974 and 1983, which affected around 12.5 million Germans. Social class no longer gives the phenomenon any meaning, Beck argues. Such systemic problems are no longer understood in the same political terms as before but are instead converted on a large scale into personal failure. What were formerly understood as social crises are therefore now perceived as having a personal origin: "The individual himself or herself becomes the reproduction unit of the social in the lifeworld."[11] One's biography becomes a reflexive project. As such,

---

[9] Ulrich Beck, *Risk society: towards a new modernity* (London: Sage, 1992).

[10] Ibid., 36.

[11] Ibid., 90.

increasingly more people will dream of a life of autonomy, but individuals are not freed from constant subjugation to social and political guidelines and are at the mercy of economic, pedagogical, psychological and medical standardized support, however much this does acquire a far more individually adapted framework.

Bauman's Liquid Modernity

The Polish sociologist Zygmunt Bauman (1925–2017) is known for his diagnosis of the contemporary era as *liquid modernity,* which he believes typifies contemporary culture's fluctuating nature, characterized as it is by non-binding ties, as opposed to the traditional, established social order.[12] The human consequences of this dissolution, for the lion's share of the population, are approximately as distant as one can get from the ideal of liberation and happiness. In 1997, Bauman published the book *Postmodernity and Its Discontents*, the title of which is a reference to Freud's original work from half a century before. Here, Freud wrote that the cultural human being had replaced a scent of happiness with a dose of security. By the end of the twentieth century, however, this cultural formula had been reversed: "postmodern men and women exchanged a portion of their possibilities for security for a portion of happiness."[13] While the dissatisfaction during the period of modernity in Freud's lifetime in the second half of the nineteenth century and first half of the twentieth stemmed from a security that tolerated far too little freedom in the search for individual happiness, the dissatisfaction during postmodernity heading into the twenty-first century stemmed from the freedom granted for the search for happiness tolerating far too little individual security. If the days of security seekers were sad and monotonous, the sleepless nights of the free human being are a curse, Bauman comments.[14] However, he reminds the hopeful but disappointed postmodern woman and man that there is no victory without loss and

[12] Zygmunt Bauman, *Liquid modernity* (Cambridge: Polity, 2000).

[13] Zygmunt Bauman, *Postmodernity and its discontents* (Polity Press, 1997), 2.

[14] Ibid.

the hope that this exists is as vain as the famous dream of a free lunch. Nonetheless, it is the case that the wins and losses associated with any type of human community must be calculated with care so each and every one of us can seek the ideal balance between them, although the postmodern man and woman have a hard time relinquishing the dream that one day a balance sheet will arrive showing benefits only.

Rosa's Social Acceleration

The fluctuating essence of modernity is also connected to acceleration. One of the most influential theories of recent years has been the German sociologist Hartmut Rosa's concept of *social acceleration*.[15] Rosa belongs to the last generation of the Frankfurt school and has an explicit objective of reintroducing Marx and the early Frankfurt school's critique of alienation. The underlying premise is an experience of acceleration shared by all humans during late modernity: "*Social acceleration* is *defined* by an increase in the decay-rates of the reliability of experiences and *expectations* and by the contraction of the time-spans definable as the 'present'."[16] Rosa's thesis is that social acceleration in its current "totalitarian" form leads to grave, empirically demonstrable forms of social alienation which prevent realization of the good life.[17] The most evident and measurable form of acceleration comprises transport, communication and production processes managed by technological objectives. This entails the shrinking of space: a trip from London to New York in the sailing vessels of the pre-industrial age took three weeks, while in the age of jet aircrafts, the same trip takes eight hours, a reduction to one-sixtieth of the former amount of time required. The next element is an acceleration of social change. In pre-modern and early modern societies, the son would inherit the father's vocation, which could potentially be passed down for generations, while today we have a choice, but we cannot expect that choice to last for a lifetime. The average American must be prepared to change jobs eleven times in the course of his or her

[15] Hartmut Rosa, *Alienation and acceleration. Towards a critical theory of late-modern temporality* (New York: Columbia University Press, 2015).

[16] Ibid., 46.

[17] Ibid.

active working life.[18] Rosa calls the third category acceleration in the speed of life, often referred to as *time pressure*. Subjectively speaking, people will experience this acceleration as a time shortage: they feel hounded, stressed and under a huge time pressure. It feels like time is moving more quickly than previously. Paradoxically, there is no logical connection between this dimension and the other two, in that the development of technological innovations should give us more time, rather than less.

Rosa situates the causes of this social acceleration in the capitalist economy's fundamental principles for profit. Beyond this, the acceleration dynamic is connected to a strong cultural promise: in the modern, secular society, acceleration functions like an equivalent to the religious promise of eternal life. The good life has become synonymous with a life that is jam-packed. And the key to achieving this is to increase the pace of life so that you can realize an infinite number of different lives within a single lifetime. But for many people in today's Western society, this takes instead the form of a tragedy: "He feels caught in a relentless hamster wheel, his hunger for life and world is not satisfied but frustrated on an increasing scale."[19] The social acceleration produces mobility and disconnection from physical space, which can be positive, but simultaneously entails an alienation from our physical surroundings which we notice less. If you move around constantly, your surroundings will no longer feel like home; they lose their history, contain no memories and are no longer interwoven with your identity, Rosa warns.

Rosa's acceleration teachings offer a convincing historical analysis of how society's orientation has shifted from *position* to *performance*. The transition from classical modernity to late modernity was informed by critical, social watersheds constituting a movement away from the struggle between generations towards a struggle within generations. Because of this it is no longer possible to rely on achieving specific positions: you are also at risk of losing these if your results are poor. And as Rosa adds: "In this way, the focus of the struggle for recognition shifts from position to performance – recognition is no longer rewarded for lifelong achievement, but is instead dependent upon a day to day investment."[20]

---

[18] Ibid.

[19] Ibid., 54.

[20] Ibid., 69.

We Are Not Thriving in Late Capitalism

In the book *Capitalist Realism*, the critic Mark Fisher asserts that although the radical philosophers of the 1960s and 1970s, including Ronald Laing, Michel Foucault and Gilles Deleuze and Félix Guattari, postulated that the most serious psychological illnesses such as schizophrenia were not to be viewed as natural states, but as products of the current capitalist system, what is needed today is a politicization of far more common conditions, such as stress, depression and anxiety:

> I want to argue that it is necessary to reframe the growing problem of stress (and distress) in capitalist societies. Instead of treating it as incumbent on individuals to resolve their own psychological distress, instead, that is, of accepting the vast privatization of stress that has taken place over the last thirty years, we need to ask: how has it become acceptable that so many people, and especially so many young people, are ill? The 'mental health plague' in capitalist societies would suggest that, instead of being the only social system that works, capitalism is inherently dysfunctional, and that the cost of it appearing to work is very high.[21]

Fisher claims thus that the incidence of psychological disorders in Western populations is a direct consequence of late capitalism's prominent position. Of central importance to Fisher and others' critical reception of late capitalism's psychological impact in the West in our times is the concept of *neoliberalism*—as the dominant political ideology of recent decades. Neoliberalism represents an economic policy in which welfare and growth are considered best provided for by facilitating individual entrepreneurship within an institutional framework of private right of ownership, free markets and free trade.[22] Historically, its breakthrough is often connected to the economic policy of Augusto Pinochet's regime in Chile in the period 1973–1990, whereupon the American social

---

[21] Mark Fisher, *Capitalist realism* (Winchester: Zero Books, 2009), 19.

[22] David Harvey, *A brief history of neoliberalism* (Oxford: Oxford University Press, 2005).

economist Milton Friedman's market liberalistic ideas were first tested, and subsequently during Ronald Reagan's terms of office in the USA in 1981–1989, Margaret Thatcher's conservative government in Great Britain in 1979–1990, and perhaps somewhat surprisingly, Deng Xiaoping's presidency of China's communist party in 1978–1997, in that at this time an opening was created for Western market liberalism within the framework of a state, authoritarian rule. This alleged worldwide ideology, which encompasses different geopolitical systems of governance, also has consequences for how one came to conceptualize the citizen, which in keeping with the principles of the political economy should be a self-governing human being, requiring a minimum of state intervention. In a speech to the British population, Margaret Thatcher and Michael Heseltine formulated it as follows:

> Wherever possible we want individuals to control, influence and determine their own destiny … the psychology of independence is to the fore [...] People should exercise their abilities (serving as authors of their own decisions, seizing opportunities, and so on) in order to help themselves.[23]

A consequence of the call for individual opportunism with the free market as a backdrop is that citizens must become entrepreneurs in their own lives, shaping their destinies through the independent choices they make and quite simply by working on themselves. The ideal citizen—*the enterprising self*—is depicted as democratic and within reach for everyone.[24] Anyone unfortunate enough to be afflicted by homelessness or unemployment can personally resolve their difficulties by reversing their fate in accordance with these ideals. On the other hand, those who cannot or will not manage themselves as entrepreneurs are excluded and marginalized. Neoliberalism's requirement of personal autonomy is often

[23] Paul Heelas, "Reforming the self. Enterprise and the characters of Thatcherism", in *Enterprise culture*, ed. Russell Keat and Nicholas Abercrombie (London: Routledge, 1991), 77.

[24] Susan Ainsworth and Cynthia Hardy, "The enterprising self: an unsuitable job for an older worker" in *Organization* 15, no. 3 (2008).

called *accountability*.[25] In keeping with the idea of individualization, it entails that the individual is held accountable by viewing social risks such as illness, unemployment and poverty not as primarily the responsibility of the state, but as situated within the individual's realm of responsibility, in the name of self-care. The democratization of psychology and the self-help culture that flourishes in the same time period gains a prominent but ambiguous role. The latter phenomena supply self-care and personal development with more or less scientific life philosophies and coping strategies, all the while risking disclosure of society's actual structures of power.[26]

Dufour's Anthropological Mutation

The most indignant critics of neoliberalism don't stop there, but claim that neoliberalism even has an ambition of creating a new human being in its image, as the French philosopher Dany-Robert Dufour does in his book with the hard-hitting title *The Art of Shrinking Heads: On the New Servitude of the Liberated in the Era of Total Capitalism*.[27] Here Dufour depicts the development of *the postmodern subject* as radically different from that of influential predecessors, such as Immanuel Kant's critical nineteenth-century subject and Sigmund Freud's neurotic twentieth-century subject. Dufour asserts that under neoliberalism, both of these subject types are under threat of extinction when everything becomes a commodity. Neither the critical nor the neurotic subject possesses the requisite flexibility to connect with the constant flow of new goods, experiences and identities in the economy of desire. Neoliberalism's ideal human being, on the other hand, whom Dufour christens an uncritical subject with psychotic tendencies, contains a subjective cavity ever in need of filling. Dufour is careful to emphasize that he does not mean

[25] Thomas Lemke, "The birth of bio-politics: Michel Foucault's lecture at the Collège de France on neo-liberal governmentality", *Economy and Society* 30, no. 2 (2001).

[26] Samuel Binkley, *Happiness as enterprise: an essay on neoliberal life* (Albany: Suny Press, 2014); William Davies, *The happiness industry* (London: Verso, 2015).

[27] Dany-Robert Dufour, *The art of shrinking heads: on the new servitude of the liberated in the age of total capitalism* (Cambridge: Polity Press, 2008).

psychotic in the clinical sense or that the postmodern subject is the only subject that exists; large parts of the world are still characterized by modern or even pre-modern value systems. But the postmodern subject, receptive to all kinds of fluctuating identities, represents the inevitable future, given neoliberalism's continued development.

The anthropological mutation derived from the emergence of the postmodern subject under neoliberalism in the twenty-first century should be a cause of concern for everyone, in Dufour's opinion, because the market that young people of today have at their disposal for the purpose of creating a life and an identity no longer fulfils the function Freud in his day called the work of culture—to help them resolve the existential problem of origin: Who am I? How shall I live my life? Dufour situates the shift at the moment when Western culture began abandoning the insight that the subject *is not*, and never can be, fully autonomous. Here Dufour reminds us that the word "subject" comes from the Latin *subiectus*, which describes the state of having been subjected. Being a subject means first and foremost to be subjected to something. The underlying principle of this claim is the philosophical-anthropological premise that man is a substance, the existence of which is not self-sufficient, but instead dependent upon something larger than itself. The numerous ontologies throughout history that have given human beings answers to the question of what it means to exist—nature, ideas, "God", reason, being—always constitute a first principle for being-ness. Dufour defines "God", like Nietzsche before him, as a manmade entity but equally so as a vital artefact. The human being as a speaking subject has throughout all of time unceasingly created gods to authorize his/her existence. At the centre of the human race's lifeworld, there have therefore always been one or more beings the subject believes in as if they were real: gods, devils, demons—creatures that, unlike chaos, guarantee an unchanged existence, an origin, an ending and an order. Without this Other, the meta-social guarantor, it becomes difficult for the subject to be a self. He or she no longer knows which way to turn. And all human contact becomes precarious without a common reference to the same Other, which is all that enables different individuals to belong to the same community.

It is noteworthy that Dufour addresses specifically debates typical of the times that are also taking place in Norway, about young people's loss of direction and adds that in light of his hypothesis about an ill-fated autonomy, it would be surprising if they were to have any sense of direction whatsoever: "It is therefore pointless to talk about a loss of direction, if all we mean by that is that a few old-fashioned lessons about morality can repair the damage. It is morality itself that is not working, because it can only work 'in the name of'."[28] Dufour's analysis can also explain what many have pointed out: the coming generation of young people can no longer rebel, so instead they direct their anger towards themselves. The subjects of today are free but simultaneously nowhere: because how are they to be able to resist and rebel against the Other if they have not first been alienated by it? Dufour offers a potential explanation for *the problem of revolt* under the economy of desire, which Herbert Marcuse described as far back as in the 1960s—where is one to focus one's rage when the existing order has not only colonized property and the means of production, but even language and consciousness? The rage of today's youth is not directed at exploitation and their objective is not liberation. There is no guiding ideology for it; they are *for* the consumer society and *not* alienated but concerned with *identity politics*, as Dufour had sufficient foresight to observe already at the start of the twenty-first century. In the postmodern consumer society, there is no symbolic Other in relation to which the subject may make demands, ask questions or raise objections. The postmodern subject is first and foremost confused, but without knowing it, and the indignation the subject feels from time to time is primarily focused on the self. The collapse of the central, meta-social fictional figures that formerly organized our lives sounds perhaps like a dream for all Nietzsche followers, but nonetheless the results are disappointing. We are free, but only to wish for what the products have to offer us.

[28] Ibid., 15.

The Market as a New "God"

Why then doesn't the radical freedom offered by neoliberalism fulfil its promise? In the modern Western state, "God" is dead. He has indeed always been so, but He has been fictively alive as the symbolic, meta-social guarantor. Modern democracy's most important point of reference has instead become the free individual. Dufour traces this paradigm shift back to the Swiss-French philosopher Jean-Jacques Rousseau, who in the eighteenth century actively used introspection to recover his universal nature as a means of learning to speak on behalf of the human race. Historically speaking, however, the subject gained his or her identity through reference to "God", the fatherland, or bloodlines. An external entity gave the subject existence. For the modern democracy, this hetero-reference became an auto-reference. And this auto-reference creates more problems than it solves.

The postmodern landscape is apparently characterized by an absence of the Other, but with neoliberalism, it might appear that the market is in the process of assuming this role and becoming the new Other. Under neoliberalism, the market has succeeded in becoming the ultimate rationality, because the authorities of former periods must yield to it—even the state is now willing to relinquish its guiding and regulatory role. The state becomes to a certain degree a facilitator for neoliberalism, as the social geographer David Harvey, among others, has argued.[29] This implies that the market assumes "God's" place, but the replacement has an important difference. In contrast to former symbolic structures such as religion, the market "solves" the problem of origins by bringing the subject face to face with the challenge of edification without passing through a third, meta-social guarantor. Under postmodern neoliberalism, the traditional relationship between the self and an external symbolic structure is diminished to a relationship between the self and the self. The subject's identity is no longer guaranteed through an external, symbolic connection. Dufour calls this version of neoliberalism's abolishment of troublesome structures to guarantee its continued expansion *desymbolization*. He claims to prove the existence of this process, among

[29] Harvey, *A brief history of neoliberalism*.

other places in the world economy, which acquires an ever more speculative nature, freed from the original values that money was supposed to represent. Also, the task of being parents, those who traditionally say “no”, has been made difficult because today’s parents live under a categorical imperative to be young and their ability to set limits has been undermined in that their authority is no longer as given as it once was. Authority based on pre-eminent principles is not embodied and conveyed as effectively as previously. In that the third party has disappeared as a result of desymbolization, all relationships become two-way affairs and, when conflicts break out, it is no longer possible to appeal to equally universal agreements.

The consumer culture does indeed uphold the illusion that the market, like an all-powerful God, can meet all our needs. In the economy of desire, increasingly more refined products are consumed which are not purchased primarily because of material qualities but because of their symbolic value, which enshrouds the individual with the idea that by connecting to the product, he or she becomes unique. This tailor-made marketing shall ideally take care of all manner of desires, but it cannot satisfy the subject’s greatest challenge. No matter how powerful the market becomes, it cannot provide any answers for the meaning of existence—the great strength of the religious stories. The only thing the market can do is to bring each individual face to face with himself or herself. The neoliberal human being stands alone when it comes to the most fundamental of operations: creating an identity—which Freud designated as the work of culture, as stated above. And if (the impossible) question about the origin of existence is not resolved, this will become an endless and exhausting task for the generation growing up today.

Between the Guilt and the Shame

Dufour’s analysis also explains the development of *shame* to the detriment of *guilt* as the archetypical emotion of late modernity. As stated, Freud’s neurotic twentieth-century subject is on the verge of disappearing and with it also the obsessive guilt in relation to the Other, whom the neurotic always felt he/she disappointed, or was personally disappointed with, such as one's living or dead mother or father or "God". The guilt and frustrations caused by these figures, however, could be overcome by way of a slow process of introspection and projection into an alternative future. The subject in postmodernity, on the other hand, is characterized by a feeling of omnipotence when it succeeds and total impotence when it fails. Feeling ashamed of oneself has apparently replaced feelings of guilt in relation to others. Shame is an expression of a narcissistic intolerance for frustration. In contrast to the drawn-out nature of guilt, shame requires an immediate response. We feel ashamed in the same way that we feel hunger or cold. We are thereby deprived of guilt's slow, introspective work through which one seeks to instil it with meaning, while shame compels us to find a solution here and now. We can thereby also expect the outcomes to manifest in the manner of self-harm, drug addiction and acting out as abreactions in response to a painful situation demanding a solution.

And if subjectivity is undergoing change, one must also expect the psychopathology to change. In a sense, all the *postmodern pathologies* are connected to the problem of identity and the burden of self-creation. Dufour bases his claims on the ideas of the French medical sociologist Alain Ehrenberg,[30] who has singled out depression as late modernity's archetypical psychological disorder. Ehrenberg's claim is supported by the World Health Organization (WHO), which has identified depression as the second most widespread cause of death after cardiovascular diseases. It is estimated to afflict 15–20 percent of the population in the West. WHO's estimates indicate that by the year 2030, depression will be the largest health burden in all Western nations. Ehrenberg understands depression as being the price we must pay for the radical freedom and liberation from authority in the form of the Other. The self has today become the foremost authority. This unshackling of the individual provides it with opportunities for life choices and self-realization which the majority in previous generations never had. If the individual succeeds, so much the better, but should the individual fail, the price to be paid becomes higher. The subject will not have anyone to blame but him or herself. The burden of the idea that everything is possible is a heavy one

[30] Ehrenberg, *The weariness of the self: diagnosing the history of depression in the contemporary age.*

to bear. Depression is the shame of enduring the knowledge that everything is possible, while simultaneously failing in its achievement, Ehrenberg points out. The proliferation of depression in our times is due to the postmodern form of subjectivation, which adheres to an impossible logic: we must use ourselves to become ourselves. Depression arises between the injunction of self-realization and the breakdown of identity, like a modern version of Baron von Münchhausen's "bootstrapping" trilemma, where he claimed he could pull himself and his horse out of a bog by his hair. Dufour maintains that the generation growing up today are individuals expected to create themselves by using themselves as their sole resource, and thereby they find themselves face to face with the same type of impossible dilemma.

Despite the relatively disturbing picture Dufour paints of the opportunities for living a good life under neoliberalism, his analysis also leaves a certain amount of room for hope. In many ways we are back where Nietzsche started in the 1880s, he claims, that is, the nihilistic recognition of how the old metaphysical foundation for values was never anything more than fictions spanning an abyss. The ongoing, tragic destruction of the human being, as he sees it, therefore also encompasses unexpected possibilities. We must quite simply start afresh with a new critical intelligence and a new understanding of the unconscious spiritual life. The world is open for those able to recognize the right moment to strike in the search for new, unanticipated opportunities.

Failure to Thrive in the New Millennium

The transition from one century to the next will typically engender a new-found optimism for the new, upcoming period, but the theorizing at the beginning of the 2000s does not inspire any real belief in the idea that the fundamentally critical attitude towards modernity has been abandoned. Many of the processes described here that unfolded on the brink of the twentieth century appear only to have been strengthened or to have acquired renewed currency in keeping with historical, political and technological changes. The sociologists Anthony Elliott and Charles Lemert assert that a dominant feature of life at the beginning of the twenty-first century in the West is the unavoidable social horizon of *the new individualism,* comprising four main components: (1) a ruthless emphasis on self-renewal, (2) a boundless appetite for constant change, (3) a preoccupation with the short term and transitory and (4) a fascination with speed and dynamism.[31] Further, they cite network building, short-term project work, organizational downsizing, self-help literature, compulsive large-scale consumption, cybersex, continual changes in identity and a therapeutic culture as some of the prevalent features of the global, individualist culture. The resources the individual has at his or her disposal as a means of adapting to a swift and polished new global world order by transforming themselves are exclusively about living differently, cosmetically changing their bodies or reorienting their lives according to the latest diet trend or self-help philosophy.[32] The political mentality that dominates the new individualism is "individualized solutions to global problems!"[33]

The German philosopher Axel Honneth reflects at the start of the millennium upon the paradoxes of individualization by returning to his predecessor Simmel, who, one hundred years before, reflected upon the contradictory landscape facing the modern human being:

> It is true he [the peasant at the end of the Middle Ages] gained freedom, but only freedom *from* something, not liberty *to do* something. Apparently, he gained freedom to do anything – because it was purely negative – but in fact he was without any directive, without any definite and determining content. Such freedom favours that emptiness and instability that allows one to give full reign to every accidental, whimsical and tempting impulse. Such freedom may be compared with the fate of the insecure person who has forsworn his gods and whose newly acquired 'freedom' only provides the opportunity for making an idol out of any fleeting value.[34]

---

[31] Elliott and Lemert, *The new individualism: the emotional costs of globalization (revised edition).*

[32] Ibid.

[33] Ibid., xviii.

[34] Axel Honneth, "Organized self-realization: some paradoxes of individualization", in *European Journal of Social Theory* 7, no. 4 (2004), 475.

Honneth doesn't ask whether the three to four preceding decades fully demonstrated the problem Simmel describes, since the new individualism's invitation of self-realization has gradually evolved from being a freedom-maximizing, welcome break with the tradition and conformity that curtailed the individual's development, into an instrument for economic development, whereby the standardized requirement to recreate one's life becomes in the end an emotionally rigid obligation, under which the young people of today suffer more than thrive. Like Dufour, Honneth sees Ehrenberg's explanations of depression in the West as an expression of psychological exhaustion from the unclear, yet widespread requirement to be oneself and open oneself to continuous self-development. Years after Honneth's analysis of this tipping point, however, self-realization appears only to be on the rise.

In the early 2000s, psychology was also made democratic in a serious fashion on a global scale and there is nowhere this was more clearly expressed than in the promise of happiness. Happiness is for average, ordinary human beings, for those who are not destitute, quite simply for those who want to get more out of life. The problem of happiness is the perfect mechanism for gathering all humans in the psychological fold, sociologist Sam Binkley writes in the book *Happiness as Enterprise: An Essay on Neoliberal Life*.[35] March 20 was declared the official International Day of Happiness by none other than the UN in 2012. But it is of equal significance that the Norwegian national daily *VG*'s piece in honour of the day in 2018 began with a dejected introduction:

> Last year for the first time Norway was named the happiest country in the world. This year we ended up in second place after Finland, but ahead of Denmark, Iceland and Switzerland. Nonetheless, we have a tendency to express dissatisfaction. What is that all about?[36]

Binkley makes the argument that the search for happiness reflects how community values such as moral codes of conduct and religious conceptions about humans' place in the cosmos have to a great extent

[35] Binkley, *Happiness as enterprise: an essay on neoliberal life*.

[36] Bodil Sundbye, "Kunsten å tenke seg glad" in *VG*, 20 March 2018, 25.

disappeared and what we are left with is a psychologically truncated subject who has only emotional self-manipulation at his or her disposal. "Happiness has been rendered a depthless physiological response without a moral referent, a biological potential of the individual that makes no recourse to psychic interiority, biography or social relationships of any kind, however sublimated. Happiness is the pure effect of everyday mental activities and everyday practice."[37] This limiting approach to life is sold on a large scale as psychological democratization and an invitation to life itself.

In my earlier books *The Therapeutic Turn* and *Optimizing the Self*, I have investigated how the self-help ideology finds expression and unfolds in Norway. Here I find that the circulation of the ideas about self-realization and self-optimization is by no means restricted to the commercial market. In the second decade of the 2000s, these ideas have in fact been made an institutionalized point of reference for the perspectives of the new educational framework plans for kindergartens, a long awaited part of the reform of the Norwegian National Curriculum for Knowledge Promotion in Primary and Secondary Education and Training (*Kunnskapsløftet*) and a standard for how young people in particular speak and think about themselves.[38] In her book "The Damned Freedom" (*Den fordømte friheten)*, philosopher Kaja Melsom has made the argument that the extreme consequence of modern-day culture's relentless romanticizing of the self-actualized individual is that ordinary men and women torment themselves all the more with questions of whether they are original, passionate and happy enough, and the result is often more anxiety, doubt and shame.[39] The same tendency can be discerned in the rest of Scandinavia. Psychologist Svend Brinkmann has scrutinized the *developmental imperative* that permeates the view of humanity in the Danish working life, education system and personal life in the protest trilogy *Stand Firm, Standpoints* and *The Joy of Missing Out*.[40]

---

[37] Binkley, *Happiness as enterprise: an essay on neoliberal life*, 2.

[38] Ole Jacob Madsen, *Optimizing the self: social representations of self-help* (London: Routledge, 2015); *The therapeutic turn. How psychology altered Western culture* (London: Routledge, 2014).

[39] Kaja Melsom, *Den fordømte friheten* (Oslo: Gyldendal, 2016).

[40] Svend Brinkmann, *Stand firm: resisting the self-improvement craze* (London: Polity, 2017); *Standpoints: 10 old ideas in a new world* (London: Polity, 2018); *The joy of missing out: the art of*

In Sweden, the organizational scientist Carl Cederström along with co-author André Spicer in the books *The Wellness Syndrome* and *Desperately Seeking Self-Improvement* have described, not unlike Honneth, how health, well-being and self-improvement have not just become monomaniacal goals in and of themselves, but also the expression of a contemporary ideology in which the wish to be healthy, quit smoking or lose weight is seamlessly interwoven with the free market economy and the compulsion to improve your personal market value.[41]

A unique feature of several of the diagnoses of contemporary society made in the early 2000s is also the claim that work becomes the yardstick according to which most human activities are measured. The late modern human being is by and large an employed human being, regardless of whether or not they are at work. "The Working Society" is Swedish Roland Paulsen's preferred contemporary diagnosis, with his point being that although the technological development would imply that we actually need far less manpower than previously, work appears all the more to have become a goal in its own right, regardless of what we do at work and even though burnout and stress are on the rise.[42]

In the aftermath of the global financial crisis in 2008, the Italian philosopher Franco Berardi's book *The Soul at Work* was published.[43] Here he asks how it is possible that we have apparently moved away from the working-class struggle of the 1960s, involving that class's separation from the capitalist organizations responsible for production, to the current situation in which work has become the headquarters for psychological and emotional investment, although the new economy of desire induces a series of pathologies such as attention disorders, anxiety and depression. This occurs through the colonization of the soul and desire. When the soul becomes a part of the production process, the workforce is transformed into human capital. Berardi holds that this creates the foundation for a new type of alienation—the soul is put to work—and our desire is reduced to self-administration, our involvement

---

self-restraint in an age of excess (London: Polity, 2019).

[41] Carl Cederström and André Spicer, *The wellness syndrome* (London: Polity, 2015); *Desperately seeking self-improvement: a year inside the optimization movement* (New York: OR Books, 2017).

[42] Roland Paulsen, *Arbetssamhället. Hur arbetet överlevde teknologin* (Stockholm: Atlas, 2017).

[43] Franco Berardi, *The soul at work* (Los Angeles: Semiotext(e), 2009).

regulated by economic rules, our attention imprisoned within virtual networks and every fragment of mental activity is converted into capital.

Berlin-based, South Korean philosopher Byung-Chul Han's book, published in 2010 and aptly entitled *The Burnout Society*, makes a main point that we have now abandoned the diagnostic focus of Michel Foucault's disciplinarian society. In the twenty-first century, the archetypical institutions are no longer the hospital, mental hospital, prisons, military barracks or factories, but instead fitness centres, office buildings, banks, airports, shopping malls and genetic laboratories.[44] The society of the new millennium is no longer to be considered a *disciplinary society* but instead an *achievement society*. The subjects of today are no longer *obedient subjects*, but *achievement subjects* who have become their own employers. Han refers here to the growing group of creative knowledge workers who in practical terms can work anytime and anywhere. A feature of the twenty-first century's achievement-oriented subjects is that they are free of external, ruling authorities, who either force them to work or exploit them. On the contrary, they are their own bosses. But the disappearance of ruling authorities does not lead to freedom. Instead, it would appear that freedom and coercion now coincide. Instead of foreign exploitation, we now have self-exploitation, which in reality is more efficient, since it coexists with the feeling of freedom. In practical terms, one is always at work and for many this leads to a one-track existence. The achievement society's mental illnesses must therefore be understood in light of this paradoxical freedom.

Up to now the focus has predominantly been on a faulty subjectivation which has physical or psychological consequences for the individual, although some have also viewed the tendency to revert to antisocial externalizations as reactions to the same thing. In an issue of the journal *Samtiden* dedicated to the terrorist attack that took place in Norway on 22 July 2011, literary critic Tom Egil Hverven applied Dufour's depiction of an anthropological mutation as a perspective from which to view the two different Anders, one fictive, the other real, from, respectively, the film *Oslo, 31 August* and the 22 July attack, as personifying introverted

[44] Buyung-Chul Han, *The burnout society* (Stanford, CA: Stanford University Press, 2015).

and extroverted reactions to the same self-under-threat.[45] Represented by a bloated subject's self-destruction and violence, respectively, the latter acts are viewed as sacrifices stemming from the shame over being a failure in the best country in the world, despite having every opportunity at one's disposal. The educator Per Bjørn Foros and philosopher Arne Johan Vetlesen in their book *Angsten for oppdragelsen* ("Child-Rearing Anxiety") claim that many young people in presumably well-functioning welfare states such as Norway and Denmark are recruited into extremist groups such as Islamic State (IS) in the search for meaning, identity and affiliation.[46] These lines of flight imply that many young people do not feel that their basic social and existential needs are being met. In his book *Globalized Islam: The Search for a New Ummah,* French political scientist Olivier Roy situates the development of radical Islam since 11 September 2001 in the context of an increased individualization and the self's search for authenticity.[47] Roy defines the triumph of the religious self as the situation in which secularization and sacralization meet; we have undergone a shift from religion to religiosity and from culture to identity. Religion is no longer closely integrated with the practices of local society, as was the case in traditional societies, because the *deterritorialization* entails that young men and women now live individualized lives in secular, Western cities. And if the alienation and absence of norms becomes extreme, a virtual community on the Internet is seductive, but such communities are often based on a fundamentalist belief and ruled by claims of authenticity and feelings, in contrast to former religious communities governed by customs and the intellect. A potential for radicalized groups willing to commit terrorist acts is hereby facilitated, since the late modern religiosity to a larger extent departs from the surrounding social norms, in contrast to traditional religions, which stemmed from the more deeply rooted life involving family, heritage and the local community.

Destructive men notwithstanding, there are many indications that overall it is the opposite sex who is most susceptible to the sting of late

---

[45] Tom Egil Hverven, "Megalomani og selvutslettelse" in *Samtiden* 120, no. 4 (2011).

[46] Per Bjørn Foros and Arne Johan Vetlesen, *Angsten for oppdragelsen. Et samfunnsetisk perspektiv på dannelse* (*2nd edition*) (Oslo: Universitetsforlaget, 2015).

[47] Olivier Roy, *Globalized Islam: the search for a new Ummah* (New York: Columbia University Press, 2004).

capitalism's requirements. The living-conditions health study shows that consultations with psychologists in Norway increased from 4 to 14 percent for women aged 16–24 in the time period from 1998 to 2015, while for young men during the same period, the number has remained at a stable 4 percent since 2002.[48] Why does it appear that young women to a far greater degree than young men feel the need to seek out a psychologist? Traditional explanations often focus on how it is much more difficult for men to seek help and that seeing a psychologist comes into conflict with hegemonic perceptions of masculinity allowing little room for vulnerability.[49] But this can also be turned around by asking whether women are simply more sensitive to the requirements of late capitalism. The British sociologist Rosalind Gill claims that contemporary culture is now so permeated with individualistic self-help philosophies that we have come to address the self as a project to be evaluated, advised, disciplined and improved.[50] However, what is striking is how unevenly distributed these quasi-therapeutic injunctions are between the sexes. The ideal, disciplinary subject under neoliberalism is feminine, Gill remarks. The so-called post-feminism, in which to a large extent traditional, essentialist, gender-based perceptions of men and women are abandoned, to an equally large extent meshes with neoliberalism's profiting from flexibility and plasticity—whereby the woman becomes the model for the archetypical make-over self, continually striving to optimize herself, her body and her working and private life. The stagnant, ungainly masculinity, on the other hand, is much less attractive as an object of economic exploitation and so to a larger degree is left in peace. Although engagement with therapeutic practices tends to revolve around individual strategies of self-transformation, sociologists Suvi Salmenniemi and Laura Kemppainen have shown that these strategies can also be a necessary starting place for political and social change, including addressing gender inequality.[51] Individual and social change does not always need to be mutually exclusive.

---

[48] Statistics Norway, "Levekårsundersøkelsen om helse 2015" (Oslo: Statistics Norway, 2017).

[49] Paul. M. Galdas, Francine Cheater, and Paul Marshall, "Men and health help-seeking behaviour: literature review" in *Journal of Advanced Nursing* 49, no. 6 (2005).

[50] Rosalind Gill, *Gender and the media* (London: Polity Press, 2007).

[51] Suvi Salmenniemi, and Laura Kemppainen, "Masculine performers and good girls", in *The Routledge international handbook of global therapeutic cultures*, eds. Daniel Nehring, Ole Jacob Madsen, Edgar Cabanas, China Mills, and Dylan Kerrigan (London: Routledge, 2020), 289.

Conclusion

The examples cited here are fortunately more the exception than the rule, although the genre under discussion might lead one to think otherwise. "Why, suffering is the sole origin of consciousness", the main character of Fyodor Dostoyevsky's novel *Notes from the Underground*[52] muses. If we base ourselves on diagnoses of our modern-day society, it could appear that he is right. Hartmut Rosa also views the entire origin of the genre of sociology and social philosophy as a reaction to living in modernity. What many of the reactions noted here have in common is a tendency to focus on the negative. If, on the other hand, we focus on the positive, one will perhaps not feel the same need to verbalize it on a similar scale. This also means that the distribution of the diagnoses of contemporary society can be relatively skewed and give the impression that overall, the current age is far worse off than it actually is. The sociologist Willy Guneriussen also points out that a polarization has occurred in the understanding of modernity. In the spirit of the school of the thought of the Enlightenment, there is also another tradition which views modernity's development in a far more optimistic manner, as a guarantee of increased freedom, self-realization, and expressiveness, and liberation from religious superstition.[53] Based on the World Values Survey, an investigation of human values in almost one hundred nations since 1981, German political scientist Christian Welzel has made the argument that the development of modernity has primarily been liberating, in that it has facilitated a democratic realization of human freedom and equal opportunity, both of which are also associated with increased happiness and satisfaction in the populations of a number of countries in recent times.[54] In these two chapters, I have predominantly presented the dystopian understanding of modernity. But elements of optimism can also be found in the critique of modernity: Marx predicted that capitalism would break down in the end

---

[52] Fjodor M. Dostoyevsky, *Notes from the underground*, (1864), https://www.planetebook.com/free-ebooks/notes-from-the-underground.pdf, 45.

[53] Willy Guneriussen, *Å forstå det moderne: framskrittstro, rasjonalitet, ambivalens og irrasjonalitet i diskursen om modernitet* (Oslo: Tano Aschehoug, 1999).

[54] Christian Welzel, *Freedom rising: human empowerment and the quest for emancipation* (Cambridge: Cambridge University Press, 2013).

and pave the way for the communist society, through which the individual's self-realization could come to fruition. And in his most recent works, Weber sought to identify exits from the iron cage of rationality.[55] He maintained that these were to be found in the arts, especially in music, and in eroticism. The latter spheres encompass the moments of intoxication, rapture and ecstasy formerly restricted to religious experiences. And as Guneriussen writes, these spheres represent the hope of a kind of secular salvation for the modern-day human being: "In art lies a possibility for 'redemption on this side' from a thoroughly rationalized daily life. While the rationalized spheres are fundamentally demystified, perhaps art can yet offer a form of re-mystified and enchanted life experience."[56] Weber also understood eroticism to be an area that had been differentiated through the development of modernity, becoming an independent realm of pleasure that transcended former considerations for convention, marriage and procreation. In the sublime eroticism lies, as in the arts, also a possibility for deliverance, in this life, from the iron cage of rationality. Guneriussen thus reminds us that there are sources of existential meaning to be found in modernity, which also the great theorists of modernity foresaw, but which are easily under-communicated in the dystopian descriptions. Perhaps one therefore reads the critics of modernity best if one views them as an attempt to anticipate the future and therefore as deliberately emphasizing negative features of the present day rather than giving a complete, representative image of the actual state of the world.

[55] Guneriussen, *Å forstå det moderne: framskrittstro, rasjonalitet, ambivalens og irrasjonalitet i diskursen om modernitet.*
[56] Ibid., 190.

4

Young, Privileged and Sick

THE GROWING ABUNDANCE OF THE GENRE NOTWITHSTANDING, A COMMON FEATURE OF MUCH OF THE LITERATURE endeavouring a diagnosis of the current era, a feature almost as prominent as its critique of modernity, is the lack of empirical substantiation. The absence of any basis in people's actual lives is at times sought redressed through examples from fiction. A timely example is Dufour's dramatic account of the debilitated conditions for living a good life in late modernity, where neoliberalism's purportedly psychotic subject has begun to prevail and ordinary relationships, including those between children and parents, are in a state of total dissolution. The foremost case cited to represent this desymbolization appears in a footnote, as is fitting with the above in mind, where Dufour refers to the Austrian director Michael Haneke's psychological horror film *Benny's Video* as an illustration.[1]

In this film, Haneke depicts the life of a nuclear family from the Austrian bourgeoisie, told from the vantage point of teenage son Benny, whose chief interests are cameras and videos.[2] Much of the story takes

[1] Dufour, *The art of shrinking heads: on the new servitude of the liberated in the age of total capitalism*, footnote 16.

[2] Michael Haneke, "Benny's Video" (Austria/Switzerland: Bernard Lang, 1992).

O. J. Madsen, *Deconstructing Scandinavia's "Achievement Generation"*,
https://doi.org/10.1007/978-3-030-72555-6_4

place in the boy's bedroom, which resembles something between a bunker and a TV studio. Black-out curtains prevent sunlight from entering the room, while a surveillance camera monitors what takes place outside. Benny's parents appear to be successful but there is little spontaneous warmth and genuine communication to be detected between the members of the family. The only thing that seems to awaken Benny's emotional life is a video recording of the execution of a pig with a stun gun on the family farm, which he watches virtually on a loop. One weekend when Benny's parents are away, he meets a young girl by chance at the local video shop and she accompanies him home. First, Benny shows her the film of the pig and then the stun gun which he has stolen from the farm. Benny challenges her to use it on him. She refuses. The roles are reversed. Benny sends a charge through her chest. Through his video screen, we witness how she crawls in spasms across the floor before he finishes her off with two final jolts. Benny hides the corpse in a closet and continues his weekend at home alone as if nothing has happened. When his parents come home, he fittingly unveils the misdeed by showing them the video recording of the murder. His distraught parents discuss what they should do. The father convinces the mother that since there are no witnesses of the event, nobody will suspect them. Benny and his mother travel to Egypt on holiday, while the father stays behind to dispose of the body. When the film ends, Benny, by all appearances completely unmoved by the situation, turns his own parents in to the police. In keeping with his character, he has secured evidence on video of his parents' conversation during which they decide to cover up the atrocity rather than implicate their own son.

A common theme in all of Haneke's films is how surveillance technology and a life spent in front of the screen alter the basic human condition. Haneke, who is coincidently also a philosopher by profession, presumably shares Dufour's concern for young people growing up under late capitalism, but Haneke's associated tendency to inflate signs of the times into warnings about the future does not exactly equip Dufour with any convincing case studies to support his grand-scale thesis about the ongoing anthropological mutation of human beings under neoliberalism. If there is a connection between screen time and violence, research indicates instead a decline in the latter, essentially because young people are spending more time at home and less time with each other without parental supervision.[3] The difference between Haneke and Dufour is nonetheless that all is fair in art, while in the social sciences, it is reasonable to expect a larger degree of professional accountability.

An even clearer example of an interpretation of the connection between late capitalism and the psyche on a purely fictional basis is found in the writings of theologian Ryan LaMothe, who, like Dufour, claims that the market society gives rise to social pathologies on a grand scale.[4] In the market society, the economy becomes the supporting girder of that society and it thereby also shapes relationships within the public, political and private spheres, according to the principles of the exchange of commodities. On the human level, this means that all citizens must become entrepreneurs, *homo oeconomicus*, steered by an instrumental rationality and are expected to handle social risk and uncertainty by taking sufficient precautions for themselves and their families. Today's market society creates, on the one hand, entrepreneur subjects with sociopathic tendencies and, on the other, worn out individuals who are forced to live beyond their psychological capabilities.

Fiction is rife with illustrations of this, LaMothe remarks and makes reference to well-known stories such as Charles Dickens' *A Christmas Carol*, in which Ebenezer Scrooge's relationships with people are destroyed by greed, Willie Loman's ruthless boss who fires him when he does not deliver the expected sales figures in Arthur Miller's play *Death of a Salesman,* and the investor Gordon "Greed is good" Gekko in Oliver Stone's movie *Wall Street.* But does LaMothe succeed here in convincing us of widespread, mass sociopathy in demonstrating to the reader his knowledge of the depictions of unscrupulous capitalists in Western literature, theatre and cinema throughout the past 150 years? He otherwise claims that the worn-out subjects are like the people in Plato's cave metaphor—they are unable to envision anything else because they lack a sufficiently developed critical imagination that will enable them to address the political-economic system under which they exist. They are

[3] Lars Roar Frøyland and Tilmann von Soest, "Trends in the perpetration of physical aggression among Norwegian adolescents 2007–2015" in *Journal of Youth and Adolescence* (2017).

[4] Ryan LaMothe, "The travails and tragedies of a market civilization: a psychology of faith perspective" in *Pastoral Psychology* 67, no. 2 (2017).

oppressed without knowing it. On this point, LaMothe does indeed cite a real case: 29-year-old Karen who seeks help for anxiety and depression. She has three young children and even though she and her husband both work fifty–sixty-hour weeks, they struggle to make ends meet. Individuals like Karen are exploited in late capitalist working life, in that the profits do not provide her with the adequate means to take care of herself and her family, but instead fall into the pockets of her employer.

An additional problem Karen has is that she is not able to see the true cause of her suffering. At first, Karen believed that her psychological and economic disability was due to factors from her childhood. Her self-diagnosis does not consider the political-economic system and illustrates how the exhausted subject cannot channel his or her agency towards the causes of the problem, because these have been obscured. She is not capable of what the revolutionary psychiatrist Frantz Fanon referred to in his day as enabling "[the patient] to choose an action with respect to the *real source of the conflict* [my emphasis], i.e., the social structure".[5] When, on the other hand, she receives help that enables her to see the connection to "the economic-political system that was rigged against her and her husband", she becomes more involved in the local community and in the work to bring unions into the workplace.[6] She still experiences periods of depression but feels nonetheless much better after having refocused her energies and has more faith in the future. The market society continues to pressure her to live at odds with her psychological resources but her revitalized drive helps Karen to stem the tide of this external pressure.

Although we are dealing with an actual case here, it demonstrates yet another problem with the model that LaMothe and Dufour establish: the social pathologies perspective does not sufficiently allow for individual vulnerability factors. Why are certain people, but far from all people, sick if they are all living under the same pathological social conditions? Without a satisfactory answer, the explanatory power of the social pathologies perspective alone is weak. These perspectives are also dominated by a lack of any basis in the personal illness stories of the afflicted individuals. At best, fiction is employed as an illustration, but far

[5] Ibid., 17.

[6] Ibid.

too infrequently is a reference made to people's actual experiences and illnesses. There is thereby an overhanging risk of both exaggerating how ordinary the pathologies of modernity are and depicting people as powerless in relation to the cultural, technological and political life conditions under which they are living. The argument becomes less convincing than it could have been if to a greater extent there had been an interest in how the pathologies of our times are filtered into lived life.

Illness Experiences from Life in Late Modernity

As a means of redressing some of the shortcomings of the literature offering a critique of modernity, I have in the following drawn from my own and others' qualitative studies of young people who have experienced depression in Norway, Sweden and Denmark, respectively. The studies address both unique vulnerability factors and the basic social conditions under which the individuals in question are living.

Norway: "I Get So Afraid of Missing Out on Myself"

In the following, seven Norwegian women and men, ages 20–31, were interviewed by psychologist Linn Julie Skagestad about how they experienced their depression, with the aim of investigating whether supposed social factors such as increased complexity, detraditionalization, individualization and self-realization are of key significance in terms of how they understand themselves and their illness.[7]

---

[7] The interviews were carried out by Skagestad in conjunction with the work on her master's thesis, which later also led to a scientific article co-written with the undersigned (Skagestad, 2014, Skagestad and Madsen, 2015). The issue raised on the basis of the interview materials was: What basic narratives—in other words, the story the individual tells about him or herself—do young adults employ about depression? What causes do they emphasize in these basic narratives? How do any normative contemporary ideals such as self-realization find expression in their basic narratives? The sample used in the study comprised five women and two men with an average age of 23.7 years. Five of the informants were students at OsloMet University or the University of Oslo and two were students at one of Norway's folk high schools (non-degree colleges). The inclusion criteria for

Below follows a biographical introduction to the (anonymized) informants of the study:

Thomas, 24 years old, experienced life as an uphill battle upon commencing his education at a prestigious institution of higher learning. Due to a prolapsed disc, he no longer had the strength to fully apply himself to his studies. He felt unmotivated and like a failure and became depressed. With time he started taking antidepressants.

Karianne, 27 years old, was afflicted with depression six months after moving to Oslo to pursue her studies. She struggled to develop a network, but eventually made new friends who had far stricter social behavioural requirements than she was accustomed to. She recently experienced a relapse due to a break-up, was put on sick leave, saw a psychologist and finally her doctor prescribed antidepressants.

Ingrid, 23 years old, describes an upbringing during which she was pulled back and forth between religious and non-religious environments, and how the need for self-realization emerged during her teenage years. At that time, she felt alone, without solid footing and was eventually unable to concentrate on her schoolwork. She went to see her doctor, where she received medication and was referred to a psychologist. Her situation has stabilized in recent years.

Live, 21 years old, reports periods of being bullied, experiencing loneliness and inflicting self-harm while growing up. She sought help from the Child and adolescent psychiatric polyclinic (BUP) while attending upper secondary school, told the psychologist that she smoked hash and was sent to a substance abuse treatment centre. Live experienced the focus there as being exclusively on her substance abuse and not on her depression, which she would have preferred. Things are a bit up and down for her now.

Line, 31 years old, experienced depression for the first time in her late teens, when she was struggling to fulfil the high expectations of her parents. After spending a lot of time searching in her 20s, which involved travel, work, and studies, she became exhausted. Her doctor prescribed antidepressants and referred her to a psychologist, but Line did not find

participation were (1) as a young adult at some point between the ages of 16 and 29 the participants had been diagnosed with unipolar, clinical depression by a doctor or psychologist; (2) the diagnosis must have been made at least three months ago and (3) they had to be at least 18 years old at the time of the interview. In our approach we used a semi-structured, qualitative research interview, and thematic analysis and context analysis, respectively, in interpretation of the data.

this helpful. For a period of time she lived with her parents, who now provide good emotional support.

Bendik, 21 years old, reports a difficult adolescence in the course of which he experienced bullying and had an identity crisis upon realizing he was homosexual at a time when he was living in a conservative Christian environment. He has recently moved to Oslo and thought he would finally have the chance to start the life he wanted but isolated himself and in his own words "could not make it happen". Bendik received helpful support from a friend and her mother, who helped him tell his mother and siblings about his sexual orientation. He experienced their acceptance as conditional.

Sumaira, 20 years old, was diagnosed with depression at the age of 16 after having grown up feeling lonely and being bullied. She went to see a psychologist but felt pressured to get well quickly and therefore simply pretended to feel better. Sumaira was then referred to BUP and recently she has been doing a bit better.

The Road to Depression

What causes are presented as being of central importance in the informants' basic narratives about their depressions? Not surprisingly, there were several unique responses here, but the thematic analysis also found eight recurring themes in the informants' presentations of the causes of depression. These themes were as follows:

Feeling Like a Failure In all seven accounts of the road to depression, an experience of being a failure and feeling inadequate were highlighted as significant. However, the informants described different areas in which they felt like failures. Bendik highlights an experience of not having lived up to his own expectations for how his Oslo life would be:

> I had no solution. Because I was in Oslo, then, and was so down about how I hadn't managed to make something out of my Oslo life.

Thomas describes an experience of failing to live up to own and others' expectations when embarking on a course of study he had aspired to for a long time:

> Yes, such a feeling of failure, (…). Because it was expected of me, mostly from myself, that you're sort of assessed as being intelligent enough for admission, so then you had better be very intelligent.

Karianne expresses that she has experienced it as difficult to fulfil the prevailing criteria for success of her social environment:

> I am 27 years old and single, so that becomes a measure of your success. Can't make a relationship work, can't manage to find a man.

Both Live and Line highlight an experience of failing to live up to ideals regarding physical appearance. Live describes it as follows:

> And the ideal of beauty, that you're supposed to look like this and that, and I didn't look like that (…). I like wanted to be one of those so-called Gina Tricot girls who always had cool clothes and were thin and pretty and … and I was … I had ugly clothes, was a tub of lard.

Line expresses feeling defective due to limitations in her own abilities.

> [] I feel like I'm a second-rate product.

Being Alone Six of the informants in different ways mention an experience of being alone in their understanding of own depression. Three of the participants highlight the absence of close friends in their depression narratives. Sumaira describes it as follows:

> So … I was very alone, had no friends in practical terms (…). You become very lonely.

Thomas too describes the lack of a close network:

> It was a very different life and then, having had a live-in partner for so long and suddenly having to live alone (…) I've never been the type to have a large network of friends and stuff. I know a lot of people but have few friends. So, then I ended up by myself quite a bit.

Ingrid felt alone and pulled back and forth between two different communities:

> Almost all the people around me were in one of two different communities, in a way [the school community or the church community] ... it was easy to feel completely alone then, in between these two communities.

Three of the informants also expressed not having any adults to turn to for support. For Bendik, this was about a lack of support from her family:

> But perhaps the family should be aware that it's important to follow up a bit more when a child moves out of the family home. Be the good parent who comes forward and helps with packing. Be someone who wants to be there, to help out with small things, because that means so much. (...) Because there was actually nobody who helped me.

Sumaira spoke about a lack of help from teachers and parents to put an end to the bullying she was subjected to. Two of the informants, represented here by Karianne, express how they have experienced only limited inclusion in their social environment:

> Behind the façade of being a tolerant and open community, there are actually very strict criteria for what is acceptable. And you receive a very clear response if you should end up on the outside. Then it's just that nobody can be bothered to hang out with you, nobody contacts you.

Lack of Acceptance and Acknowledgement In their stories about the road leading to depression, five of the participants in the study mentioned sensing a lack of acceptance and appreciation for who they are. Ingrid experienced a lack of acceptance because she questioned the implicit assumptions of her local congregation. For Bendik, his experience of a lack of acceptance was due to his sister's failure to fully acknowledge his homosexual orientation when he told her about it. Live experienced a lack of appreciation and inclusiveness in her class at school:

> Yes, or it started actually in first grade in primary school. Like: okay, you're not cool enough to be one of us.

Three of the informants emphasize an experience of not being able to be themselves. While for Karianne, it was about there not being space for her to share feelings of sadness with her group of friends, for Line, her parents' failure to accept her alternative lifestyle was of central importance.

Transition to Student and Adult Life Two of the informants describe how they experienced the period of upheaval between adolescence and adulthood as the beginning of identity problems in the sense of finding themselves. For Ingrid, it was solely about figuring out her own standpoint in relation to parents who had "two completely different world views". For his own part, Thomas describes an insufficient ability to cope with his studies as difficult:

> I felt it was very frustrating not to measure up. I had broken up with my live-in partner right before I started (my studies) and thought that now I can like dedicate my life to that.

Karianne found it difficult to establish a social network as a new student. For Line, insufficient realization of her expectations for adult life seemed to be of key significance:

> The fact that I was now done [with secondary school] and finally an adult, in a way, and could do what I wanted. And then it didn't turn out quite in the way I imagined it would, I think.

Loss of Close Relationships Four of the interviewed individuals cite a loss of close relationships as important in their understanding of their depression. While for Line, this entailed girlfriends who pulled away, Sumaira highlights the loss of her little brother as an important cause. Karianne for her part connects her second depression to a breakup:

> When I was in a relationship, I felt very much taken care of and supported, then you don't carry everything all alone, right ... (...) You could sort of change course before you slide off track then.

In Live's view, not being allowed to have contact with her best friend was one important reason why the depression appeared when it did:

> A lot of what caused me to become very depressed was that suddenly my parents found out that she [my friend] smoked [hash]. (...) And suddenly I wasn't allowed to spend time with her any longer (...). So, I just sat there all alone and didn't know what to do and then it just got even worse.

Bullying Live, Bendik and Sumaira began their stories about depression by highlighting the significance of having been bullied. Sumaira explains this:

> After having been bullied for ten years. And then ... well, I didn't manage to do well in school, because I was very depressed and couldn't remember anything (...) Yes, then there was a period that lasted for ten years. That I started to react. And yes, then I got depressed.

Predisposition Towards Depression This was a theme which three of the informants cited as important. Both genetic disposition in the form of depression in the family and a personality-based tendency towards existential brooding were stressed. Thomas emphasizes the latter:

> I don't know if you've seen Sopranos? But the guy, the main character there, claims to have a genetic predisposition to depression ... I think I have it. I can easily get buried by my own thoughts. Back to the business of complexity, then, I like to dwell on my thoughts and stuff.

Depression as Something Self-Inflicted Three of the participants maintain that they have personally contributed to bringing on depression, either by having pushed themselves beyond the limits of their abilities, or as a result of a negative cognitive bent. Live describes the latter as follows:

> I think that a lot of it is self-inflicted. Many of the thoughts I have I maybe come up with myself. Like: 'Now I don't have anything to do, so then I get depressed and go around crying' or 'now I'm bored, now I'll go cut myself.' or just lame things like that.

Self-Realization's Exhausting Downside

The purpose of the interviews was also to study how the basic narratives could be predicated on the normative ideals of our times. As a means of illuminating this, we wanted first to investigate which explicit norms and ideals in our times are recurring and appear to influence the informants' self-perceptions and living conditions. A normative ideal was defined as explicit if the informants made direct reference to it in their accounts, without any prior suggestion. The analysis of context shows that four explicit norms and ideals are of key importance.

Successfulness Some components mentioned as defining successfulness would appear to be recurring: an attractive physical appearance, completion of higher education with good marks, a large circle of friends, efficiency, flexibility in terms of behaviour and image, a good career and high ambitions, settling down with a partner and children and coping with and demonstrating control over one's existence. Karianne summarizes this as follows:

> That you are attractive, both intellectually and physically. But perhaps in a slightly different way [than when she was younger], now you're supposed to be more secure and more grown up. Have control over your life. Know where you're headed, where you are.

About career she says:

> Career is a big one, I would say (…) I mean, successfulness, that you can cope. Have a good job, get good results.

Line mentions a conflict between the experience of an expectation that she must appear successful and her own needs as being directly related to her depression:

> I can get all dressed up and attend family parties and balls and those kinds of fancy events, blend in and be the way I am expected to be. So that has certainly had a big impact [on her depression], that I haven't felt that I could be myself.

Individualism This norm is presented with different nuances. Karianne appears to express scepticism:

> It's very individualized, the socialising is limited to scheduled meetings, often at a bar or a club, with a beer in your hand (...). There's like no place, no space (...) where people can just meet either. There are specific places where you can be, with specific things you can do. Because of this, people are very alone.

On the other hand, Ingrid appears to have a more positive perception:

> There's something very attractive, I think, about individualism.

Social Support Although individualism is perceived as a prevailing norm, three of the participants describe explicitly positive experiences in terms of the significance of social support. Bendik acknowledges the importance of how his friend and her mother helped him when he was feeling the worst:

> So, I called a friend who lived just down the road and her mother lived there too. And so, I just said 'listen, I can't take any more, I'm on the edge now. I have to come down and see you.' And I was of course allowed to do that. So, I went right over there and went inside and cried and was totally messed up. And they welcomed me, took me in, they saved me, that family.

Self-Realization A desire for self-realization was explicitly highlighted as important by three of the informants, either in the form of being able to pursue their interests and lives in accordance with personal orientations, take advantage of all the opportunities life has to offer or anxiety about missing out on something or making the wrong choice. Ingrid describes the latter as follows:

> I didn't know what to do at all. And at the same time, you feel that time is passing, that you don't want to miss out on yourself or the group or God [laughs], in a way. But at the same time, you don't know where to start (...) I believe it's the times, a bit, there is a lot of focus on your own self-realization. You become so afraid of missing out on yourself, at least I was, very much so.

Optimization of the Self

How do current normative ideals, such as self-realization, find expression in their narratives? Are some of these norms and ideals expressed in an implicit, internalized way and how are these in turn contingent upon the informants' self-perception and living conditions? The analysis of narrative context revealed the recurrence of five implicit normative assumptions.

Individualization and Self-Realization Five of the informants implicitly expressed an idea about being responsible for where you are in life. For Live, this seemed to be about taking responsibility for her depression by attributing the disorder to her own, negative cognitive style rather than to external experiences or frameworks. Bendik explains the difficult situation he was in psychologically and socially in terms of his inability to cope, which can indicate an underlying norm of personal accountability:

> So, I lay in bed and couldn't breathe and was completely apathetic and was unable to collect my thoughts and (...) all I could see were all my failures.

Sumaira describes how she would sometimes wonder about whether the bullying was her own fault:

> Then you also think about what if I hadn't committed that blunder, maybe then they would have stopped? So, you end up always blaming yourself.

Karianne speaks of how she wished she had taken the social environment into account when she became depressed, but instead, she only blamed herself. Line also explains that she went to work when she was depressed even though she did not really have the energy. This can be interpreted as implying the existence of an underlying assumption that one must manage independently of others, even during illness.

Little Room for Vulnerability For four of the interview subjects, a central normative assumption seems to be that there is little room for vulnerability. Line describes how she wants to shield a future partner from being with her due to the risk of another depression:

> But I remember when I met boys, then I thought: 'Poor guy, you'll be spared having to be with me.'

Thomas for his part expresses how he resumed his studies too soon after his illness due to what he experienced as an expectation to excel. This can be interpreted as an assumption of there being not only little room for vulnerability in the education system, but also little internal room. Two of the participants explicitly express how they have experienced it as important to keep up an appearance of coping, which can be understood as an indication of an underlying norm of limited acceptance for showing vulnerability. For Sumaira, it was about maintaining the façade of being "above it all" in response to bullying. Line admits that despite having an open personality she has found it difficult to speak about her own vulnerability. Karianne describes an experience of there being little tolerance for mistakes within her gang of teenage friends.

Instrumentalization of the Self In the accounts of three of the informants, there appears to be an underlying implication of an instrumental relationship to the self, whereby the self becomes a means to an end outside the self. In Live's narrative, such instrumentalization appears in connection with her school environment, whereby a social strategy of forgoing own impulses to associate with whomever she wanted and restricting herself instead to certain popular pupils, was utilized as a means to the end of social status:

> The [cool kids] probably wanted to be friends with kids who weren't in the popular group, but for sure they just had to tough it out.

Karianne also describes an expectation of a specific way of being in her social environment that was required in order to achieve social status. The method for accomplishing this appears to be to abandon aspects of her personality she experienced as her own and instead try to show other characteristics that were valued more:

> And there was the time when she [a friend] said 'Karianne, you never smile, what's wrong with you, can't you just try to smile a bit?' and then I'd been going around trying to be so cool, right. I am actually a happy person and so it was a matter of trying to find a balance between being cool and edgy (...). I couldn't manage to find that balance.

Conditional Self-Worth and Community A normative assumption regarding the conditional nature of self-worth and recognition from oneself and others is recurring in the stories of four of the informants, as is the experience that in-group inclusion is contingent upon a specific type of behaviour. In the following quote from Thomas, self-actualization appears to be connected to having accomplished something:

> You are supposed to accomplish something. That's important to me, for my self-realization, you could say (...). If I haven't done that [accomplished something], then I feel guilty when I go to bed at night. Then I feel like I've wasted a day.

Along the same lines, Karianne expresses satisfaction with herself because of external results:

> To manage things, when I haven't done that, then it piles up, sort of (...). I completed my master's degree a short while ago and I will be extremely upset if I don't get an A, basically.

Bendik experienced that while unconditional acceptance from his family depends on him being heterosexual, external success gave another type of recognition, which could "compensate" for his homosexual orientation:

> [I wanted] to be the best I could be before I told them. Because I was so afraid that I wouldn't, like, handle it well. So, it was important to be as successful as I could.

Karianne expresses how she has always "tried to play a bit on her intellect" because she "hasn't achieved very much otherwise". This can be interpreted as meaning that the unconditional value of simply existing is not enough; the underlying norm is the necessity of having something to "play on" to gain recognition and be of value.

Self-Optimization A normative expectation both from oneself and others that one should strive to become the optimal version of oneself appears in the accounts of three of the informants. While Karianne, as stated, aspires to do her very best scholastically, Line describes an expectation to become the best possible version of herself:

> We have (...) every opportunity before us. And so, everyone around you expects you to become the person you can be, because the opportunity is there. And that puts an enormous amount of pressure on young people.

Thomas' thoughts would appear to be based on the same self-optimization norm when he describes having high standards:

> I think I will never feel that I am good enough, but I have simply recognized that. But some days it feels as if it's the only thing that's important (...). I set high standards for myself.

Sweden: "You Should Really Make the Most of What You've Received"

There is reason to believe that the above results are reasonably representative, in that similar interview-based studies from comparable nations such as Sweden and Denmark have revealed some of the same ideas in depressed adolescents' self-perceptions. The Swedish psychologist

Hanna Bornäs has done semi-structured qualitative interviews with young adults 20–30 years of age who at the time of the interviews were taking antidepressants such as selective serotonin reuptake inhibitors (SSRIs) or serotonin–norepinephrine reuptake inhibitors (SNRIs). Bornäs consistently finds a variety of causal explanations which the informants apply to depression, but in her materials, another recurring theme is how the pressure of expectations to succeed becomes boundless and exhausting, as Eli relates here:

> I wanted to do better at everything. But there wasn't like any limit, that's how it was, I was just supposed to be the best in everything, that was like impossible and then I had no choice but to feel bad about it. Both about how I couldn't be the best and the realization of that, was just extremely frustrating.[8]

Bornäs herself comments here on how depression acquires the character of being a challenge that arises after a long period of intense, external pressure to achieve. She also highlights how the idea of the strong and superior individual who has every possibility for success can suddenly turn into an experience of requirements and the feeling of not measuring up in relation to an unattainable standard, as Erika describes:

> Mummy and daddy have always been very much like that … which is fantastic, which I love them for, but like this: 'You can do anything Erika, you manage everything, you should be able to do whatever you want to do … you'll manage it.' They've also been like 'You're so smart and accomplished that you can, it doesn't matter if you don't get the best marks in everything and you're so fantastic that you should really take advantage of this … make the most of what you have received.[9]

Bornäs highlights how the informants shift between "you can" and "you have to", between encouragement and commands and between praise and discipline. And she also points out how it seems virtually impossible

[8] Hanna Bornäs, "'Att inskolas som vuxen' – medikaliseringen av. unga vuxnas psykiska lidande i Sverge", in *Snart er vi alle pasienter. Medikalisering i Norden*, Hilde Bondevik, Ole Jacob Madsen, and Kari Nyheim Solbrække, eds. (Oslo: Scandinavian Academic Press, 2017), 162.

[9] Ibid.

for Erika to express anything but her gratitude to her parents, which paradoxically only increases her feelings of guilt and of being a failure.[10] In Bornäs' sample, we also find Lovisa, who highlights her ideal, Swedish middle-class background, free of both alcoholism and sexual abuse, so she is left with nothing to blame but herself in her explanation for her depression:

> If I wasn't depressed then I could have done anything! Then I could have pursued any kind of education! Then I could have done so many wonderful things, because then I would have had such a tremendous amount of energy to do this and that and that![11]

Lovisa appears to have completely internalized the all-or-nothing essence that characterizes postmodernity, where one has every opportunity, and therefore nobody to blame but oneself if one fails at self-realization.[12]

Denmark: "You Bloody Well Better Perform Well in This Society, Right?"

In Denmark, the sociologist Anders Petersen has also done a series of qualitative interviews with depressed 20-year-olds in which many of his informants relate their depression to a normative ideal of self-realization particular to our times. When Catherine is asked whether there are things other than purely personal factors that can explain her depression, this is her response:

> Yes. There are many requirements to be like this and like that. That you must be an exceptional person, for the labour market, etc. But what if you can't be that person? What if you don't manage to be that way? Then you

[10] Ibid.

[11] Ibid., 163.

[12] Ehrenberg, *The weariness of the self: Diagnosing the history of depression in the contemporary age.*

> are simply a loser. There's no room for people who don't want to compete and don't want to be career-oriented.[13]

Regardless of whether one reads Catherine's perception of the cut-throat requirements imposed on young people as truthful or an exaggeration, the quote clearly illustrates how many young people today perceive the expectation as very real. A number of Petersen's other interview subjects also express feeling under constant pressure to perform and achieve results, among them Iben:

> Being young is stressful. Again, because so many things are piled on top of us from the outside world. What you must do and what you mustn't do. There are so many requirements for what you must do ... so I think that's stressful and confusing.[14]

Solveig also communicates well how feeling pressured leads to a downward spiral as one aspires to fulfil the requirements but is drained of more and more strength as the discrepancy between what one personally experiences as achievements and what one feels one should manage to achieve becomes too great:

> So, there's the pressure. It has of course been a contributing factor, when you are a bit pressed for time at the outset and so much is expected of you, and you feel, you have to just give 120% all the time, just to keep up. Then you just become even more drained ... You bloody well better perform well in this society, right? At least if you want to get somewhere in the world and then it all just comes to a head, there are just more and more bad days and you sleep more and more poorly, and your state of mind gets worse and worse.[15]

The distance between the ideal and the reality grows, and the recognition of this disparity becomes more and more painful. Studies from Norway's

---

[13] Anders Petersen and Ole Jacob Madsen, "Depression: Diagnosis and suffering as process" in *Nordic Psychology* 69, no. 1 (2017), 23.

[14] Ibid.

[15] Anders Petersen, *Præstationssamfundet* (Copenhagen: Hanz Reitzel, 2016), 65.

closest neighbouring countries in the east and south indicate at the very least that a normative ideal associated with self-realization and the pressure to perform well is in no sense unique to Norway but has become a shared social horizon for young people throughout all of Scandinavia.

Where Are We Now?

All the informants mentioned the experience of feeling like a failure in their stories about the road to developing a depressive disorder. A necessary condition for feeling like a failure must be a standard, imagined or real, in relation to which one has an experience of not measuring up. The participants report that they are aware that this is just an external ideal, while several of their statements indicate that they have nonetheless internalized it. The findings can also imply that the informants personally accept a large part of the responsibility for the task of living up to their own or others' ideal standards and expectations, in keeping with the theory about increased individualization.[16] There appears to be a relative consensus among the interview subjects on the areas where it is important to succeed and where they have personally experienced not measuring up. This would support, for example, Honneth's postulate from the previous chapter about a standardization of self-realization that is attached to specific values such as efficiency, personal accountability, performance, independence, initiative and flexibility.[17]

Being alone, in the sense of an absence of supportive, reliable adults or friends, was a recurring factor mentioned in all the analyses and appears as such to be one of the study's main findings. In the narratives, depression does not appear to be predominantly connected to the life challenges in themselves but rather to having to face these alone. For example, Karianne and Bendik in their accounts about commencing their education in a new city specifically relate depression to difficulties in finding a network and nobody being there for them, respectively. Or when Live neglects to

[16] Ulrich Beck and Elisabeth Beck-Gernsheim, *Individualization: institutionalized individualism and its social and political consequences* (London: Sage, 2002).

[17] Honneth, "Organized self-realization: some paradoxes of individualization".

place importance on a turbulent adolescence per se in her understanding of depression, but instead on being alone after contact with her friend was severed. Or finally, when Ingrid experienced that it was having to make choices all by herself that was a strain, and Sumaira explains that the worst part of bullying was the loneliness and absence of supportive friends or adults. This can imply that a pertinent preventive measure in this context could be a better organized system of social support for vulnerable groups of adolescents.

Another finding is that several of the identified causal explanations and several of the identified explicit and implicit norms and ideals appear to reflect the supposedly normative features of late modernity outlined above here. Among other things, the causes of feeling like a failure and a lack of acceptance and recognition can be connected to the above-mentioned, apparently standardized norms for self-realization and successfulness and reflect how it is not always easy to live up to these. The identified theme of being alone also seems to reflect features asserted as characteristic of our current society, such as individualism, loss of community and detraditionalization.

Although we find considerable congruence between the causal explanations that the interview subjects offer about their depression and social theoretical models, it remains the case that more unique biographical factors can be identified in many of the informants' lives that cannot be simply explained by the living conditions of late modernity. For example, three of the informants mention periods of bullying while growing up, while four cite the more unique and biographical factor of a loss of close relationships. Explanations such as a predisposition towards depression do underscore the necessity of supplementing the sociocultural theoretical framework with more unique, individual, biological factors, in that from a psychosocial perspective[18] people always exist in an interactive tension between individual and social factors. Why explanatory models such as bullying or a predisposition towards depression are chosen can naturally be related to relatively widespread attribution mechanisms at work in our times. An example of this is the tendency to explain human factors using

[18] Stephen Frosh, "Psychososial studies and psychology: is a critical approach emerging?" in *Human Relations* 56, no. 1545–1567 (2003).

biological factors.[19] Or that a phenomenon such as bullying can also be understood through factors extraneous to an individual context, factors such as normative categorizations related to gender, ethnicity and identity and shifting cultural perceptions of success and social exclusion.[20] If one proceeds on the basis of such a perspective, factoring in Honneth's postulate of a standardized, restricted self-realization, bullying can be understood as a potential expression of how more young people must of necessity be excluded when the cultural perception of what is considered successful, and therefore worthy of inclusion, becomes narrower.[21]

A third finding is that both the disassociation from and the embracing of what are perceived as the prevailing norms and ideals of the culture can constitute a source of psychological strain for the informants. For example, Line rejects the norm of settling down with a husband and children but nonetheless experiences panic when confronted with that same norm. Karianne is sceptical about an explicit individualism which entails that people are very alone, but she feels affected by it all the same. This can indicate that the cultural ideal of late modernity, despite the present day's exaltation of its unique freedom, is inevitably informed by a number of fixed norms which one is obliged to address. Or as I have expressed previously: "the individual's freedom and autonomy are fundamental values, but the freedom to contest the fundamental values of the consumer society is not a real alternative."[22] These underlying norms hereby entail that some aspects of human life are held in less esteem and experienced by the participants as being off-limits. For example, to experience and have the opportunity to live one's own vulnerability does not appear to be included as a creditable alternative. In accordance with Honneth's observations, this can contribute to the reinforcement of standardized and unrealistic requirements for self-realization, not to mention increasing the pressure and stigma triggered by a failure to live up to them.

---

[19] Fernando Vidal, "Brainhood, anthropological figure of modernity" in *History of the Human Sciences* 22, no. 1 (2009).

[20] Robin May Schott and Dorte Marie Søndergaard, eds., *School bullying: new theories in context* (Cambridge: Cambridge University Press, 2014).

[21] Honneth, "Organized self-realization: some paradoxes of individualization".

[22] Madsen, *The therapeutic turn. How psychology altered Western culture*, 27.

However, a limitation of the study is that in qualitative research interviews, one will typically understand statements that emerge during an interview as information arising in a specific, interpersonal context and not as neutral findings originating from within the informant.[23] Whether or not we have discovered anything universal about depression in young people today is in other words uncertain, since the results will inevitably be coloured by the interviewer's procedure and manner of questioning, along with the particular interests of the study. It must also be added that an experience of inadequacy is a common symptom of depression,[24] and consequently, the possibility that the feelings of inadequacy reported by the informants can be explained by depression and not normative ideals in society cannot be ruled out. The same caution should also be exercised with respect to the reported feeling of being alone, which both corresponds with prevailing theories on increased individualization and is a common symptom of depression. Presumably, there will always be an extremely complex interaction between a unique vulnerability specific to an individual and the general living conditions that affect everyone. It should also be pointed out that since the study investigates the explanatory narratives of young adults who have experienced depression as a psychological disorder, this cannot be directly compared with studies that find an increase in depressive symptoms in this group. Simultaneously, we cannot rule out that the findings can be relevant to an understanding of depressive symptoms in young people.

Somewhere Over the Rainbow

Another reservation concerning these studies is that the majority of the informants are living in large Scandinavian cities such as Oslo, Stockholm, Lund, Malmö and Aalborg. In all three studies, the majority of the participants are students at institutions of higher learning. It is possible that students have a greater than average familiarity with at least some of

[23] Steinar Kvale, and Svend Brinkmann, *Interviews: learning the craft of qualitative research interviewing (2nd edition)* (Los Angeles, CA: Sage).

[24] Ulrik F. Malt, Nils Retterstøl, and Alv A. Dahl, *Lærebok i psykiatri (2nd edition)* (Oslo: Gyldendal Akademisk, 2009).

the theories in circulation about individualization and identity in late modern society and because of this are more aware of how these may manifest in their own lives. Although the participants express many mutually shared conceptions, it is far from certain that all young people share this understanding of the social landscape. A classical study in this regard is the social psychologist Per Olav Tiller's investigation of school compositions in the 1960s, where he found clear differences between the values of schoolchildren in the cities versus the villages of Norway.[25] Urban children appeared to be more concerned about material values and the status of owning things, while rural children seemed to have a greater focus on finding work in and having a close affiliation with the local community. In a follow-up study done in the early 2000s, sociologist Mariann Villa found that the differences between urban and rural adolescents in Norway in terms of materialism are now virtually non-existent, while urban youth nonetheless appear to be more globally oriented than rural youth and more focused on career or success in their depictions of the future.[26] These distinctions also correspond with the British journalist David Goodhart's analyses of sensational political events of recent years, such as Brexit and the election of Trump, which Goodhart holds can be understood to a large extent as the expression of a widening value gap between so-called *anywheres* and *somewheres*.[27] The former refers to the cosmopolitan, urban middle class in possession of higher education and liberal values, while the latter refers to people who have roots in one place and often more traditional values and ways of life. The informants in the interview studies are to a large degree "anywheres", and it is very possible that their descriptions of the exhausting work of self-realization and optimization do not necessarily epitomize the most pressing challenges for "somewheres", the voices of whom are not well represented here. It is also conceivable that the latter to a greater extent are protected from the strain of being alone.

---

[25] Per Olav Tiller, "Verdiorienteringer hos tre grupper av norske skolebarn" in *Sosialpsykologi I. Familie, ungdom og kjønnsroller*, Lars Hem and Harriet Holter, eds. (Oslo: Universitetsforlaget 1978).

[26] Mariann Villa, "Materialistisk ungdom? Verdiorienteringar hos by- og bygdeungdom" in *Tidsskrift for Ungdomsforskning* 2, no. 1 (2002).

[27] David Goodhart, *The road to somewhere* (London: Hurst, 2017).

Despite these reservations, there is nonetheless on the whole cause to believe that the stories of the informants are to a certain extent an expression of common conceptions acquired from the historically and culturally determined living conditions of many young, urban people in Norway, Sweden and Denmark today. Statements such as "I get so afraid of missing out on myself" can be interpreted from an individual psychology perspective as a component of depression's symptomatic make-up, but at the same time, such sentiments illustrate how many young people of today, starting in childhood, are met with the adult culture's expectations of self-optimization. I have previously found self-optimization ideals such as "becoming the best version of yourself" in the educational framework plans of several Norwegian kindergartens.[28] It is unlikely that these children are required to demonstrate their aspirations with regard to this expectation to their kindergarten teachers, but the example nonetheless demonstrates the degree to which Norwegian society is permeated by this mentality. Depression can accordingly be understood as the Janus face of self-realization. Or as Honneth described the paradox of individualization: "the permanent compulsion to draw the material for an authentic self-realization from their own inner lives requires of individuals an ongoing form of introspection which must sooner or later leave them feeling empty."[29] Ten years down the road, it can appear as if the trend evidenced by this study has only continued, in the sense that some of today's young people are not only at risk of feeling empty, but are now also afraid of missing out on themselves.

Conclusion

There is an abundance of sociological and socio-philosophical literature that addresses the problem of how macro-structures typical of late modern society can be pathology inducing, but up to now, much of this research has been insufficiently grounded in the experiences of the individual. A qualitative interview study that investigated young adult Norwegians'

---

[28] Madsen, *Optimizing the self: social representations of self-help.*

[29] Honneth, "Organized self-realization: some paradoxes of individualization", 475.

narratives about the road to depression was therefore carried out. The results can indicate that features of late modernity such as increased complexity, loss of traditions and community and a greater emphasis on individualization, personal accountability and self-realization are norms that can have a negative impact on the informants' life conditions, identity construction and self-concepts. In spite of this, it also appears that several of the informants have experienced more unique negative life events in childhood, such as bullying, or claim to know that they are genetically predisposed to depression. As always, the preliminary conclusion here must therefore be: more research is needed that investigates the interactions between unique individual and general social factors in the development of depression in young people. This is particularly true for groups of young people who do not necessarily live in big cities and will pursue higher education and are first and foremost concerned about finding permanent, paid employment in the places where they grew up.

We have seen how a sample of young people in Norway, Sweden and Denmark understand their depression. Qualitative studies of illness case histories can accordingly provide us with a useful indication of how illness is experienced and how young people at all times must carry out the work of interpretive negotiations between internal, bodily signals and external, social frameworks to give their suffering meaning. However, a limitation of such qualitative studies is that they do not tell us much about how representative such experiences are, in other words, how widespread they are in the general population. In the next chapter, I have therefore chosen a more quantitative approach to how it is to be young today, in which I review the best available research and living condition statistics, which can give us other indicators and insights on how young people are actually doing.

5

Youth Under Pressure

On 9 May 2017 the headmasters of the primary schools in Trondheim sent a letter to all parents and guardians in the district advising them to go out of their way to ensure that they are taking good care of their children. The writing of the letter was triggered by several recent cases of suicide and suicide attempts. In the letter the Trondheim headmasters write:

> May is a particularly challenging month, offering many arenas in which young people are exposed to different kinds of pressure, such as exams, substance abuse and perhaps crushed hopes about belonging. All young people have a need for additional care during this emotionally difficult period and it is for that reason you are receiving this letter now.[1]

Several experts praised Trondheim municipality for sounding the suicide alarm, stressing that it could have a preventive effect.[2] A few weeks later,

[1] Trygve Strand Joakimsen, "Ber foreldre være på vakt etter selvmord i Trondheim", (2017), https://www.nrk.no/trondelag/ber-foreldre-vaere-pa-vakt-etter-selvmord-i-trondheim-1.13509097, paragraph 4.

[2] Frank Haugsbø, "Eksperter roser Trondheim kommunes selvmordsalarm" (2017), http://www.vg.no/nyheter/innenriks/psykisk-helse/eksperter-roser-trondheim-kommunes-selvmordsalarm/a/23995106/

O. J. Madsen, *Deconstructing Scandinavia's "Achievement Generation"*,
https://doi.org/10.1007/978-3-030-72555-6_5

a similar situation report of three registered cases of suicide among young people surfaced in the Lillehammer region. Here too, the causes were pondered. The headmaster of Lillehammer upper secondary school Torbjørn Ljones gave the following explanation: "We are in a period of exams and graduation celebrations, when people are supposed to be joyful and happy. The contrasts are great."[3] A few weeks later, 600 invited guests attended a garden party at Maihaugen on the occasion of the Norwegian royal couple's anniversary trip through the inland region of Norway. Eighteen-year-old Marte Sklet Johansen from Lillehammer upper secondary school addressed the dramatic recent events in her speech to the royal couple as follows:

> And the challenges are about pressure, a pressure to be perfect and fit in. And today we also have many kinds of social media that intensify this. For example, Instagram, Facebook, Snapchat, VSCO, and many others. In many ways, we live under the constant pressure of expectations to be the best in every realm. Our parents, teachers, families and friends all have their own expectations of us. And last, but not least, it is perhaps our own expectations of ourselves that constitute the greatest pressure. For some, this can become such a burden and so demanding that they choose to end their lives. Here in Lillehammer several teenagers and young adults have done just that.[4]

Is it really the case that the evolution of society has reached the point where the ramifications of the pressure many young people in Norway feel they are under are manifesting in a suicide trend? This was the question many people asked themselves in the aftermath of these tragic events. Can topical research and statistics on the living conditions of young people confirm or disprove this growing concern?

---

[3] Runa Røed, "Bekymring etter flere selvmord og selvmordsforsøk på Lillehammer" *VG* (2017), http://www.vg.no/nyheter/innenriks/psykisk-helse/bekymring-etter-flere-selvmord-og--selvmordsforsoek-paa-lillehammer/a/24007585/, paragraph 19.

[4] Knut Storvik, "Her er Marte Sklet Johansens tale til kongeparet" in *Gudbrandsdølen Dagningen* (2017), https://www.gd.no/kongehus/maihaugen/tale/her-er-marte-sklet-johansens-tale-til-kongeparet/s/5-18-463522, paragraph 6.

Suicide in Norway

Every year 500–600 suicides are registered in Norway.[5] If we look at the historical development of suicide in Norway, there was a doubling in the suicide rate for both men and women from the end of the 1960s up to the end of the 1980s. For young people under the age of thirty, during the same period, the incidence of suicide increased three to four times over. In the period 1991–2005, the suicide rate among men decreased and subsequently levelled out. The suicide rate has also decreased among women and remained reasonably stable over the past twenty years. In 2018 a total of 673 suicides were registered in Norway; of these, 471 were men and 202 women.[6] This amounts to a suicide rate of 12.9 out of 100,000 for both genders, with 18.1 for men and 7.8 for women. The number of suicides in Norway in 2018 was somewhat higher than in the preceding years but still within the anticipated year-to-year fluctuations, and it is too early to say whether it represents a significantly rising trend.[7] There are a number of bright spots here. Compared to 1990, when there were 16.4 suicides per 100,000 inhabitants, the risk of suicide has dropped by one-fourth in the course of one generation in Norway. The decrease is particularly pronounced among men. It is also noteworthy that the suicide statistics do not provide any basis for the claim that suicide is most prevalent among young people. The majority of those who took their own lives were in the 50–54 age group. In the under-20 age group, there were 31 registered suicides in 2018, which amounts to 4.6 percent of the total.[8]

[5] Norwegian Institute of Public Health, "Fakta om selvmord og selvmordsforsøk", (2017), https://www.fhi.no/fp/psykiskhelse/selvmord/selvmord-og-selvmordsforsok%2D%2D-fakta/

[6] "Selvmordsrisikoen redusert med en firedel på én generasjon", (2017), https://www.fhi.no/nyheter/2017/selvmordsrisikoen-redusert-med-en-firedel-pa-en-generasjon/

[7] Ibid.

[8] Ibid.

Suicide Among Young People

In the autumn of 2017 the Norwegian Broadcasting Corporation (NRK) aired a documentary about twelve-year-old Mia Næss from Kolbotn who had taken her own life.[9] Many people asked themselves how something so tragic as a child committing suicide could occur, an appropriate question since suicide in the under-15 age group is extremely rare.[10] On the other hand, if we look at the 15–24 age group, there is a larger basis for comparison. The figures for this age group coincide with the suicide rate in Norway in general. Not only was there a doubling, the suicide rate for young people increased three to four times in the period from 1970 to the end of the 1980s, at which point the incidence once again showed a downturn until the mid-2000s and subsequently plateaued.

The suicide statistics provide no basis for the claim of a dramatic rise in the suicide rate, neither for young people nor for adults, in recent years in Norway. The total number of registered suicides in Norway for 2018—673 recorded cases—was higher than the preceding year, with 595 cases, but simultaneously, there were fewer suicides than the previous year among children and young people under the age of twenty: 31 suicides. Chief Physician Christian Lycke Ellingsen at the Norwegian Cause of Death Registry made the following statement about the total number of suicides in this context: "We have no basis for claiming that the change is greater than the fluctuations we see from year to year" and he states that this would be a plausible interpretation of suicide incidence among young people also.[11]

The statistics for the number of suicides among young people for the year 2020 were not available at the time of this writing, but the figures for the total number of deaths in the 0–19 age group for 2018 show no indication of a suicide trend.[12]

[9] NRK TV Brennpunkt, "Arnar og Mia" (Oslo: NRK, 2017 https://tv.nrk.no/serie/brennpunkt/MDDP11001117/19-09-2017).

[10] Norwegian Institute of Public Health, "Fakta om selvmord og selvmordsforsøk".

[11] Lisbeth Nilsen, "Færre unge tok sitt eget liv" in *Dagens Medisin* (2016), https://www.dagensmedisin.no/artikler/2016/11/02/farre-unge-tok-sitt-eget-liv/

[12] Statistics Norway, "Døde, etter region, alder, kjønn, statistikkvariabel og år", *SSB* (2018), https://www.ssb.no/statbank/table/08426/tableViewLayout1/?rxid=ed401dfe-

Suicide Internationally

How does the international picture look? If we use the available statistics from the Organization for Economic Co-operation and Development (OECD) for suicide among teenagers aged 15–19 in 35 nations throughout the world for the period 1990–2015, these indicate a slight downward trend.[13] In 1990, there were on average 8.5 suicides per 100,000 teenagers in OECD nations, and in 2015, the average had dropped to 7.4. In the 1990s, the incidence of teenage suicide was relatively stable, while most of the decline occurred in the early 2000s.[14] The lowest average of 6.3 suicides per 100,000 was in 2007. With the exception of 2008, the average remained below 7.0 until 2014 and then rose slightly again in 2014 and 2015.

If we break this down to look at individual nations, the incidence of suicide among young people varies. In the USA, the suicide rate for the 15–24 age group was relatively stable during the first decade of the 2000s, 10.1 per 100,000 in 2000, but since 2014 there has been a discernible annual increase reaching 14.45 in 2018.[15] In England and Wales, the curve for a long time showed a gradual drop from a peak in 1998 for the 10–24 age group, however since 2012 for females and since 2017 for males the tendency has been negative, with 3.1 female and 8.2 male suicides in 2019.[16] If we look to Norway's Scandinavian neighbours, the suicide statistics for Denmark for the 15–19 age group and 20–29 age group show a clear downturn from the 1980s and 1990s, with a fairly stable level in the 2010s, with 4.6 and 5.9 deaths per 100,000 in 2018 for the two groups.[17] In Sweden, the curve is more stable within the 15–24

2d0d-4b38-8c37-6dd8f1d0ee88

[13] OECD, "CO4.4: Teenage suicides (15–19 years old)" (2017), https://www.oecd.org/els/family/CO_4_4_Teenage-Suicide.pdf

[14] Ibid.

[15] American Foundation for Suicide Prevention, "Suicide statistics" (2020), https://afsp.org/suicide-statistics/

[16] Office for National Statistics, "Suicides in England and Wales: 2019 registrations" (2020), https://www.ons.gov.uk/peoplepopulationandcommunity/birthsdeathsandmarriages/deaths/bulletins/suicidesintheunitedkingdom/2019registrations

[17] Centre for suicide research, "Statistik" (2020), http://statistik.selvmordsforskning.dk/

age group, where the suicide rate has been relatively stable since the early 1990s, with 14 per 100,000 in 2019 for this age group.[18]

Overall, the OECD average for more than 35 nations shows a stable, but slight downturn in the number of suicides among young people over the past ten years. In Scandinavia and partly in England and Wales, there has been a decrease following relatively high incidences of suicide in the 1980s and 1990s. On the other hand, when a nation such as the USA shows an increase in suicide among young people since 2014, this should be duly noted, because the country wields considerable power of definition, which can lead to the erroneous impression that the increase in teenage suicide in the USA is representative of the situation for the rest of the world.

Suicide and Psychological Disorders

It has been established that people with psychological disorders are at greater risk of suicide than the population otherwise, although psychological disorders are seldom the sole cause of suicide.[19] The percentage of people with psychological disorders who take their own lives is low—the lifetime risk of suicide with serious depression is estimated to be 3–6 percent.

Suicide can also occur even though a person does not suffer from a serious psychological disorder. Some physiological illnesses can also increase the risk of suicide, such as neurological, degenerative diseases and conditions involving extreme physical pain. Other known risk factors, according to the Norwegian Institute of Public Health, are:

> [N]egative life events in the form of physical, psychological and sexual abuse in childhood, loss of a spouse and other close interpersonal relationships, unemployment or change in social status or other events that feel defamatory. Flagging self-esteem, perfectionism, high personal performance standards, debilitated problem-solving abilities in conflicts with

[18] National Centre for Suicide Research and Prevention of Mental Ill-Health, "Självmord i Sverige" (2020). https://ki.se/nasp/sjalvmord-i-sverige-0

[19] Norwegian Institute of Public Health, "Fakta om selvmord og selvmordsforsøk".

other people, low tolerance for psychological pressure and the experience of inner loneliness can also be of significance.[20]

Perfectionism and high personal performance standards combined with a low tolerance for psychological pressure are highlighted here as risk factors that can be significant to the risk of suicide. But the statistics on cause of death from the period up to and including the year 2018 provide no basis for making the claim that an increase in performance requirements is reflected in an increase in suicide among young people in Norway in recent years. However, another approach would be to look at the incidence of the most common psychological disorders in young people, such as anxiety and depression, in which any increase can be viewed as a warning of a potential increase in the risk of suicide among young people.

Psychological Disorders and Complaints

It is common to distinguish between psychological disorders and psychological/mental health complaints. *Psychological complaints* are mental health problems that are troublesome, but not to the extent that they qualify for diagnosis as a *psychological disorder*. On the question regarding an increased incidence of psychological complaints and disorders, the Norwegian Institute of Public Health holds that a change in the living conditions of society will probably influence mental health complaints to a greater extent than it will psychological disorders.[21] Mental health complaints are thought to be more contingent upon living conditions than are psychological disorders, which are more closely associated with factors such as genetics, biology and individual vulnerability.

The Norwegian Institute of Public Health points out that changes in society over time will potentially have an impact on such assessments, since both language and forms of expression change, the social

[20] Ibid., paragraph 20.

[21] "Forekomsten av psykiske plager og lidelser i befolkningen – stabil eller i endring?", (2015), https://www.fhi.no/globalassets/dokumenterfiler/moba/pdf/forekomsten-av-psykiske-plager-og--lidelser-i-befolkningen%2D%2D-stabil-eller-i-endring-pdf.pdf

acceptance of speaking about psychological problems changes; what is considered to be a psychological problem changes, and the clinical treatment for these conditions undergoes constant development.[22] The idea that mental health complaints in the population are more affected by changes in living conditions in society than psychological disorders corresponds well with the impression produced by the available statistics on the incidence and evolution of psychological disorders and complaints among young people in Norway.

In 2010, the two psychologists Ann Kristin Knudsen and Arnstein Mykletun produced a status summary on the incidence of psychological disorders in Norway.[23] Knudsen and Mykletun state that there are a number of factors that can give the impression of a growing incidence of psychological disorders in the population, factors such as the number of disability pensions granted for psychological disorders over the past fifteen years and a dramatic increase in treatment of psychological disorders in the same time period. However, these are so-called indirect indicators of the incidence of psychological disorders, since they also involve how we, as a society, choose to address psychological disorders. As regards a possible direct increase, Knudsen and Mykletun summarize the status of knowledge as follows:

> Most of the studies that have directly addressed this find no increase in the incidence of psychological disorders: The replication study of the National Comorbidity Survey in the USA found no significant changes in the incidence of psychological disorders in general for the period 1990 to 2003. The question of whether there has been an increase (or reduction) in the incidence of psychological disorders in Norway has not been adequately clarified and will be the subject of further research. But the best documentation we have available today does not provide sufficient findings to establish an increase or decrease in psychological disorders in the population.[24]

[22] Ibid.

[23] Ann Kristin Knudsen and Arnstein Mykletun, "Det du trenger å vite om forekomsten av psykiske lidelser i Norge" in *Tidsskrift for Norsk psykologforening* 47, no. 4 (2010).

[24] Ibid., 343.

The latest report from the Norwegian Institute of Public Health in 2018 offers the following status update on the incidence of psychological disorders in the population:

> A number of factors can give the impression of a growing incidence of psychological disorders in the population. The number of disability pensions granted for psychological disorders has increased in recent years and there has been a slight increase in sickness absenteeism due to psychological disorders. A dramatic increase in the treatment of psychological disorders has also occurred. These are however only indirect indicators of the incidence of psychological disorders, which also reflect how society handles such disorders. Most studies comparing incidence figures in the population over time find no increase in incidence.[25]

The conclusions here are based on different studies on the incidence of psychological disorders from the USA and Western Europe for the time period 1980–2009, and no direct increase was found, but factors such as a population growth entail an increase in the absolute number of people with psychological disorders. In a study addressing the incidence of psychological disorders in Australia in the period 2001–2014, the prevalence of the most common psychological disorders was also found to be relatively stable.[26] The number of people who received disability benefits due to psychological disorders did indeed increase dramatically in this period, but this primarily says something about the incidence of treatment, which can be based on wholly different factors, even though it may seem counter-intuitive that the number of disabled individuals with psychological disorders increases without any increase in the actual incidence of the same.

A review article from 2014 summarizing scientific studies of children's and young people's psychological health, predominantly from Europe, as well as some studies from the USA and China, finds no increase for

---

[25] Norwegian Institute of Public Health, "Psykisk helse i Norge" (Oslo: Norwegian Institute of Public Health, 2018), 32.

[26] Samuel B Harvey et al., "Is the prevalence of mental illness increasing in Australia? Evidence from national health surveys and administrative data, 2001–2014" in *The Medical Journal of Australia* 206, no. 11 (2017).

children, but an actual increase in self-reported internalization ailments for teenage girls.[27] Also another review article from 2015 that summarizes studies from Norway, Iceland, Finland, Sweden, Great Britain, the Netherlands, Greece, Brazil, the USA and New Zealand finds an increase in psychological complaints among young people in recent decades and particularly in girls.[28] There are some findings indicating a related trend among young women also in Norway. Statistics Norway's (SSB) living conditions survey, which uses a self-report inventory, shows that the percentage who reported considerable mental health complaints decreased in the period 1998–2005, but increased slightly again in the period leading up to 2012. Here an increase was also found among young people aged 16–24, and in particular young women.[29] The most recent survey done by the Norwegian Institute of Public Health from 2018 concludes that while the total load of psychological symptoms is stable, or even slightly on the decline for most children and young people, it is rising in teenage girls.[30] There is an increase from 5 to 7 percent in psychological disorders such as depression, anxiety and eating and adaptive disorders among young girls, age 15–17 years, and the percentage of girls who report experiencing a significant symptom load due to mental and physical health complaints has risen steadily from 14 percent in 1998 to 25 percent in 2015.

Psychological Complaints in Young People

Previous summaries have reported a gradual increase in the incidence of depressive symptoms for both boys and girls in the time period between 1992 and 2002 and a plateau and decline in symptom incidence between

27 William Bor et al., "Are child and adolescent mental health problems increasing in the 21st century? A systematic review", *Australian & New Zealand Journal of Psychiatry* 48, no. 7 (2014).

28 Stephan Collishaw, "Annual research review: Secular trends in child and adolescent mental health" in *Journal of Child Psychology and Psychiatry* 56, no. 3 (2015).

29 Norwegian Institute of Public Health, "Psykisk helse i Norge".

30 Ibid.

2002 and 2010.[31] For self-reported psychological complaints and symptoms among young people in Norway for the period following 2010, we have comprehensive data from the Ungdata local youth surveys, which are offered free of charge to Norwegian municipalities and county authorities. The database contains the responses of 666,000 young people from 412 different municipalities in Norway, including Svalbard. The results are believed to provide a good understanding of how young people experience growing up in Norway today. The main image of Norwegian youth that emerges from the Ungdata study up to the present day is that of a well-adjusted and home-loving generation of young people. The most recent national report at the time of writing, released to the public in August 2020, describes the main features of the 211,500 responses from pupils in lower and upper secondary schools as follows:

> The survey shows that Norwegian youth are doing well. 85 % of young people are satisfied with their lives, and 80 % believe that they have everything they want. Most youth are happy with their parents, with the school and their teachers and with the local community where they live. Nine out of ten have close and confidential friends – and almost everyone has friends to be with both at school and in their free time. Most youth live an active leisure time, where social media, computer games, training, organized leisure activities, schoolwork and being with friends characterize their everyday life. The majority report good physical and mental health. Optimism about the future among Norwegian youth is considerable.
>
> All in all, this shows that the vast majority of young people have good conditions for growing up and a life characterized by a good quality of life.[32]

This depiction of how it is to be young in Norway in the year 2020 must unquestionably be described as relatively positive, with respect to both young people's actual daily lives and their thoughts about how their future lives will be. But some alarming signs disturb the harmonious image.

---

[31] Tilmann von Soest, "Tidstrender for depressive symptomer blant norske ungdommer fra 1992 til 2010" in *Tidsskrift for Ungdomsforskning* 12, no. 2 (2012).

[32] Bakken, "Ungdata. Nasjonale resultater 2018, NOVA Rapport 8/18", 2–3.

Thirty-eight percent in lower secondary school and 49 percent in upper secondary school report that they have "worried too much about things" and 33 percent in lower secondary school and 43 percent in upper secondary school report having felt that "everything is hard work".[33] Another clear trend in the Ungdatas reports is that self-reported mental health complaints continue to show a marked increase for both boys and girls throughout the 2010s. As stated by way of introduction, the percentage of self-reported depressive symptoms, particularly among girls, has increased since the Ungdata surveys were initiated in the beginning of the 2010s. In 2011, 15.9 percent of lower secondary school girls reported a high level of depressive symptoms, while in 2017 this had risen to 20.7 percent.[34] In upper secondary school one also sees a clear increase: 29.3 percent of the girls now report a high level of depressive symptoms.

For the boys, in 2011, 6.9 percent in lower secondary school reported a high level of depressive symptoms. In the next four years, the percentage of boys who responded affirmatively to being disturbed by depressive symptoms went down, while in the last two surveys, this trend was reversed, and the percentage rose again to 6.7 percent.[35] In upper secondary school the increase is even clearer for boys: 10.8 percent report a high level of depressive symptoms. For the question of whether they suffer due to loneliness, a similar trend can be discerned: a gradual increase each year since the surveys started for girls who report that they "suffer very much" due to loneliness. The results of self-reported loneliness for boys have been fairly stable since the surveys began, but here also the results of the last two years indicate an increase in keeping with the overall pattern.[36]

Starting in 2017, surveys were also carried out on the experience of stress and pressure among young people, in which a large variation was found primarily in terms of the amount of pressure young people experience and the areas in which this occurs: "71 percent of the boys and 45 percent of the girls have not experienced so much pressure that they've had problems handling it. But 6 percent of the boys and 16 percent of the

[33] Ibid.

[34] "Ungdata. Nasjonale resultater 2018, NOVA Rapport 8/18".

[35] Ibid.

[36] Ibid.

girls have often had problems handling pressure."[37] School is the arena where the majority experience pressure; half the girls report this, while gaining recognition on social media is associated with the least amount of pressure. Twenty-five percent of the young people in the survey experience pressure in at least two areas, and again, the problem clearly appears to be the most pronounced among girls.

Overall, the recent Ungdata reports provide a picture of a clear deterioration in mental health measured as depressive symptoms and loneliness for both boys and girls in recent years compared to previous years. A considerable number of young people, girls in particular, are also experiencing a lot of pressure and stress. What must be emphasized, however, is that it is not possible to state with certainty whether the rise in the reported incidence implies that increasingly more young people are struggling with psychological problems whether it is an outcome of how young people report health complaints.

Why the Increase in the Reporting of Psychological Complaints?

What reasons can be found to explain why young people, and girls in particular, are reporting more psychological complaints than previously? NOVA researchers Mira Aaboen Sletten and Anders Bakken have produced a knowledge review which covers different, well-known explanations, such as an increase in drug use, changes in the relationship to the body and appearance and different requirements in relation to school and education.[38] As for drug use, research shows that there has been a positive development in Norway up to the present day since the turn of the new millennium, so this explanation is no longer relevant in Norway. von Soest and Wichstrøm have previously done a study of the body image, slimming habits and psychological problems of Norwegian youth which shows a connection between these, but it has not been clearly established

[37] Ibid., 73.

[38] Mira Aaboen Sletten and Anders Bakken, "Psykiske helseplager blant ungdom – tidstrender og samfunnsmessige forklaringer. Notat nr 4/16" (Oslo: NOVA, 2016).

whether slimming habits and dissatisfaction with their own body leads to mental health complaints. However, the possibility that a depressive emotional state leads to dissatisfaction with one's body and appearance cannot be ruled out.[39] Sletten and Bakken also mention the role of social media as a potential added strain in the experience of body-related pressure, particularly in girls. Performance-related stress in school also appears to be a possible explanation, in that a number of studies from the Nordic region have found a connection between the experience of stress in school and mental health complaints, and consistent gender differences in the experience of school-related stress were evidenced.[40] Sletten and Bakken show how some developmental trends can have contributed to this: school and education appear to play a more important part in young people's lives than previously, in that more of the jobs that typically were within reach for young people with little education and a low level of formal competence have disappeared in recent years. The Programme for International Student Assessment (PISA) surveys that entered into force at the start of the millennium have also contributed to an enhanced focus on performance assessments in the school system, which may also be an underlying, contributing factor in the experience of school-related stress.[41] The significant increase in experienced pressure among school children, especially in nations such as Norway, Denmark, Sweden and Germany between 1998 and 2002, can be connected to these nations scoring the most poorly on the PISA studies, while countries such as Finland and Canada, which ended up at the other end of the scale, do not show the same surge in terms of school-related stress in this period.[42] In a British study of Scottish fifteen-year-olds for the period 1987–1999, it was found that girls were more worried about school performance than boys, while the girls' reported mental health complaints increased

[39] Tilmann von Soest and Lars Wichstrøm, "Secular trends in depressive symptoms among Norwegian adolescents from 1992 to 2010", *Journal of Abnormal Child Psychology* 42, No. 3 (2014).

[40] Sletten and Bakken, "Psykiske helseplager blant ungdom – tidstrender og samfunnsmessige forklaringer. Notat nr. 4/16".

[41] Ibid.

[42] Don A. Klinger et al., "Cross-national trends in perceived school pressure by gender and age from 1994 to 2010", *European Journal of Public Health* 25, no. suppl_2 (2015).

significantly more than the boys during this period.[43] A later study of Scottish youth concluded that the increase in psychological difficulties from 1987 to 2006 could be best explained by arguments between parents, the young people's engagement in school and worries about school performance.[44] But as always: the conclusion of NOVA's knowledge review is that more research is needed to establish whether the findings from Scotland can be generalized. In their conclusion, Sletten and Bakken make the argument that we must presumably view more risk factors in context, in that they also clink the deterioration of young people's health to developments in society, such as increased individualization, due to which the requirements for self-realization and self-discipline can constitute a strain, especially for girls who experience a *two-fold pressure* to perform well at school and to meet conformist gender role requirements related to appearance, the body and social success. This is confirmed by this year's Ungdata report. In the next chapter, we will look at how such a problem is frequently labelled, dubiously, the "good girl syndrome".

The Public Health Agency of Sweden has also produced a knowledge review which investigates why ill health has increased among young people in the period between 1985 and 2014.[45] Family circumstances are not accepted as an explanation for the changes, nor economic vulnerability, but an increase in socio-economic differences is cited as a potential cause, though some uncertainty remains regarding the latter. While the research on digital media is inconclusive and shows both a negative and a positive impact on young people's well-being, this illustrates the need for further research on digital media as a possible contributing factor for ill health in the 2010s. On the other hand, problems at school are highlighted more unambiguously, as reflected in sinking performance levels coupled with increasing school-related stress.[46] A more uncertain labour market is also cited, in combination with higher requirements for education and exper-

[43] Patrick West and Helen Sweeting, "Fifteen, female and stressed: changing patterns of psychological distress over time", *Journal of Child Psychology and Psychiatry* 44, no. 3 (2003).

[44] Helen Sweeting et al., "Can we explain increases in young people's psychological distress over time?", *Social Science & Medicine* 71, no. 10 (2010).

[45] Folkhälsomyndigheten, "Varför har den psykiska ohälsan ökat bland barn och unga i Sverige?", Folkhälsomyndigheten ed. (Stockholm 2018).

[46] Ibid.

tise than previously to secure inclusion in that market, which has contributed to the development of a number of psychosomatic symptoms in young people in Sweden.

Which Group of Young People Is Hardest Hit?

Based on the "Young in Oslo" (Ung i Oslo) surveys done between 1996 and 2015, Mira Aaboen Sletten has demonstrated an apparent trend showing a greater increase in depressive symptoms specifically among Oslo girls with an ethnic Norwegian background and who are from affluent neighbourhoods, have an average to large amount of books in the home and who have average to good marks.[47] But if comparisons are to be made on a national basis, it is still the case that the lower the socio-economic background, the greater the overall number of reports of mental health complaints. Among those who score the lowest on objective measures of family economic well-being, 27 percent report four to six health complaints compared to 15 percent for those with the highest scores on objective measures of family economic well-being.[48] In contrast to this, with regard to subjective measures of family economic well-being, 55 percent of those who feel that "the family is hard up all the time" report four to six health complaints, compared to only 12 percent of those who feel that "the family is financially well-off all the time". In cases where neither of the parents has completed higher education, 20 percent of the young people report four to six health complaints compared to 15 percent in cases where both parents have completed higher education.[49]

If we were to evaluate the relation between the two groups, it is still the case that youth with traditional risk characteristics are the main problem. This group, however, appears reasonably stable, while the psychological complaints appear to increase most in the group with the most

[47] Mira Aaboen Sletten, "Psykiske plager blant ungdom – og hva ungdom selv tror er årsaken [PPT-presentasjon]", (2015).

[48] "Psykiske plager blant ungdom: sosiale forskjeller og historien om de flinke pikene", *Oppvekstrapporten 2017* (2017).

[49] Ibid.

resources.[50] The problems of the achievement generation will also have an impact on the group with fewer resources, a cultural narrative they are also confronted with, and which can be a source of additional strain if they feel they don't satisfy these requirements and the gap between "them" and "the others" only widens.

Use of Medication

If we turn to so-called indirect measurements, such as the use of medication among young people, especially antidepressants and over-the-counter painkillers, they paint a more disturbing picture of the development, if viewed in isolation, than of the incidence of psychological disorders and mental health complaints in the young population. The most recently publicized statistics on young people's consumption of antidepressants in the period between 2010 and 2016 states that, "Among girls in the 15–19 age group there has been an increase of 85 percent in the use of antidepressants over the past seven years. The increase has been significantly less among boys."[51] In 2015, there were 4565 girls in the 15–19 age group who were taking antidepressants in Norway.

The summarized findings for consumption of pain-reliefs medication show a corresponding pattern. Overall, for the entire Norwegian population there has been a clear increase since over-the-counter sale of certain pain-relief medications in pharmacies was legalized in 2003. The total consumption of pain-relief medication such as paracetamol and Non-Steroidal Anti-Inflammatory Drugs (NSAID) increased by 25 percent from 2003 to 2014. The consumption of NSAID has not changed to any degree worthy of mention since 2003, but paracetamol has increased by 75 percent and ibuprofen (Ibux) has increased by 80 percent.[52] There has also been a marked increase in the number of reported poisoning-related cases and here the abuse has been most widespread among young

[50] "Psykiske plager blant ungdom – og hva ungdom selv tror er årsaken [PPT-presentasjon]".

[51] Norwegian Pharmacy Association, "Unges bruk av antidepressiva fortsetter å øke", *Apotekforeningen* (2017), https://www.apotek.no/Default.aspx?ID=8444

[52] "Bruken av paracetamol og NSAID i Norge 2003–2014", (2015), https://www.apotek.no/Files/Filer_2014/Nyheter/150213%20Faktanotat%20paracetamol%20og%20NSAID.pdf

women.[53] In a Norstat survey from 2015 on young people's use of paracetamol, 40 percent of the girls participating in the survey from the 15–24 age group responded that they take paracetamol several times a month.[54] This is twice as many as boys in the same age group. Forty percent of the girls in the survey stated that they take paracetamol to enable them to go to school or work, a percentage three times greater than the boys. A third of the girls in the survey carry paracetamol at all times. And 34 percent of the girls in the 15–18 age group take paracetamol as a preventive measure.

If we combine the findings for consumption of prescription antidepressants and over-the-counter pain relievers, they indicate that to a growing extent young girls experience a need for mood regulation and pain alleviation. We don't know for certain whether this is due to an actual exposure to greater stress and pressure in their daily lives, or because the threshold for taking happy pills or pain relievers is lower, or that such medication is more easily available than previously; presumably all explanations indicate contributing factors. In the last Ungdata survey, however, the percentage of boys and girls who take over-the-counter medication on a weekly basis went down in lower secondary schools between 2015 and 2017. In upper secondary school consumption has also stagnated for girls while there has been a slight increase for boys.[55]

Self-Harm

Self-harm entails inflicting pain or injury to one's own body but without the intention of taking one's own life. The estimates of the scope of self-harm among young people in Norway in recent years are somewhat inconclusive, but it is conjectured that around 10 percent of Norwegian youth in the ninth and tenth grade and the first year of upper secondary

[53] Elisabet Høye and Ida Louise Rostad, "Paracetamol-misbruket. NRK", (2016), https://www.nrk.no/livsstil/xl/paracetamol-misbruket-1.12755817

[54] Apotekforeningen, "En undersøkelse om ungdommers forhold til paracetamol", (2015).

[55] Bakken, "Ungdata. Nasjonale resultater 2018, NOVA Rapport 8/18".

school have at one time or another attempted self-harm.[56] Internationally, the figures vary between 13 and 23 percent; an average estimate for self-harm gives a lifetime prevalence of around 18 percent.[57] Self-harm appears to manifest for the first time at 12–14 years of age and is most widespread in the 15–17 age group, after which it again drops. With regard to gender differences, there is also some uncertainty, but some findings have indicated that there can be three times as many girls as boys who carry out this type of self-destructive behaviour.[58]

Is self-harm a growing problem among young people? In the Norwegian Directorate of Public Health's most recent knowledge status report for Norway from 2017 they respond as follows: "An increase in self-harm was reported for the past decade, but it remains uncertain whether this is due to an actual increase, a greater focus on the phenomenon, or more research and better registration practices. The incidence level has been stable for the past five years."[59]

Internationally, several alarming developmental trends have been reported in the past year alone, such as in Great Britain where one finds a 68 percent increase in self-harm among girls 13–16 years of age, from 45.9 per 10,000 in 2011 to 77 per 10,000 in 2014.[60] Also in the USA one finds an increase among young girls 10–19 years of age in acute hospital admissions for self-inflicted, non-fatal injuries in the period 2001–2015.[61] Up until 2008, no statistically significant increase was registered, but from 2009 to 2015, the registered acute cases of self-harm

---

[56] Julie Nybakk Kvaal, "Ny behandling reduserer selvskading hos ungdom", *Suicidologi*, no. 1 (2017).

[57] Helsedirektoratet, "Veiledende materiell for kommunene om forebygging av selvskading og selvmord", (2017), https://helsedirektoratet.no/folkehelse/psykisk-helse-og-rus/selvmord-og-selvskading/veiledende-materiell-for-kommunene-om-forebygging-av-selvskading-og-selvmord#om-selvskading

[58] Anita Johanna Tørmoen, "Self-harm among adolescents: From identification to tailored treatment", (Oslo: University of Oslo, 2017).

[59] Norwegian Directorate of Health, "Veiledende materiell for kommunene om forebygging av selvskading og selvmord", n.p.

[60] Catharine Morgan et al., "Incidence, clinical management, and mortality risk following self-harm among children and adolescents: Cohort study in primary care", *BMJ* 359 (2017).

[61] Melissa C. Mercado et al., "Trends in emergency department visits for nonfatal self-inflicted injuries among youth aged 10 to 24 years in the United States, 2001–2015", *JAMA* 318, no. 19 (2017).

among girls 10–14 years of age increased by 18.4 percent annually and girls in the 15–19 age group by 8.4 percent annually.[62] For boys the development was relatively stable for the entire period.

Whether the same trend can be expected among young girls in Norway is uncertain. Young people report that the motives behind self-harm are a need to release internal pressure, gain control over difficult emotions, express non-acceptable feelings and make contact with others.[63] If we base our interpretations on other behaviour, we can speculate as to whether the increase in consumption of pain relievers and antidepressants indicates a greater need for control over painful emotional states, which entails that perhaps we will also see an increase in self-harm. At the same time, a strong correlation between the suicide rate and the self-harm rate in the population has been found previously,[64] and in this case the relatively stable suicide rate in Norway in recent years would imply that one can also expect a similarly stable incidence of self-harm.

Externalizing Behaviours

How are today's youth doing if we now shift our focus to acting-out behaviour? In terms of sexuality, statistics show that teenage births have been reduced by half from the time of the early twentieth century to the beginning of the twenty-first.[65] The number of teenage abortions is also generally low, and it is natural to view this in the context of greater knowledge and improved access to birth control. Also the sexual debut age in Norway falls into the same pattern, having gradually declined since record-keeping of related statistics commenced in the end of the 1920s to

[62] Ibid.

[63] Line Indrevoll Stänicke, Hanne Haavind, and Siri Erika Gullestad, "How do young people understand their own self-harm? A meta-synthesis of adolescents' subjective experience of self-harm", *Adolescent Research Review* 3, no. 2 (2018).

[64] Galit Geulayov et al., "Epidemiology and trends in non-fatal self-harm in three centres in England, 2000–2012: Findings from the Multicentre Study of Self-harm in England", *BMJ Open* 6, no. 4 (2016).

[65] Bakken, "Ungdata. Nasjonale resultater 2018, NOVA Rapport 8/18".

becoming reasonably stable since the early 2000s: 17 years of age for girls and 17.9 years of age for boys.[66]

The most recent Ungdata survey from Oslo even shows that the percentage of first-year upper secondary school students who report having had intercourse has decreased: in 1996, 46 percent of the boys and 39 percent of the girls reported having had sexual intercourse, while in 2018 the percentage had dropped to 37 percent for the boys and 27 percent for the girls.[67] Also in the USA a similar pattern of later sexual debut than previously has been documented: 54 percent, a majority, of high school students had had sexual intercourse in 1991, while those who had had sexual intercourse in 2015 constituted a minority of 41 percent.[68]

If we look at tobacco, alcohol and drug use, it is a fact that the number of smokers among young people has declined dramatically from the turn of the millennium up to today. In 2011, 4.4 percent of boys in lower secondary school reported that they smoked daily or weekly, while in 2016 the number had dropped to 2.6 percent.[69] Correspondingly, 4.2 percent of the girls in lower secondary school reported that they smoked in 2011, while in 2016 the percentage was 1.6. The percentage of young people who take snuff has indeed increased during the same time period, but overall, the use of tobacco is still declining. The year's Ungdata figures, however, show a plateau in the trend and even a small increase again among boys who report that they smoke.[70] A possible explanation can be that this is related to an increase in consumption of cannabis. Although alcohol consumption among young people is still relatively widespread and the scope does not show the same dramatic decrease as smoking, the summarized findings for alcohol consumption in lower secondary school from 2011 to the present day also show a relatively clear downward trend. In 2011, 15.3 percent of boys in lower secondary school reported having

[66] Hein Stigum, Sven O. Samuelsen, and Bente Traeen, "Analysis of first coitus", *Arch Sex Behav* 39, no. 4 (2010); Bente Træen, Sven Ove Samuelsen, and Katrina Roen, "Sexual debut ages in heterosexual, lesbian, gay, and bisexual young adults in Norway", *Sexuality & Culture* 20, no. 3 (2016).

[67] Bakken, "Ung i Oslo 2018. NOVA Rapport 6/18".

[68] Jean M. Twenge and Heejung Park, "The decline in adult activities among U.S. adolescents, 1976–2016", *Child Development* (2017).

[69] Bakken, "Ungdata. Nasjonale resultater 2017, NOVA Rapport 10/17".

[70] "Ungdata. Nasjonale resultater 2018, NOVA Rapport 8/18".

been visibly intoxicated in the past year, while in 2016, this had dropped to 11.7 percent.[71] Girls also show a corresponding decline in drunkenness from 16.7 percent in 2011 to 12.3 percent in 2016. But here as well, in this year's Ungdata report, the downturn in alcohol consumption among lower secondary school students has now come to a halt, while in upper secondary school a certain increase in the percentage who have been intoxicated can again be discerned, especially for boys.[72] The use of narcotic substances such as hash and marijuana has been relatively stable throughout all of the 2010s, showing a slight, gradual decline until 2015. However, in the past couple of years there has again been a slight upturn, while the increase in use among boys in upper secondary school is quite marked: "from 13 percent in 2015 to 16 percent in 2017".[73]

The Ungdata scores for the 2010s for rule-breaking showed a stable or downward trend until 2015. However, this trend has reversed in the surveys of the past two years, especially for boys. There has been a 2 percent increase in both lower and upper secondary school boys who have committed at least ten rule violations in the past year.[74] Again, whether this can be viewed as correlated with use of cannabis is under discussion, since we know there is a connection between cannabis use and different types of rule-breaking behaviour, especially for those who are frequent users. The results for shoplifting and vandalism show the same tendency: a gradual decline until around the year 2015, then a marked increase again for boys, particularly in the last two years of secondary school.[75]

Although this trend of the past couple of years provides some cause for concern, the big picture nonetheless shows that violations of the law committed by youth under the age of 18 has dropped considerably in Norway since the beginning of the 2000s.[76] In 2002, 9956 adolescents under the age of 18 were charged with different violations of the law,

---

[71] "Ungdata. Nasjonale resultater 2017, NOVA Rapport 10/17".

[72] "Ungdata. Nasjonale resultater 2018, NOVA Rapport 8/18".

[73] Ibid., 103.

[74] Ibid.

[75] Ibid.

[76] Bård Amundsen, "Kriminaliteten nesten halvert blant ungdom – mer enn doblet blant eldre", *forskning.no* (2017), https://forskning.no/samfunn-barn-og-ungdom-kriminalitet--samfunnskunnskap/2017/07/kriminaliteten-nesten-halvert-blant

while in 2015, only 5925 young people were charged with violations of the law. This corresponds to a reduction of around 40 percent. A current study established that juvenile violence has been reduced by half between 2007 and 2015.[77] The Oslo police have reported an increase again for the period 2015–2017, but in fact, this amounts to only 3 percent of all 10- to 17-year-olds responsible for most of the juvenile crime in the Norwegian capital.[78] Ninety-seven percent of Oslo's 50,000 young people have never been under suspicion. A widening gap appears to have arisen between the majority of "respectable" young people and an increasingly violent, marginalized minority.[79]

The drop in criminality in recent years, incidentally, is not unique to Norway but a familiar phenomenon in other Western nations such as the USA, where violent crime has decreased dramatically in the period 1993–2015. The percentage of Americans who report having been the victim of a violent crime in the course of the past half year shows a dramatic decrease of 77 percent for the past three decades.[80]

The incidence of bullying in Norway is relatively stable, but for girls in lower secondary school, the percentage of those subjected to bullying has increased from around 6 percent to a stable 8 percent in recent years.[81] For the percentage of lower secondary school students who have been subjected to threats of violence or violence that has resulted in cuts or injuries, the figures indicate a slight decrease for both sexes since the beginning of the 2010s, but this year's survey shows a slight increase, especially for lower secondary school boys.[82]

[77] Frøyland and von Soest, "Trends in the perpetration of physical aggression among Norwegian adolescents 2007–2015".

[78] Runa Victoria Engen and Tormod Strand, "Politiet om 150 tenåringer: – Vi greier ikke å stoppe dem", (2018), https://www.nrk.no/norge/politiet-om-150-tenaringer_-_-vi-greier-ikke-a-stoppe-dem-1.14029325

[79] Lars Roar Frøyland and Tilmann von Soest, "Ungdomsvold halvert på åtte år. Mindre alkohol og mer skjermbruk kan være forklaringer", *Aftenposten* (2018), https://www.aftenposten.no/viten/i/8wQA8W/Ungdomsvold-halvert-pa-atte-ar-Mindre-alkohol-og-mer-skjermbruk-kan-vare-forklaringer

[80] Amundsen, "Kriminaliteten nesten halvert blant ungdom – mer enn doblet blant eldre".

[81] Bakken, "Ungdata. Nasjonale resultater 2018, NOVA Rapport 8/18".

[82] Ibid.

Overall, the combined parameters paint a picture of a respectable and well-adjusted generation of youth throughout the first half of the 2010s. Acting-out and extreme, over-the-line types of behaviour became less common than before. However, it would appear that a departure from the respectability trend commences around 2015, at which time criminality and problem behaviour again began to increase, after several years of decline. It is too early to draw any conclusions about the cause of this. If we combine these findings with increased reports of depressive symptoms, loneliness and stress and pressure, a picture emerges that possibly shows a greater incidence of problems in today's youth compared to previous generations, although one cannot rule out the impact of changes in norms due to which problems are reported to a greater extent than before.

The New Digital Existence

Surveys of young people's use of time in Norway show a clear trend of spending increasingly more time in their daily lives on digital activities. More than half of 15- to 16-year-olds surveyed spend more than three hours a day in front of the screen and there has been a significant increase just since 2015.[83] There are also clear gender differences: girls on average spend more time on social media, while boys spend most time on online computer games.[84] It is for that reason, perhaps not surprisingly, that when depressive symptoms increase, especially in girls, many people have pointed the finger at social media as a source of mental health complaints. And when time use surveys show that young people spend less time out together with friends than previously, since more socializing takes place online and entails physical separation, while depressive symptoms and loneliness are on the increase, an obvious conclusion drawn is that online communities can never replace the rewards of interpersonal, physical contact.[85] A number of studies have also confirmed what many

[83] Ibid.

[84] The Norwegian Media Authority, "Dataspill: Fortsatt store kjønnsforskjeller", (2018), http://www.medietilsynet.no/om/aktuelt/dataspill-og-kjonnsforskjeller/

[85] Bakken, "Ungdata. Nasjonale resultater 2018, NOVA Rapport 8/18".

have already suspected: the more time young people spend on a social medium, the greater the probability of their reporting depressive symptoms.[86] A possible explanation can also be so-called *social comparisons*—humans have the tendency to compare themselves with others—but media such as Instagram and Facebook provide a distorted picture of how rich the lives of one's circles of friends are, in that most users are more likely to post status updates when they experience positive life events. In a British survey, young people were asked how diverse social media platforms influenced their well-being and mental health, and here the photo-based, colour-filtered Instagram medium was assessed as one of the worst, followed by Snapchat, Facebook, Twitter and YouTube, in that order.[87] For that reason it has been alleged that the use of social media increases the risk of not only depression, but also suicide. Last year the American psychologist Jean Twenge's book *iGen* was published, along with a related study in the journal *Clinical Psychological Science*, in which Twenge and colleagues claim that the greater the number of hours that young people spend in front of the screen, the more they are at risk of developing depression and suicidal thoughts.[88] The basis for this claim is an increase in self-reporting of depressive symptoms and suicide among young Americans in the period between 2010 and 2015, particularly for girls. Young Americans, who report spending more time on social media and smart phones, report more psychological complaints than young people who spend more time on activities that are not screen-based, such as activities involving face-to-face contact with others, sports and exercise, homework, reading and religious activities. These alleged connections have received a great deal of international attention, among other things through the much shared excerpt from Twenge's book in the *Atlantic*

[86] Mai-Ly N. Steers, Robert E. Wickham, and Linda K. Acitelli, "Seeing everyone else's highlight reels: How Facebook usage is linked to depressive symptoms", *Journal of Social and Clinical Psychology* 33, no. 8 (2014).

[87] Royal Society for Public Health, "#Status of mind. Social media and young people's mental health and wellbeing", (2017).

[88] Jean M. Twenge et al., "Increases in depressive symptoms, suicide-related outcomes, and suicide rates among U.S. adolescents after 2010 and links to increased new media screen time", *Clinical Psychological Science* 6, no. 1 (2018); Jean M. Twenge, *iGen: why today's super-connected kids are growing up less rebellious, more tolerant, less happy – and completely unprepared for adulthood – and what that means for the rest of us* (New York: Atria Books, 2017).

article "Have Smartphones Destroyed a Generation?"[89] and in Norway, through Conservative Party Member of Parliament Mathilde Tybring-Gjedde's feature article in the Norwegian national daily *Aftenposten* with the attention-grabbing headline: "The cell phone is young people's new drug of choice."[90]

An objection that has been voiced in response to these assumed connections is that Twenge and colleagues do not document a chain of cause and effect between social media and depressive symptoms and the risk of suicide. It is basically possible that the alleged connection that Twenge highlights is a so-called spurious or random connection, which in contradistinction to a causal connection shows two tendencies that correspond in time but need not have anything to do with one another. The sale of yoga pants has also increased dramatically in the same time period, but there are few who would hold this responsible for the increase in mental health complaints or suicide.[91] Psychologist Amy Orben has also criticized Twenge's study for postulating flimsily substantiated, grand-scale connections, in that social media can only explain 0.36 percent of the co-variance of girls' depressive symptoms.[92] Depressive symptoms of 99.64 percent of girls do *not* appear to have anything to do with their use of social media. Twenge's co-variance is so miniscule that it can just as probably be due to statistical noise and erroneous reporting, Orben states.

There is also a great deal of other research on social media, including Norwegian online users, demonstrating that those who are avid social media users are also more likely to have more friends in real life and that social media use is a practical means of communicating with and staying in touch with others, which can have a positive impact on personal well-being.[93] It must be said that a group of large-scale users, predominantly

[89] "Have smartphones destroyed a generation?", *The Atlantic*, September (2017), https://www.theatlantic.com/magazine/archive/2017/09/has-the-smartphone-destroyed-a-generation/534198/

[90] Mathilde Tybring-Gjedde, "Mobiltelefonen er ungdommens nye rusmiddel", *Aftenposten*, 24 February 2018.

[91] Psycritic, "About that Jean Twenge smartphone article", *Psycritic* (2017), http://www.psycritic.com/2017/10/about-that-jean-twenge-smartphone-article.html

[92] Amy Orben, "Social media and suicide: a critical appraisal", *Medium* (2017), https://medium.com/@OrbenAmy/social-media-and-suicide-a-critical-appraisal-f95e0bbd4660

[93] Petter Bae Brandtzæg, "Social networking sites: Their users and social implications – a longitudinal study", *Journal of Computer-Mediated Communication* 17, no. 4 (2012).

men, reported an increase in loneliness. In a recently written research report for UNICEF that addresses the connection between screen time and children's mental health, a U shape is employed as an image: no use and extreme use both appear to have a slightly negative impact on children's well-being, while moderate use appears to have a slightly positive impact.[94] On the whole, the research therefore provides no obvious substantiation for describing social media and smart phones as "young people's new drug of choice". Coffee, in fact, is a more plausible culprit, since the research in both cases is inconclusive as to whether it has a positive or negative effect on health. But as long as one's daily consumption is not extreme, or one does not indulge just before turning in for the night, both coffee and social media would appear to be compatible with a normal quality of life. To explain why some people nonetheless use online technology in an extreme manner, we must consider the individual vulnerability factors.[95]

Why then the great concern about social media? The general alarm is naturally related to how the Internet and social media have quickly changed our lives in a virtually unprecedented fashion in recent years, and thereby also a number of wholly legitimate concerns arise that are beyond the scope of this book, ranging from protection of privacy and surveillance to the aggregation of power in the hands of large, global corporations to the emergence of a digital self, in which self-presentation is of far greater importance than it has been for previous generations. Not to mention how one becomes perpetually accessible to others. The philosopher Øyvind Rabbås has pointed out how Sartre's "hell is the other"—the self-conscious shame of being seen by others—now acquires a wholly new dimension with and through social media.[96] But without seeking to trivialize these legitimate concerns, it is also important to keep in mind that this is virtually a ritual occurrence whenever new technology is intro-

[94] Daniel Kardefelt-Winther, *How does the time children spend using digital technology impact their mental well-being, social relationships and physical activity? An evidence-focused literature review. Innocenti Discussion Paper 2017–02* (Florence: UNICEF Office of Research – Innocenti, 2017).

[95] Fulvio Castellacci and Vegard Tveito, "Internet use and well-being: A survey and a theoretical framework", *Research Policy* 47, no. 1 (2018).

[96] NRK P2, "Selvrealiseringens tyranni", in *Debatt i P2* (2018 https://radio.nrk.no/serie/debatt/KMTE82010518/09-04-2018), 45:11.

duced. Just look at how Ludvig Holberg in 1748, in a book, ironically enough, expressed concerns about the impact of the art of printing on the overall mental powers of human beings:

> On the other hand, the objection can be made that the facility and comfort, which printing entails, cause considerable inconveniences. The world is hereby encumbered with an unheard-of quantity of useless documents and studious individuals fill their brains with abstruse erudition, without giving themselves the time or means to reflect upon what they read. Beyond this, one does not see in our time the kind of rare geniuses, as one did in the old days, when studious men instead sharpened their minds through perpetual meditation rather than filling them with voluminous reading and the thoughts and opinions of others, for in the same manner that one can fill one's house with so many guests that one has no room to turn about, so can one fill the brain with so many foreign ideas that one has no space for own thoughts.[97]

A discipline such as psychology appears also to possess a certain affinity for pessimism about technology, due to which the concerns quickly surface about the impact of "artificial" new media and digital technologies on the individual's "natural" emotional lifeworld and authentic patterns of human socializing, while down the road one seldom finds any evidence to speak of in support of such concerns.

Generational Differences

The final source I will employ to understand today's young people is the study of generational differences. And I do so even though some have questioned whether it is meaningful in any sense to highlight allegedly distinctive, shared characteristics for a given cohort.[98] The labels placed on generations will in many cases reveal just as much about how the adult generation prefers to view their successors.

[97] Ludvig Holberg, *Epistler* (Copenhagen: Ludvig Holberg, 1748–1754), 14–15.

[98] Runar Døving, "Generasjon A", (2016), https://kristiania.no/artikkel/media/generasjon-a

A somewhat common characterization of today's young people in the West, and in the USA in particular, is the label the "Me generation", which, in contrast to previously well-known epithets for generations, such as the "1968 generation" implies that today's youth have less of a collective and political orientation than their predecessors and are more individualistic and concerned about self-development. A central contributor of assertions underpinning this image of the generation is the abovementioned Twenge, who in 2006 published the book *Generation Me.*[99] Twenge comments here how the generation following the now-established "generation X", from 1980 onwards, has not yet been assigned a generation label with staying power, although there are many suitable proposals, such as "generation Y", "millennials" and "iGeneration". Her own suggestion is the "Me generation", which is intended to capture the freedom and individualism that characterizes the lives of young people born after 1980, in that they have been encouraged by their parents and teachers to put their own needs and feelings first.[100]

In the sequel, *The Narcissism Epidemic*, co-authored with psychologist W. Keith Campbell, Twenge continues to cultivate this portrait of a generation. Twenge and Campbell paint a picture of the USA in which loving oneself is an even more fundamental creed.[101] Among 11- to 13-year-olds in the 2000s, 93 percent score higher on self-esteem than the average for their predecessors in 1980. However, Twenge and Campbell see dark clouds on the horizon and ask whether this ego bolstering hasn't been taken too far, in that the result is not merely high self-esteem, but a thriving narcissism, characterized by a fundamentally unbalanced self with a grandiose, bloated self-image and inadequately developed ties to other human beings. The narcissism is manifested in every nook and cranny of American contemporary culture: on a reality TV show, a girl plans her sixteenth birthday party and wants the traffic to be rerouted so a marching band can lead her entrance on the red carpet; it is now possible to hire paparazzi when you go out on the town so after-

[99] Jean M. Twenge, *Generation me – why today's young Americans are more confident, assertive, entitled – and more miserable than ever before* (New York: Free Press, 2006).

[100] Ibid.

[101] Jean M. Twenge and W. Keith Campbell, *The narcissism epidemic: living in the age of entitlement* (New York: Free Press, 2009).

wards you can order a fake celebrity magazine with your own photograph on the cover; people buy expensive homes by taking on mortgages far beyond their means; American women and men strive to promote themselves as a personal brand and high school students attack classmates and seek attention for their violent behaviour by posting videos of it on YouTube.[102]

Twenge and Campbell emphasize how the underlying narcissism must be understood on a level with the obesity epidemic in the USA, which has become dramatically worse among young Americans since the 1980s. They base this view on the Narcissistic Personality Inventory (NPI), which contains forty scales in which trial subjects must choose the one of two alternatives they agree with most: 1. A – "The thought of ruling the world scares the hell out of me. | B – If I ruled the world it would be a better place"; 2. A – "I prefer to blend in with the crowd. | B – I like to be the center of attention"; 3. A – "I can live my life any way I want. | B. People can't always live their lives in terms of what they want." NPI measures seven sub-factors: authority, exhibitionism, exploitativeness, entitlement, self-sufficiency, superiority and vanity. Through comparison with data from as far back as 1979, Twenge and Campbell find that American college students in the early 2000s were significantly more narcissistic than baby boomers and generation X, who grew up in the 1970s, 1980s and 1990s. In 2006, two-thirds of American college students scored higher than the scale's average for the period 1979–1985, while in 2006 one-fourth chose predominantly the alternatives indicating narcissism. And even though men on average score higher than women, the changes are especially associated with an increase in narcissism in young women.

However, developmental psychologist Jeffrey Jensen Arnett has challenged the fundamental pillars of Twenge's portrait of a generation.[103] The first objection concerns the NPI questionnaire, which contains points of relevance for assessing narcissism such as "I like to show off my body" and "If I ruled the world it would be a better place" but also fea-

---

[102] Ibid.

[103] Jeffrey Jensen Arnett, "The evidence for generation we and against generation me", *Emerging Adulthood* 1, no. 1 (2013).

tures that Arnett holds up as being far more socially desirable such as "I am assertive" and "I like to take responsibility for making decisions." The increase in the NPI score in recent decades is negligible and corresponds only with more responses on one or two of the questions, but because Twenge only operates with a total score, we don't know which points the increase pertains to, Arnett points out. We do know, however, that gender roles have changed in recent decades: young women increasingly demonstrate traditionally masculine personality traits such as assertiveness. As such, the increase in narcissism reported by Twenge can essentially stem from a change in gender roles, due to which young women today are more confident and assertive than previously. There are even other studies showing an increase on the NPI for women alone, Arnett adds.

The second main objection concerns the fact that those whom Twenge refers to as young Americans are in reality white, affluent college students accepted into four-year college programmes and who comprise around 20 percent of all young people in the USA in the 18–25 age group. Arnett's third objection is based on competing studies that utilize data different from what Twenge uses and show both the narcissism and self-esteem of American college students to be relatively stable in the period 1976–2005. And if Twenge is correct in her theory about increased narcissism in young people and narcissism predicates a series of negative outcomes, it should be possible to detect these outcomes. For example, one could expect to see an increase in impulsive risk-taking behaviour, because many young people would lack sufficient self-control and they would feel entitled to immediate gratification. But as Arnett substantiates, the incidence statistics for fatal car accidents, teenage pregnancies and juvenile delinquency, for example, have all decreased in the past twenty years in the USA. A plausible explanation can basically be, contrary to Twenge's theory, that crime has gone down because young people's impulsiveness has decreased. Arnett also cites an increase in presumed positive actions in the same period, including volunteer work among college students. The young people of today have a more positive attitude towards people from another ethnic background or sexual orientation than before, which is consistent with their being neither more egocentric nor narcissistic. On the whole, young people would appear to be better off than Twenge gives them credit for, is Arnett's conclusion.

The youth researchers Kristinn Hegna, Guro Ødegaard and Åse Strandbu have asked more matter of factly if we are perhaps dealing with "A 'pathologically serious' generation of youth?"[104] Based on the trends presented here, they speculate about whether the price today's respectable, hard-working and dutiful young people are paying is an increase in psychological stress. They point out how young people from the 1960s found freedom through work, while the 2010 generation finds its freedom through education. *The Schooled Society*, as sociologist David Baker has christened the educational revolution of the past 150 years, entails that youth must administrate their childhood starting from a relatively early age, which results in a more conformist generation of youth, since within the parameters of an education the permitted margin of error is more restricted.[105] It has also been commented that the education system appears to be increasingly cultivating another type of ideal student than previously. The Swedish ethnologist Jonas Frykman's apt formulation about this is as follows: "Before one went to school to become something, learn a certain profession, but today one goes to school to become successful."[106] This educational pressure and on the whole, the entire *disciplined future-orientation* in which not only is school to be mastered, but the body trained and the health tended, and you have only yourself to blame if you fail, can take its toll on young people's mental health in the form of worries, feelings of hopelessness, insomnia and stress.[107] Grown-up requirements lead to growth in a number of complaints. And for some, the grown-up complaints appear earlier than before in the form of physical and mental health complaints.

[104] Hegna, Ødegård, and Strandbu, "En 'sykt seriøs' ungdomsgenerasjon?", 374.

[105] Ibid., 376.

[106] Miriam Lund Knapstad, "Sykt flinke", *Aftenposten*, 17 August 2013, 25.

[107] Hegna, Ødegård, and Strandbu, "En 'sykt seriøs' ungdomsgenerasjon?".

Conclusion

To summarize, the statistics indicate that young people in Norway are doing relatively well in most areas. Although psychological disorders in the population are not on the rise, mental health complaints do appear nonetheless to be increasing among young people, both boys and girls. And some behaviour, including the consumption of both prescription and over-the-counter medications such as painkillers and antidepressants, presumably speaks to a development in which especially teenage girls are seeking to alleviate pain and regulate their moods to a far greater extent now than was the case just a few years ago, in keeping with the idea of a disciplined future orientation and the schooled society, which demands more from them. Perhaps the increase in cannabis consumption, especially among boys in secondary school between 2015 and 2018, in Oslo showing the greatest increase in affluent districts, can also be understood as an abreaction strategy in response to pressure.[108] But is it exclusively features of the societal development that imply that young people supposedly suffer from more complaints and are sicker today than before? Or must we also consider the possibility that we have applied specific ideas about youth that we constantly confuse with the reality and which young people will also eventually try to live up to?

[108] Bakken, "Ung i Oslo 2018. NOVA Rapport 6/18".

6

Social Representations

After religion, we had science and politics and psychology and the welfare state. This is our faith, although we choose to call it reason and rationality. And one could claim that it is a faith equally strong and equally flammable as the belief in a God once was in this country.
—Sara Stridsberg *(Sara Stridsberg, "Et åpent ansikt"* Klassekampen, *11 February 2017, 4)*

A DEFINING FEATURE OF MODERNITY'S TRANSITION from a vertical order with "God" at the top to a horizontally arranged cosmos is the shift from collective to social representations. According to Émile Durkheim, *collective representations* were religions, myths and legends that existed independently of individuals and used to explain life in the pre-modern society. *Social representations,* according to Durkheim's successor, the French-Romanian socio-psychologist Serge Moscovici (1925–2014), are more dynamic and replaceable images, values, ideas and practices shared by a group or social forms that function as a common code of

O. J. Madsen, *Deconstructing Scandinavia's "Achievement Generation"*,
https://doi.org/10.1007/978-3-030-72555-6_6

understanding.[1] Social representations are quite simply necessary conditions for all communication in modern society. Beyond this, they are a means of converting that which disturbs us—that which is on the outside looking in from the distance and threatening our universe—into something familiar. Moscovici describes two processes in particular through which new social representations can arise: objectification and anchoring.[2] *Objectification* involves making something abstract into something more concrete. *Anchoring* is a means of giving new phenomena meaning, whether these be objects, relations, experiences or practices, by integrating them into an existing worldview and thereby enabling their interpretation and comparison with already familiar elements of established interpretive frameworks. The unknown and alien aspects of these objects will thereby be experienced as less threatening.

An important element of Moscovici's modernization of Durkheim's collective representations is that the latter exists within a magical and religious understanding of reality, a role fulfilled by science in late modern society. The early sciences of the nineteenth century, before professionalization, were inspired by common sense, while today it is instead the opposite—common sense is often based on science. The research filtered through the media appears to have become a key ingredient of the spiritual diet of modern human beings: "Researchers have now discovered that" or "I read in the newspaper that".

In this chapter, I will therefore look at key concepts such as "the achievement society", "the achievement generation" and "the good girl syndrome" as social representations and ideas in circulation in the media that function as equivalents to myths.

---

[1] Serge Moscovici, "The phenomenon of social representations" in *Social representations: explorations in social psychology*, ed. Gerard Duveen (Cambridge: Polity Press, 2000).

[2] Ibid.

The Achievement Society

A key, recurrent idea found in many accounts about our times is the claim that we live in an achievement society. The German theologian Heinz Zahrnt in his book *Warum ich glaube. Meine Sachem mit Gott* from 1977 provides an easy-to-understand definition of the achievement society that remains relevant to this day:

> As a model case, I choose the issue of the *achievement society* of our time. Here I am making reference to the fact that the achievements demanded from the individual by our society are to an increasing extent experienced as pressure, not solely by the losers, who hereby feel pushed out into the margins of society, into 'asociality', but also by the winners, found in the midst of this society and holding sway within it.[3]

In today's cultural climate, it is not unusual to postulate that the achievement society comes at a huge human cost if the outcome is exhaustion and psychological disorders such as depression, as held by the Danish sociologist Anders Petersen in his book "The Achievement Society" (*Præstationssamfundet*):

> [T]he explosion of the depression epidemic must be viewed in light of the ideal status achievement has acquired with respect to the good life. Depression is a seismograph for ongoing trends stipulating that it is critical to assert oneself and perform well both at work and in one's private life. It isn't important what one is good at, but it is of decisive importance to perform optimally in one field or another. The societal pressure which individuals of today must manage and address is the cornerstone of a depression epidemic.[4]

Here Petersen makes clear how what is currently designated as the achievement society denotes a time period in the West in which accomplishment in all arenas has become an unquestioned value that imposes a substantial and incessant pressure on individuals. The human

[3] Heinz Zahrnt, *Hvorfor jeg tror* (Oslo: Gyldendal, 1977), 185.

[4] Petersen, *Præstationssamfundet*, back cover.

cost is a virtual epidemic of depression. Petersen makes a case for how the achievement society rests on the vision of the *competition state*—the idea that the traditional welfare society has outlived its usefulness in the global economy of market liberalism.[5] In Denmark, the term competition state was introduced by the political scientist Ove Kaj Pedersen at the Copenhagen Business School in 2011 and quickly gained currency in the political arena—among others, Denmark's former Minister of Finance Bjarne Corydon under Helle Thorning-Schmidt's social democratic governments wholeheartedly embraced the concept. The term competition state has not been incorporated to an equal extent in Norway. In the past three years it has appeared several times in the Norwegian media, but in several of the articles reference is made to Danish sources and dissemination of the term is still relatively modest in scope. A possible explanation can be that the construct is experienced as a less fitting description of the Norwegian state than of the Danish. Of the Scandinavian nations, Denmark is often singled out as the best example of a political shift to the right in the 2000s, through which the welfare state and its values of equality are abandoned.[6]

The affiliated metaphor *the competition society*, however, is found in Norwegian, denoting a political and cultural climate in which goal rationality, efficiency and achievement have become defining values. One of the most influential and indefatigable critics of such a social development in Norway was the professor of social medicine Per Fugelli (1943–2017). In his book "Radical medicine: Essays on perfection, achievement and health" (*Rød resept: Essays om perfeksjon, prestasjon og helse*), he takes issue with the spirit of the times on the brink of a new millennium, a spirit which he maintains will have a negative impact on our health. Fugelli explicitly singles out both *perfectionism* and *achievement*. He understands the achievement requirement as a direct outcome of the competition society, the society towards which he holds that Norway is headed. In this context, Gro Harlem Brundtland's famous statement "It is typically

---

[5] Ibid.

[6] Bue Rübner Hansen, "Danmark-koden" *Manifest tidsskrift* (2016), http://www.manifesttidsskrift.no/danmark-koden-13/

Norwegian to be good" from her New Year's speech as prime minister, on 1 January 1992, heralds such a transition.[7]

This, in fact, is one professor of social medicine's critique of another for prescribing the incorrect remedy for Norway. Fugelli reads the new national slogan as a kind of final farewell to the solidarity-based welfare society of the 1950s and a covert adaptation to the tougher competition society of the 1990s, which promotes an *achievement culture* he maintains will lead to the freezing out of human beings who do not function optimally and produce an increase in stress, fear and fatigue-based illnesses for those in greatest demand and best able to perform within these frameworks, the requirements of which in reality "exceed the bounds of natural human capacity".[8] To encourage this development will accordingly affect Norwegians at both ends of the achievement culture's performance spectrum. Fugelli here anticipates subsequent discussions about both market-based social differentiation and the achievement society.

But if we read Gro's famous slogan in its actual context, it is reasonable to interpret the statement as an attempt on Brundtland's part to live up to her role as mother of the nation by endeavouring to renew the Norwegian people's faith in themselves and their country. The New Year's speech began with a retrospective on "the dramatic year of 1991" and recalled "the feelings and reactions provoked by the death of King Olav".[9] It can appear that doctor of social medicine Brundtland wanted to surmount this national trauma and the pervasive collective insecurity related to issues such as increased unemployment, social welfare benefits, the banking crisis, political upheavals leading to the dissolution of the former Eastern Bloc, war in the Middle East and increased foreign competition and lay the foundation for the new era that had already commenced: "The 1990s are simultaneously a decade of great opportunities in international relations."[10] In Brundtland's defence, she also mentions the traditional values which Fugelli calls for, such as solidarity, the welfare society, equal rights and belonging. At the same time, Brundtland's

[7] Per Fugelli, *Rød resept: essays om perfeksjon, prestasjon og helse* (Oslo: Universitetsforlaget, 1999).

[8] Ibid., 81.

[9] Gro Harlem Brundtland, "Statsministerens nyttårstale" (NRK TV1992 https://tv.nrk.no/serie/statsministerens-nyttaarstale/FAKN70000191/01-01-1992), 0:03.

[10] Ibid., 1:29.

speech is implicitly based on ideas about competition and achievement—such as in the analogy drawn between sports performances/elite athletes and high culture and expectations for Norwegian trade and industry as a means of an understanding of the spirit of the times, which can be said to correspond with the achievement society: "The girls' soccer teams, girls' handball teams, our men on skis and the Oslo Philharmonic Orchestra. They are excelling in the company of the world elite. In the same manner we will show that Norwegian trade and industry can succeed internationally. Perhaps we need a new slogan? It's typically Norwegian to be good."[11]

It is also possible to detect the source of inspiration for Brundtland's speech as *the third way*,[12] a newly staked out balance between market liberalism and state control based on initiative and entrepreneurship, which would soon come to power through Bill Clinton's presidential terms of office in the USA from 1993 to 2001 and Tony Blair's new Labour government in Great Britain from 1997 to 2007, both of which critics understood as typical of a more neoliberalist perspective on human life in which individual accountability played a central role. It is possible to discern the contours of these ideas in Brundtland's modernized social democratic appeals:

> We must then also question the welfare schemes we have developed […] help for self-help […] new opportunities for the individual […] Solidarity entails our making demands on everyone […] Assuming responsibility for our fellow man does not mean taking responsibility away from them.[13]

The term that Fugelli, among others, connected to the alleged shift in values—the achievement society—appears to have had its breakthrough in the Norwegian press in 1999, according to the media archive Atekst Retriever. Before this point, only a few, sporadic mentions are found and in the years before the period 1995–1998, the term is not used on a single occasion. In the year 1999, however, the Norwegian term for "achievement society" (*prestasjonssamfunnet)* appears more than eleven times in

[11] Ibid., 09:06.

[12] Anthony Giddens, *The third way: the renewal of social democracy* (London: Polity Press, 1998).

[13] Brundtland, "Statsministerens nyttårstale", 10:30.

Norwegian print media. And it is of particular interest to note who has found fit to use the term in these less than one dozen articles. In contrast to Denmark, the term in Norway does not yet bear any obvious connotations and neither are there ideological architects and political agitators flirting with what could be called neoliberal ideas,[14] nor any of the kind of outward enthusiasm for the term that might be expected from heads of private industry, leaders in the public sphere or coaches and motivators—on the whole, people who are interested in results—and who now claim that the achievement society has become a virtue of necessity if Norwegian employees aim to stay competitive in the global labour market at the turn of the new millennium.

Without exception, the term "achievement society" is embraced by individuals in the eleven articles in question who are fond of presenting themselves as critical of this alleged development. In the first piece of the year, the beloved philosopher Arne Næss, eighty-seven years of age at the time, was interviewed by the newspaper *Dagbladet* about the meaning of life. Here Næss warns Norwegians against believing that achievement will bring happiness: "Yes, because one hears so often that one must become something. As if we are not already something to begin with [sic]. That we are nothing, sort of, until we dive into the achievement society."[15] Næss offers a diagnosis of the times as he dissects the prevailing social morality in Norway, in which happiness has become synonymous with achievement. The consequences are, according to the enthusiastic philosopher, countless depressions in young, resourceful human beings seeking help from the university health services: "They are 20 years old and already walk around frowning."[16]

The Norwegian Commission for Human Values, appointed by the Bondevik government to strengthen the positive community values of society, also appears in a number of news reports that year, since the Commission has identified five areas in which they want to promote a socio-ethical mobilization, "where the Commission itself will step forward to submit an opinion and encourage society to take action. This

[14] Arild Utaker, "Michel Foucault om liberalisme og nyliberalisme" *Sosiologi i dag* 35, no. 2 (2005).
[15] Pål Mathiesen, "Livet som filosofi" *Dagbladet*, 24 January 1999, 4.
[16] Ibid.

pertains to the schools, violence, consumption and justice, traffic mortality rates and the achievement society."[17] One item on the Commission's project list of all of thirty-eight items reads: "Values under fire: the achievement society. Write a situation description; What does the requirement for efficiency and the requirement to be strong do to us as human beings? What happens to those who fall through the cracks?"[18] The inclusion of the achievement society along with target areas such as schools, violence and traffic mortality rates implies that already at this time it was experienced as a prevailing requirement with extremely real consequences for the individual—both for those who master the requirements and for those who do not. The "achievement society" along with the "consumer society" is otherwise highlighted in a critical rebuttal of the Commission's work in which the question is asked whether the use of such terms discloses a Leftist orientation.[19]

In 1999 the newspaper *Dagbladet* interviewed the above-mentioned Fugelli who was omnipresent in the media even back then. He advises readers to dial it back a bit: "The escalating differences must be resisted, that benefits everyone – also the winners. The achievement society produces more poverty, but the strain will also be substantial for the winners. Driving the distance in fifth gear is not a normal state."[20] In another piece from the newspaper *Aftenposten* the same man gives advice for improved public health by unmasking the sports analogy of the Norwegian people's Brundtland: "When cultural life is functioning, you gain a vibrant and playful society. It's a matter of removing the jacket of the achievement society's gold medal winner before it becomes a straitjacket."[21]

In another article from *Dagbladet* the same year, sexologist Ken Purvis speculates about why Norway is a world leader in Viagra use, according to a new study: "The achievement society demands peak performance from us at all times and we are influenced by the ideals."[22]

---

[17] Geir Salvesen, "Verdikommisjonen liv laga?" *Aftenposten*, 13 March 1999, 35.

[18] Hans Petter Aass, "Kommisjonens 38 punkter" *VG*, 30 January 1999, 4.

[19] Salvesen, "Verdikommisjonen liv laga?", 35.

[20] Trude W. Strømman, "Fugelli vil ha politikk mot hodepine" *Dagbladet*, 4 November 1999, 6.

[21] Terje Wiig, "Naturen styrker kropp og sjel" *Aftenposten*, 22 August 1999, 20.

[22] Frode Hansen and Asbjørn Svarstad, "Kvinnene krever bedre sex – Og bidrar til at Norge er i Viagra-toppen" *Dagbladet*, 7 October 1999, 8.

The same year *Aftenposten* prints an article about the alcohol consumption habits of Norwegians in which researchers Bente Træen and Arild Hovland from the Norwegian Institute of Public Health are interviewed about why Oslo's urban residents consume alcohol: "It is well known that alcohol is used to create a breather or a time-out from daily life's activities and the achievement society."[23]

At the other end of the spectrum, the national Christian daily *Vårt Land* prints an interview with unit nursing officer Marie Aakre from the cancer ward at the National Hospital in Trondheim, who sees many obstacles in our times that get in the way of the work of providing care for other human beings:

> I see many counterforces at work in our times that affect both the congregation and diaconal work in general. The work of caring for others takes time and is curtailed by the pace, efficiency, rationalization, technology, the achievement society and status, both in the health care sector and otherwise. I am afraid we are unable to achieve enough closeness and we don't take the time to understand. Our meeting places are so easily marked by indifference and superficiality.[24]

Those responsible for the eleven examples of the term "achievement society" found in the newspapers in 1999 are one unit nursing officer, two alcohol consumption researchers, one doctor of social medicine, a sexologist, a philosopher and the Commission for Human Values. There is not a businessperson or a person on the street in sight—the term comes exclusively out of the well-intentioned mouths of experts—all of whom warn against the achievement society in different areas of life. But here a question arises, and this is whether the well-intended warnings help to usher the concept into everyday speech.

As for the frequency of the use of the term "achievement society" in the media after the year 1999, the statistics tend to imply that the concept was sought introduced two decades too soon for Norway. In the years that follow, the "achievement society" appears on only a handful of

[23] Anne Hafstad, "Drikker for å finne seg selv" *Aftenposten*, 26 October 1999, 2.

[24] Vårt Land, "La oss oppmuntre hverandre til gode gjerninger!" *Vårt Land*, 24 November 1999, paragraph 5.

occasions in the course of a newspaper year. As late as in 2011, the term was used only once: the local newspaper *Tønsbergs Blad* printed an interview with Bishop Laila Riksaasen Dahl in which she speaks about the continued significance of the church in today's society, despite declining membership, and alleges that it must be a counter-culture, offsetting "the achievement society, consumer society and market-driven social exclusion".[25] In the subsequent period, however, something happens—and the "achievement society" becomes a more frequently applied term—for example, in 2016 it appears seventy-six times. And in the course of these five years, the achievement society has apparently managed to establish itself as a more central point of reference in the social debate. In the first hit, Tove Ytterbø, leader of the Norwegian Association of Pharmacists, is interviewed by *Ukeavisen Ledelse* who asks "Are there any developmental features that worry you?" to which she replies: "the achievement society, which ensures that you always feel inadequate and excludes many".[26] In a commentary a few days later Vilde Bratland Hansen of *Oppland Arbeiderblad* describes the life of young people: "In the achievement society, 'ordinary' jobs have become something to be avoided at all costs."[27] In *Adresseavisen*, Associate Professor of sports sciences from NTNU Anne Thorild Klomsten answers the question of whether it isn't parents rather than the school who are responsible for making young people feel secure: "They aren't capable of doing that, because they are also victims of the achievement society."[28] *Aftenposten*'s weekend supplement *A-magasinet* prints a long feature article about Norwegian youth, including Martin, who suffers from a condition of chronic pain: "The 17-year old is one of several young people suffering from inexplicable pains. Is the achievement society responsible?"[29] The newspaper *Trønderavisa* announces a record increase in the number of students enrolled at Sund Folk High School (a non-degree college) and functioning headmistress Astrid Moen states in a comment: "The folk

---

[25] Lars Døvle Larssen, "Ber deg ta ansvar" *Tønsbergs Blad*, 15 March 2011, 11.

[26] Ukeavisen Ledelse, "Egenmeldingen" *Ukeavisen Ledelse*, 15 January 2016, 38.

[27] Vilde Bratland Hansen, "Jakten på den uoppnåelige sikkerhet" *Oppland Arbeiderblad*, 19 January 2016, 14.

[28] Grete Holstad, "Forsker anbefaler kjønnsdeling" *Adresseavisen*, 21 January 2016, 8.

[29] A-magasinet, "Gåten Martin" *A-magasinet*, 12 February 2016, front page.

high schools offer young people a hiatus from the achievement society."[30] Even in a letter to the editor by Arne Sauar in the newspaper *Agderposten* about something as essentially unrelated as municipal reform, the term now pops up: "We have the achievement society which a child encounters as early as in primary school, maybe already in kindergarten."[31] Sauar reminds us that the aim must be to create a warmer society, irrespective of whatever the general consensus might be.

Based solely on the first two months of 2016 we see that the "achievement society" has apparently established itself as a central idea in the public discourse and become a term now frequently connected to the living conditions of young people, in the form of an expanding and exhausting external standard to be lived up to. This assumption is however also challenged from time to time. In the newspaper *Fædrelandsvennen*, eighteen-year-old Bendik Dalen from Tangen Upper Secondary School in Kristiansand speaks out: "I seldom experience being an adolescent as stressful, sometimes I actually think it's a bit too laid-back [...] The media focus on how young people are subjected to far too much pressure seems a little exaggerated. Clearly life is hectic in periods but not all the time."[32] Also among the experts there are a few opposing voices. Psychologist Peder Kjøs, known from the Norwegian television series *Jeg mot meg* (Me against Myself), in response to the question of whether the situation is worse now than before, replies: "It is an exaggeration to claim that the achievement society causes psychological problems. Those who are hurting the most are those who are completely excluded."[33]

Despite sporadic comments questioning the veracity of the depiction of our times implied by the "achievement society", the tendency in 2016 is for the term to pop up as the preferred explanation for psychological illness in young people. In connection with the publication of the report

[30] Trønderavisen, "Rekordsøkning til Sund" *Trønderavisen*, 13 February 2016, 33.

[31] Arne Sauar, "Verken ja eller nei til kommunereformen" *Agderposten*, 29 February 2017, 19.

[32] Kari Byklum and Christine Gulbrandsen, "–Jeg kjenner meg ikke igjen i ungdomspresset" *Fædrelandsvennen* (2016), https://www.fvn.no/familieogoppvekst/%2D%2DJeg-kjenner-meg-ikke-igjen-i-ungdomspresset-8883b.html, paragraph 3.

[33] Lene Skogstrøm, "TV-psykologen gråt da han tok avskjed med de åtte: – Jeg ble så glad i alle sammen" *Aftenposten* (2016), https://www.aftenposten.no/osloby/i/ddRyo/TV-psykologen-grat-da-han-tok-avskjed-med-de-atte%2D%2D-Jeg-ble-sa-glad-i-alle-sammen, paragraph 13.

from the Ungdata survey of secondary schools in Aust-Agder, Stein Kristiansen, the assistant director of education for the county authority, employs terms such as "the success generation" and the "achievement society" as an explanation for why 24 percent report having attempted self-harm and 40 percent report having suffered due to worries in the past week.[34] On World Mental Health Day, Line Karlsvik, vice-chairman of the Socialist Party for Møre and Romsdal, writes in the Kristiansund newspaper under the fitting title "Requirements of Our Times" (*Tidens Krav*): "Is it any wonder that one becomes depressed? The achievement society. The society for the successful. Those who can handle demanding studies and jobs and do volunteer work for both this and that."[35]

The Achievement Generation

The idea of the achievement society in Norway appears to have also produced at least one legitimate child, specifically, the label "the achievement generation" to define the young people of today who supposedly are growing up in the achievement society and internalizing the current demands to excel both in school and out. The first case of the Norwegian term for "achievement generation"—*generasjon prestasjon*—found in Atekst Retriever is in an article in the newspaper *Morgenbladet* from December 2011, written by former journalist and now physician Charlotte Lunde, who addresses the trend of performance-enhancing medication being taken by students, academics and night-shift workers to improve their performance—so-called smart drugs.[36] In Lunde's essay, the term "achievement society" is not used directly, but it is nonetheless just beneath the surface since she connects the use of Ritalin to the pressure to perform and the Western competition society. In her interpretation, the performance requirement Lunde describes is closely bound up with a medicalization thesis: "In a society of increased economic requirements, the outcome will potentially be an expectation from both working

[34] Carl Christian Engstad, "–Ungdommene trives" *Lillesands-Posten*, 29 July 2016, 7.
[35] Line Karlsvik, "Verdensdagen for psykisk helse" *Tidens Krav*, 21 October 2016, 8.
[36] Lunde, "Generasjon prestasjon".

life and school that people take medication to enhance their performance."[37] In other words, for the time being, the term "achievement generation" applies exclusively to those who take chemical aids to enhance performance. Later the concept would be disassociated from the medication aspect and live its own life as a description of the expectations, imagined or real, of contemporary society for the lives of young people, which for many lead to exhaustion, stress and depression.

The next time the term appears two and a half years later, it is in a less artificial setting and employed more as a natural description of the current day's imperative to accomplish something. In a commentary written by the journalist Marit Bromark in May of 2014 and published on the website *foreldre.no*, a critical focus is directed towards the trend of talent programmes for children, such as the Norwegian television channel TV2's *Idol Junior* and *Norske talenter* ("Norwegian Talents"). Here the labels "achievement generation" and "achievement society" appear both in the headline and in an admonitory statement from Professor May Britt Drugli from the Regional Centre for Child and Youth Mental Health and Child Welfare at NTNU: "We are living in an achievement society, this is absolutely not the age of mediocrity. It has been claimed that that [sic] we are in the process of producing so-called achievement children, in other words, that children believe they have to excel in everything all the time."[38] However, the term "achievement children" has a rather brief shelf-life as a media phenomenon, while the "achievement generation" enters the public discourse in a serious fashion starting in 2014.

In the months following this introductory discussion, the term "achievement generation" begins to appear little by little in media content characteristic of the times about young people's quality of life. In the newspaper *Romsdals Budstikke,* journalist Solveig Oterhals Landsvik writes a few weeks later that, "Perhaps we can call them the 'achievement generation', those who are teenagers today."[39] A few days later, a similar

---

[37] Ibid., 13.

[38] Marit Bromark, "Prestasjonsbarna: – I dag er det ingen arena for det vanlige, bare for det som er best" *foreldre.no* (2014), http://www.klikk.no/foreldre/barn/prestasjonsbarna-1447809.ece, paragraph 12.

[39] Solveig Oterhals Landsvik, "–Ikke la samfunnspress og en hashtag ta styringen" *Romsdal Budstikke* (2014), http://www.rbnett.no/nyheter/article9808306.ece, paragraph 4.

statement was printed in the newspaper *Trønderavisa*, "Comments, likes, and sharing on social media occupy a large part of the daily life of the coming generation – the 'achievement generation'. There are many who hold that this is reflected in the mental health of children and young people."[40] In the late autumn of the same year, the term experiences its national breakthrough in earnest when Norway's most read national daily newspaper *VG* puts the trend under a microscope in an article series. In the weekend edition's feature entitled "The Achievement Generation" ("*Generasjon prestasjon*") the reader meets 15-year-old Annika Solstad Vogt who "works out up to fifteen hours a week, attends an advanced math course four hours a week and aspires to be the best in everything". The lead paragraph makes the claim that "Three out of ten Norwegian girls make themselves sick with stress".[41] The article presents the following portrait of a generation:

> They are hard-working and future oriented. They have a good relationship with their parents, do well in school, have lots of friends and exercise several times a week. They are the children of the oil generation, who enjoy all manner of privilege in a time offering great opportunities. Despite this, more and more young people are struggling with their lives.[42]

In the article the veracity of this description of today's youth in Norway is substantiated by a statement from Anders Bakken, head of research at NOVA. In response to a question from the weekend edition *VG Helg* about whether "Norwegian girls are being so good that it's making them sick?" Bakken replies: "Previously alcohol and drug problems and family conflicts were the cause of depression in young people. Now successful youth are also struggling."[43] Bakken speculates about whether this stems from "the requirement for perfection".[44] The newspaper follows up on

[40] Monica Irén Solberg Susegg, "'Galskap å si at det der er en tjukk jente'" *Trønder Avisa*, 20 June 2014, 10.

[41] Hanne Kreutz-Hansen, Kari Mette Hole, and Christine Rian Johannessen, "Generasjon prestasjon" *VG+* (2014), http://pluss.vg.no/2013/09/13/1359/1759_23293421?order_id=101848081&code=42f41cbdabd17a52fa3a85c20246e851d15be3f4

[42] Ibid., paragraph 8.

[43] Ibid., paragraph 11.

[44] Ibid., paragraph 12.

the article on several platforms during the following week with yet another online piece and a debate held at the Parkteater in Oslo, which is broadcast on VGTV. The newspaper *Dagsavisen* prints a feature article entitled "The Achievement Generation" the same week, which makes reference to the *VG* week-end feature article.[45] And on the following week-end, columnist Hanne Skartveit writes in *VG*'s Saturday edition about the young people of today who take their anger out on themselves rather than their parents, citing "what many refer to as 'the achievement generation'".[46] Skartveit links this to a culture that tells the coming generation that they can achieve anything:

> Parents and the media have told children that everything is possible. Everyone can achieve whatever they wish. That is a difficult message for those who don't succeed, or don't know what to choose. What we are indirectly telling young people is that if they should fail then they are personally responsible.[47]

In weeks that follow, there is a veritable explosion in the use of the term in the Norwegian media, at first with a qualifying "what some have called",[48] but eventually more and more without this phrase, as if it has now become a reality. In just a few months, the media coverage of the achievement generation has moved from the question "Maybe we should call them the 'achievement generation'" to the verifying "what many call 'the achievement generation'".

Statistically speaking, the evolution of the use of the term in the Norwegian media shows how use of the characterization takes off in a big way in the course of a relatively short time period. The first time it appears, is as stated in 2011, but in both 2012 and 2013 it does not appear at all, while when it is reintroduced in 2014, it figures 95 times, in 2015, 252 times, in 2016, 507 times and in 2017 there are 516 unique occurrences of the term in Norwegian newspapers. A competing label for this generation, such as "the obedience generation", had more than one

---

[45] Marit Øimoen, "Generasjon prestasjon" *Dagsavisen*, 17 September 2014.

[46] Hanne Skartveit, "Det tause opprøret" *VG*, 20 September 2014, 2.

[47] Ibid.

[48] Romerikes Blad, "Ros for åpenhet" *Romerikes Blad*, 27 September 2014, 2.

hundred hits in 2015, but after several months of debate about sociologist Gunnar Aakvaag's take on the coming generation, the label scored only seven hits in 2017 and appears to have disappeared. One possibility might be that "the achievement generation" encompasses "the obedience generation". For example, in Skartveit's above-mentioned commentary entitled "The silent rebellion" (*Det tause opprøret*), the "achievement generation" is not merely a characteristic of the younger generation of today, but a common strategy comparable to those of previous youth rebellions. However, it is a rebellion that is not primarily directed outward; instead, it is directed inward, at the self: "An invisible youth rebellion is underway in Norway. Unfortunately, it is not adults who are under fire. While previously young people rebelled against society and their parents, today many young people vent this anger on themselves."[49] Skartveit's opinions receive the support of psychology specialist Per Are Løkke, who in the Norwegian Psychological Association's journal *Tidsskrift for Norsk psykologforening* argues that anger directed at the self is an unavoidable consequence of the diagnosis culture:

> While their parents grew up in a culture in which the expression of rage directed at the authorities and false ideals was legitimate, the logic of self-realization and the diagnosis culture have contributed to closing off these channels. When disorders become privatized, the collective responsibility for finding solutions for cultural issues, such as a hysterical focus on mastery, a pathological investment in an ideal body, and the divorce epidemic, is rendered invisible. The diagnosis culture contributes to this cover-up and thereby supports the conclusion that the 'fault' lies in the girls and not in society.[50]

Løkke also writes a feature article version for *Aftenposten*, entitled "Diagnoses hide girls' rage" (*Diagnoser skjuler jenters raseri*),[51] and the message of an introverted rebellion is spread by a number of other articles

---

[49] Skartveit, "Det tause opprøret", 2.

[50] Per Are Løkke, "Jenters stumme raseri – i diagnosenes tidsalder" *Tidsskrift for Norsk psykologforening* 51 (2014): 771.

[51] "Diagnoser skjuler jenters raseri" *Aftenposten*, 14 September 2014.

during the same time period.[52] The "achievement generation" is now being disseminated by a number of traditional media genres. *VG*'s popular self-help series "How to handle…" ("*Slik takler du…*") is standing by, ready to connect with the "achievement generation". "Experts: This is how parents can handle 'the silent rebellion'."[53] And the description which initially was used by the adult generation's columnists is now also appropriated by young people in their own self-depictions. "We are the children of a generation so motivated for success that it is making us sick", Karoline Rekaa writes of her peers in *Aftenposten* the following week.[54] The consolidation appears to be complete. What is unique about a number of the self-depictions that now appear is how the contradictions of pathological goodness, grandiose ambitions and exhaustion, performance excellence and suicidal dreams about escaping the pressure once and for all, are seamlessly interwoven. Below I have quoted an article from *Si ;D, Aftenposten*'s online debate forum for young people, in its entirety. Written by nineteen-year-old Mia Olea Vettestad, the article entitled "The Achievement Generation" ("*Generasjon prestasjon*") illustrates this ambivalence:

> I have everything. I know it. I am painfully aware that appearances can be deceiving. But I am exhausted. I am angry. I am disappointed. Most of all, I am frightened, afraid of failing, afraid of not living up to the expectations. Afraid of myself. My greatest fear is that the bubble will burst. That others will realize that my life is just a facade. An upholstery covering up all the darkness inside that I am trying so hard to hide. A protection from myself. The online newspapers are overflowing with accounts of people making an honest effort to break out of this vicious circle. I know that I am just one of many, one of several thousand good girls out there, who don't understand how this world can be called a home. Because I am tired of being misunderstood. I am tired of forcing myself to smile, when my entire self

[52] Se Øimoen, "Generasjon prestasjon"; Eli Skjeseth, "Digitale misjonærer", *Aftenposten*, 21 September 2014; Eirin Eikefjord, "Prestasjonspikene" *Bergens Tidende* (2014), https://www.bt.no/btmeninger/kommentar/i/852gx/Prestasjonspikene

[53] Camilla Bergland, "Eksperter: Slik kan foreldrene takle 'det tause opprøret'" *VG* (2014), https://www.vg.no/nyheter/innenriks/skole-og-utdanning/eksperter-slik-kan-foreldre-takle-det-tause-opproeret/a/23301970/

[54] Karoline K. Rekaa, "Det er ok ikke å være best i alt" *Aftenposten*, 24 September 2014, 11.

> wants only to scream and let the tears come. But I am scared to death. What if nothing good comes of it? There are many who don't see the joy of waking up to a new day. Who hold themselves to such a high standard that the only solution becomes the dream of escape. Escape from waking up, from new opportunities that seem so insurmountable. Escape from the pressure. I am 19 years old. I have just been accepted into the study programme of my dreams. But all I'm capable of doing is lying curled up in a ball on the floor, staring at the wall and hoping that this state between living and not existing will soon come to an end. So, what am I trying to say? Well, it hit me that a part of what is keeping this feeling of suffocation alive, is that nobody talks about the problems while they are experiencing them. The formula for how to handle daily life comes from those who have already done so. But the achievement generation also needs to hear the stories about those of us who can't see the light at the end of the tunnel. Because I can't promise that things will get better. I cannot, with my hand on my heart, say that your perception of the world is only a misunderstanding. But I can offer comfort. I can demonstrate that coping with life is difficult and there's no shame in that.[55]

Not many days pass before the adult generation starts using "the achievement generation" as the main explanation for why many young people are struggling psychologically. In an editorial in the newspaper *Romerikes Blad* that appeared one week later, reference is made to Skartveit's comment and the achievement generation, where the claim is summarily made that "Very many young people are struggling psychologically. The diagnoses are often vague. But a common feature can presumably be identified. Young people hold themselves to a high standard and do their best; they want very much to excel in everything they do."[56] In a letter to the editor that appeared in *Harstad Blad* on the same day, special needs teacher Edvin Eriksen also makes reference to Skartveit and goes to great lengths to explain the defection from secondary school and lack of access to working life as a consequence of an education policy, including Gudmund Hernes' Reform 94, dictating that everyone perform according to the same theoretical standard:

[55] Mia Olea Vettestad, "Generasjon prestasjon" ibid., 26 September, 15.

[56] Romerikes Blad, "Ros for åpenhet", 2.

> It is the 'Achievement Generation' with an exaggerated focus on performance and success. Both in their free time and at school, children and young people's appearance and performance are to be assessed and measured. When will there be a focus on all those unable to master the theory and requirements for success in all areas of life?[57]

A few days later, Camilla Klovning Strømø, Head of the Childhood and Youth Services Committee (*Oppvekststyret*) in Haugesund municipality, expressed the following in an article in *Haugesunds Avis*:

> The exact number of children and youth in Norway who are struggling has not been determined conclusively, but the public authorities hold that approximately twenty percent of all children are experiencing psychological difficulties. The most widespread complaints are anxiety, depression, loneliness, eating disorders, behavioural disorders, self-harm, suicidal thoughts and/or difficulties in school. Another study also shows widespread use of medication in young people. This is a consequence of the 'achievement generation'.[58]

Finally, it is interesting to note that the Church of Norway does not waste much time in embracing the perception and interpreting it as meaning that we are dealing with a generation that has quite simply forgotten that they are a part of God's Creation. In her comment "Fully Achieved" ("Ferdig Prestert") printed in *Dagen*, Maria Celine Lundeby, the youth group leader for the Norwegian Lutheran Mission in Oslo, offers hope for today's youth:

> Our Maker Himself speaks to us; there is freedom and refuge to be found in His words. You were created in His image. You are infinitely valuable merely on the force of being human, the pinnacle of His creation, the crown on His kingdom. This is what the achievement generation needs to hear.[59]

---

[57] Edvin M. Eriksen, "Generasjon prestasjon" *Harstad Tidende*, 27 September 2014, 22.

[58] Camilla Klovning Strømø, "'Generasjon prestasjon' med psykiske konsekvenser" *Haugesunds Avis*, 3 October 2014, 13.

[59] Maria Celine Lundeby, "Ferdig prestert" *Dagen*, 1 November 2014, 37.

In a short period of time, the "achievement generation" has become the appropriate reference, irrespective of whether the messenger wants theory taken out of the schools again or for youth to return to the church. The retro ska band F5, who allegedly found the inspiration for their Eurovision Song Contest Junior entry in the contest itself,[60] therefore appeared to hit the nail on the head more than once when during the final at Telenor Arena in 2017 they sang: "The achievement generation, this is a strange situation" ("*Generasjon prestasjon. Dette er en rar situasjon*").[61] The reflexive modernization is opportune, though F5 doesn't win on this occasion. And to paraphrase Baudrillard: what we have on our hands is a generation with no myth other than themselves.

Good Girl

Another remarkable, gendered expression that is used in Norway to capture the essence of a generation of industrious but stressed-out youth is the *good girl syndrome.* "Being a good girl is now a syndrome. A medical condition. How did this come to pass?"[62] laments *Aftenposten*'s news editor Håkon Borud, on behalf of his own and others' daughters in 2015. His disavowal "Being a good girl is no illness" can be understood as a reaction to how the term "good girl" has acquired a prominent position in our understanding of ambitious and psychologically tormented young women. His concern was wholly understandable in that the term, or more precisely its Norwegian equivalent *flink pike,* appeared 1220 times in the Norwegian media in 2014. An important voice here was the filmmaker Solveig Melkeraaen's autobiographical documentary *Flink pike* ("Good Girl") in which moviegoers could experience her struggle with anxiety and depression:

---

[60] NRK Presse, "Finalistene i MGPjr 2017 er klare" (2017), https://www.nrk.no/presse/finalistene-i-mgpjr-2017-er-klare-1.13492215

[61] F5, "Generasjon prestasjon" in *MGP Jr. 2017* (Oslo: NRK, 2017).

[62] Håkon Borud, "Å være flink er ingen sykdom" *Aftenposten* (2015), https://www.aftenposten.no/meninger/kommentar/i/2XA4/A-vare-flink-er-ingen-sykdom., paragraph 7.

> It's fine to be good, but not if it is just in relation to the expectations of others. I remember standing in the shower and how much anxiety I had. [...] Perhaps it's because your best qualities can also be your worst?[63]

With time Melkeraaen's "goodness" apparently becomes such a problem for her and assumes such enormous proportions in her life that in the end it leads to a paralysing psychological disorder. A number of people have wondered about how such a thing is even possible, among them the psychologist Torunn Espe, who in his master's thesis *Kvifor vert nokon sjuk av å vere flink?* ("Why does being good make some people sick?"), investigated the incidence of the term "good girl syndrome" (*flink pike syndrom*) in Norwegian newspapers in the database Atekst Retriever and found a striking increase in the incidence of the term in the new millennium and with a particularly explosive development in the 2010s.[64]

The results of Espe's searches clearly demonstrate that the male equivalent "*flink gutt*" is far from unknown to us and is in fact used more frequently than the female "*flink jente*" or "*flink pike*". But if the word "syndrome" is added, there are only 11 hits for "*flink gutt syndrome*", while "*flink pike* syndrome" scores 301 hits. Hence, it would appear that being good as a boy or girl, respectively, has, linguistically speaking, extremely disparate outcomes, in that the need for a semantic term as a symptom for illness in men arises only as an exception, while it is much more widespread in reference to women. About one half of the "*flink gutt* syndrome" hits also occur in contexts addressing how there *isn't* any commonly used term for such a phenomenon. I will now illustrate the historical development of the use of term *flink pike* in the Norwegian media, as a means of investigating how something that in principle is positive, could end up becoming something associated with morbidity. And apparently only for one of the sexes.

---

63 Solveig Melkeraaen, "Flink pike. En feelgood film om depresjon" (Norge: Tour de Force, 2014), 00:16.

64 Torunn Espe, "Kvifor vert nokon sjuk av å vere flink? Ei undersøking av flink pike-syndrom sett i lys av sosial representasjonsteori og identitetsprosessteori" (University of Oslo, 2015).

The Good Girl: A Media History

The archives of the Norwegian National Library attest to the existence of the term "*flink pike*" as an expression as far back as in the early 1900s. The following advert appeared in the newspaper *Trondhjem's Adresseavis* in 1903: "Seeking a good girl to fill the post of maid-of-all-work as of April 15 or before at Koller & komp., Kongens gate 12."[65] In *Aftenposten* in 1907, there is an advert seeking: "A nice, good girl for a domestic position to begin immediately in Nordstrand, next to the railway station. Mark the envelope '4 adults 124'."[66] The term also seemed to have been incorporated in the contemporary literature of the day. In Sigrid Undset's novel *Jenny*, for example: "You are very good girl, Miss Winge."[67] And in Knut Hamsun's novel *Children of the Age*, he writes: "You are a good girl, the mistress has use for you."[68] As the examples demonstrate, "good girl" ("*flink pike*") in this time period is synonymous with an attractive quality that was sought after in female employees working in service.

The very first use of the term *flink pike* found in the Atekst database was in the newspaper *Verdens Gang* in 1952, where the term appears in the comic strip *Cappy and the new cook*. The sailing ship Krakk is praised for its seaworthiness in bringing the crew to America. "The Krakk is a good girl!"[69] In 1959 the same newspaper covered the largest high society event of the year: the wedding in southern Norway of the billionaire Steven Rockefeller Jr. and the fishmonger's daughter Anne Marie Rasmussen from Søgne. Anne Marie, whose nickname is Mia, receives glowing references from everyone around her: "Also her teacher in Søgne and her housekeeping teacher [sic] can confirm that Mia is an enthusiastic, good girl."[70] It comes as no surprise that with respect to the housewife role of the 1950s, being a "good girl" seemed to be exclusively a boon—in the sense of someone who excels in the performance of her duties. Ten

---

[65] Trondhjems Adresseavis, "[Advert]" *Trondhjems Adresseavis*, 16 March 1903, 4.

[66] Aftenposten, "[Advert]" *Aftenposten*, 6 November 1907, 4.

[67] Sigrid Undset, *Jenny* (Kristiania: Aschehoug, 1911), 189.

[68] Knut Hamsun, *Børn av tiden* (Kristiania: Gyldendalske forlag, 1913), 159.

[69] VG, "Cappy og den nye kokken" *VG*, 19 August 1952, 7.

[70] "Sint veps ville stikke Anne Marie" *VG*, 5 August 1959, 5.

years later, Norway's chances of winning the upcoming Eurovision song Contest in Vienna in 1967 are assessed, where the following is written about Norway's contestant Kirsti Sparboe: "We have a resident of Tromsø – and she is a good girl."[71] Even in the entertainment industry of the 1960s, being a "good girl" appears to have had nothing but positive connotations.

In 1969 *VG* prints a report of a sex crime in which a man was charged for having forced a woman into prostitution. According to the woman's explanation, he was full of praise if the night had been profitable: "If I'd made a lot of money, he said I was a good girl and gave me a pat on the cheek. 'You are my best good girl,' he said sometimes."[72] In the Norwegian translation of an Agatha Christie series published in *VG* two years later, Dr. Quimper instructs Lucy: "But be on your guard and keep your mouth shut, there's a good girl."[73] In both of these cases, from real-life and fictional criminal environments, there is a sense of the term "good girl" having a clear patriarchal undertone: the expression is used by men as an implicit warning for women. The latter are expected to do as they are told; if not, they must expect sanctions.

In 1978 the limitations of the term are more visible in legal contexts as found in a film review of Karen Arthur's *Legacy*, a portrait of a stay-at-home, upper class woman's restricted lifeworld: "Still, Bissie is an impoverished person. She grew up as a sweet, good girl, who did as the grown-ups said and never complained."[74] In 1984 *Aftenposten* published a feature article about beauty contests for children in the USA where five-year-old Janie receives praise from her mother because she hasn't risked getting any scrapes on her knees. "And she has been a good girl and left her roller skates alone."[75] The context implies that "good girl" is an ambiguous expression for something many Norwegian readers presumably feel to be a disturbing development in which the freedom of children's playtime is infringed upon by the condemning gaze of the adult world.

---

[71] Espen Eriksen, "Kirsti på medaljeplass?" ibid., 8 April 1967, 15.

[72] Jan Schjelderup Mathiesen, "'Satte meg på to skift på Rådhusstrøket'" ibid., 26 September 1969, 8.

[73] Agatha Christie, "4.50 fra Paddington" ibid., 30 August 1971, 13.

[74] VG, "Anmeldelse: Mot stupet" ibid., 2 October 1978, 40.

[75] Nina Bratt, "Minimisser i rampelyset" *Aftenposten*, 3 November 1984, 23.

The first time the term was explicitly addressed in Norway was in 1987, when the journalist Anne Lise Stafne in the *Aftenposten* column "Just between us" ("*Oss i mellom*") sheds light on the theme of performance anxiety and concedes that it manifests differently in men and women but that the differences are not substantial in that both sexes are afflicted by the goal of perfect performance in all arenas. "The milk cups of our childhood had the words '*Kjekk gutt*' (Fine Fellow) and '*Flink pike*' (Good girl) on them and those of us who grew up with such imperatives are still trying, more or less, to live up to them."[76] Although boys are included here, the messages on the milk cups can nonetheless be said to demonstrate a certain inequality between the sexes: the adjective *kjekk* can mean: "cheeky, outspoken, or fearless", "bold, courageous, brave", "to have good physical vigour, healthy and hearty" or "easy-going and pleasant; friendly and funny".[77] The Norwegian word *flink*, on the other hand, has fewer meanings and is primarily used as a synonym for "capable; hardworking" and "especially in areas where no special abilities are required".[78] There are in short underlying differences in the available latitude of these categories—boys have a number of ways in which they can be *kjekk*, while for girls, being *flink* is closely tied to achievements and carries connotations of being a climber, presumably to compensate for a shortage of gifts. A similar pattern can be discerned today in the ideas of Norwegian children down to the age of four who will correct adults who say something "wrong" by reciting traditional aphorisms such as "boys are cool and girls are sweet". "Coolness" can imply all manner of things, while "sweetness" is inexorably wrapped up in one's appearance.

In the newspaper year of 1988 a new journalistic trend appears—in-depth interviews. In *Aftenposten* the film director Berit Nesheim and the Conservative Party of Norway's MP Kaci Kullmann Five were both interviewed in articles presented under the headline: "Good Girls" ("*Flinke piker*").[79] Some people experienced such compliments as evidently confining. Four years later, *Aftenposten*'s recently hired news editor Anne Lise

[76] Anne Lise Stafne, "Oss i mellom: Må vi alltid lykkes?" ibid., 29 August 1987, 25.

[77] Ordnett.no, "Kjekk" (2018), https://www.ordnett.no/search?language=no&phrase=kjekk

[78] "Flink" (2018), https://www.ordnett.no/search?language=no&phrase=flink

[79] Per Egil Hegge, "Kaci Kullmann Five: Pen, flink pike fra Bærum" *Aftenposten*, 23 January 1988, 7; Kaja Korsvold, "Profilen: Flink pike" ibid., 14 June, 9.

Gjetvik was interviewed. When Gjetvik is confronted with her friends' description of her as "ambitious", "studious" and "diligent Lise", she takes issue with this judgement:

> I don't see anything wrong with being ambitious. I am ambitious in terms of doing a good job – but not in terms of position and title. It seems like many people think that I MUST be ambitious, since I have this job. Strange that nobody says the same thing about my male colleagues. It is seldom one hears about men who excel in their career being characterized as ambitious, studious, diligent, conscientious young lads. I am studious and am not ashamed of it. And I am hard working – isn't that the same as being diligent? This 'good girl syndrome' is quite stereotypical and I am starting to grow weary of it.[80]

Notwithstanding the objections to the term, the 1990s also brought rise to another tendency: women interviewees used the term in their depictions of themselves. Up until 1993 the term *flink pike* had exclusively been used by men about women or by journalists about interviewees. It is incidentally ironic that it was Norway's first female Prime Minister Gro Harlem Brundtland who was the first to do this, when visiting the graduating class at Ledaal Secondary School in Stavanger, at which time she told them about her own modest graduation celebrations: "Personally I was a good girl and probably a bit prudish."[81] And the choreographer Jane Hveding makes the following admission in reference to her latest dance production: "I have been a 'good girl' for so long. The time has come to create something provocative, something that asks questions and departs from received notions within dance and the performing arts."[82] Both the opposition to *flink pike* and its internalization reflect that the term has at this point been incorporated into the language for a long period of time.

In the years that follow we also find examples that foreshadow what was to come two decades later. In 1995 one of the letters to psychologist Sissel Gran's column "On the Inside" ("På innsiden") in *Aftenposten*

[80] Signy Fardal, "Blått blikk i gul sofa" *Dagens Næringsliv*, 5 September 1992, 16.
[81] Eirik Ramberg, "'Grillet' av førstegangsvelgere" *Aftenposten*, 17 April 1993, 4.
[82] Anne Lise Stafne, "Frekk dans på Black Box" ibid., 3 May, 15.

signed "Best wishes, Good girl", was written by a woman struggling with performance anxiety at work.[83] The suspicion that good girl-ness can be a problem also runs just beneath the surface of a number of articles in the following years. In 1997, the thirty-five-year-old Oil and Energy Minister Marit Arnstad was interviewed and like so many other successful women before her, she was confronted with others' description of her as being "hard-working", "capable", "idealistic" and "loyal": "Isn't it tiresome having to be such a good girl all the time?"[84] Arnstad dismisses the issue out of hand. In another in-depth interview in *Dagens Næringsliv* two years later, she nonetheless employs the term, although in reference to others' opinions of her: "On the outside I can perhaps appear serious, aloof, and reserved. A little good-girlish."[85] While being a good girl may be tiresome, forgoing the use of the expression would appear to be even more difficult.

The Good Girl Syndrome

The first occurrence of a direct coupling of the term *flink pike* with "syndrome" in the Norwegian media archive Atekst is in an interview with crime fiction author Pernille Rygg by *Dagbladet*'s Hege Duckert from 2000, when Rygg describes the main character of her new book, the psychologist detective Igi Heitmann: "Heitmann is a kind of well-educated, reflective heroine. Her stomach is perpetually in knots and she is driven by a good girl syndrome. She leads group therapy sessions at a psychiatric hospital as part of her daily work. As Jung said: Whatever is rejected from the self, appears in the world as an event."[86] It is however remarkable that in the interview Rygg personally reflects upon the fact that psychology functions as a myth in our times. To a question from Duckert about whether she is afraid of what psychologists will have to say about her book, she answers as follows:

---

[83] Sissel Gran, "På innsiden" ibid., 19 August 1995, 38.

[84] Liz Buer, "Kvinnfolk: Itj så lætt-skræmt" *Dagbladet*, 19 October 1997, 3.

[85] Cecilie Enger, "Eneste høne i kurven" *Dagens Næringsliv*, 13 February 1999, 32.

[86] Hege Duckert, "Smerte uten hjerte" *Dagbladet*, 8 July 2000, 13.

> I am more worried about the S&Mers. I haven't studied psychology but have always been interested in it. Psychology is the big myth of our times; it occupies a lot of space. We psycho-analyse ourselves and our surroundings all the time, use psychology to answer questions when the explanation is perhaps in the body. It amazes me that antidepressants are considered so dodgy compared to how fabulous it is supposed to be to speak with a psychologist, as if he or she could not be potentially manipulative.[87]

Ironically, many people will hold that the term "good girl syndrome" represents a psychologizing of the pressure to perform well that afflicts young girls. A syndrome, according to the Norwegian Medical Dictionary (*Medisinsk ordbok*), is defined as "a group or set of symptoms, features and findings that in combination indicate or constitute a clinical entity and represent an illness or condition".[88] The paradoxical example of Rygg is not unique. As I will illustrate through another example in the next chapter, there are many indications that the "good girl syndrome" with time became a self-fulfilling prophecy although the intention of many of the cultural architects discussing it was to liberate young women.

In the early 2000s, the incidence of the use of both the terms *flink pike* and *flink pike* syndrome increases. The newly appointed group managing director of the radio station P4 Cecilie Nordland says about being the boss: "It was especially in the beginning that I was severely afflicted by the good girl syndrome. I believe I'm doing better."[89] Author Tale Næss expresses herself along similar lines in an interview with *Adresseavisen*: "I have suffered from the good girl syndrome for a long time", Tale says. "It is only now that I am able to shake it off – only now that I have started not giving a damn."[90] The "good girl syndrome" has now clearly become a common term for a specific disorder: to go overboard in one's endeavours to fulfil the role of a conscientious individual. And as the above statements attest to, this thereby also becomes something women must regulate themselves. From being a figurative expression used by successful

[87] Ibid.

[88] Ordnett.no, "Symptom", (2018), https://www.ordnett.no/search?language=no&phrase=syndrom

[89] Therese R. Ridar, "Skal få P4 til å sprudle" *VG*, 20 May 2001, 34.

[90] Alexandra Beverfjord, "Under overflaten" *Adresseavisen*, 16 February 2001, 11.

Norwegian women to describe their personalities or the lifestyles of fictional characters, the good girl syndrome in this period also gains a closer connection to serious illnesses that afflict ordinary people. In *Dagbladet* in 2002, it appears as a caption for a picture of a girl who got As in all subjects, but who started dieting as a thirteen-year-old, in an otherwise serious article about a new form of treatment for anorexia.[91] In an article from *Hamar Dagblad* in 2003, we meet one of the participants of a self-help group for dealing with anxiety who states: "I have suffered a bit from the 'good girl' syndrome. The demands on people today are so exacting, especially when it comes to education and working life. I developed performance anxiety."[92] In 2004 the term is used in a headline in *Aftenposten* about Kari Hånsnar Rinne, who was an active, elite indoor bandy player, who wore herself out "because her ambitions were too high".[93] The discussion of the good girl syndrome in this article nonetheless implies that this is still relatively unusual: "She has trained obsessively, filled her daily life with so many tasks that in the end she collapsed. 100% sick leave. And a type of diagnosis that Kari herself refers to as the 'good girl' syndrome."[94] Based on this account we understand that Rinne is using the term in reference to herself. Whether it was a doctor or psychologist who in fact gave her the label is not stated.

In the following period, Norway would appear to be looking to Sweden for assistance, given that the latter country had apparently made more progress in identifying the phenomenon. *Dagsavisen* features an interview with the Swedish journalists Jennie Sjögren and Tinni Ernsjöö Rappe, both of whom experienced burnout at an early age and later published the book: "Diagnosis: Gifted. A handbook for overly ambitious girls and everyone else who should care" (*Diagnose: Dyktig. Håndbok for overambisiøse jenter og alle andre som burde bry seg*).[95] Even before the era of Facebook and other social media, here they warn readers against comparing themselves too much with others:

[91] Kine B. Hertz, "Spiser på kommando" *Dagbladet*, 27 July 2002, 14.

[92] Hamar Dagblad, "Starter angstgruppe" *Hamar Dagblad*, 26 September 2003, n.p.

[93] Mette Bugge, "Lider av 'flink pike'-syndrom" *Aftenposten*, 6 February 2004, 6.

[94] Ibid.

[95] Bente Bakken, "Hvordan unngå 'flink pike'-syndromet" *Dagsavisen*, 18 October 2004.

> When one reads interviews with famous women, incredibly often they talk about how they usually prepare bread dough after work. And then they serve delicious dinners with a handful of sweet basil from their own herb gardens. How in the world do they have time for this? Such things only lead to so-called stress addition: One adds stones to one's own burden by constantly comparing oneself to others and thinking about all the things one should have been doing rather than focusing on the things one achieves.[96]

Their destiny is viewed in the context of a dramatic increase in long-term sickness absenteeism in Sweden for women under the age of thirty-five in high-salary positions. There is no shortage of related examples from Norway. In the newspaper *Vårt Land* the story is told of Member of Parliament May-Helen Molvær Grimstad, who finally had to acknowledge that she was burnt out at the age of thirty.[97] Here the observation is made about how women now appear to be following men's example in running themselves into the ground. The cause is allegedly the pressure to achieve success in working life combined with traditional female virtues dictating that they are supposed to do everything right and take care of others around them. The final consolidation of the good girl syndrome appears to occur a few months later in 2005, when a number of Norwegian news media outlets, including the radio station P4's news programme, discuss the scientific "discovery" of the syndrome from Sweden:

> High-salaried women become ill because they impose overly exacting requirements on themselves. This is what researchers at the Karolinska Institute in Stockholm claim, who maintain that they have discovered a 'good girl' syndrome. It is because such good girls strive for perfection and fail to speak up when they feel overlooked that women struggle with depression and burn-out more often than men in corresponding jobs.[98]

The radio station's chosen heading, "Women's own requirements are making them sick", is a tragic indication of what lies ahead: a

---

[96] Ibid., 18.

[97] Marianne Lystrup, "Knus koppen, ta vare på kroppen" *Vårt Land*, 10 October 2004, n.p.

[98] P4, "Kvinner syke av egne krav" (P42005).

pseudo-scientific term that explains women's and young girls' vulnerability by making them personally responsible for their own misery in that they are incapable of reining in their own ambitions. The Karolinska Institute study done by Monica Renstig and Hélène Sandmark shows that it is no longer primarily low-salaried women in Sweden who are experiencing the greatest increase in sickness absenteeism, but instead women in high-salary professions.[99] Working too many hours a week, striving for perfection, internationalization, the expectation that they should work longer hours, the wrong job and a lack of equality in the home are mentioned as possible causes. All the same, it is striking how what is highlighted in the introduction in *Stavanger Aftenblad*'s version is specifically that "women's own requirements for perfection constitute a health strain". In an article in the magazine *Arbeidsmiljø*, this possible cause is also emphasized first, while the four other hypotheses are not mentioned until the end.[100] An explanation can be that the solution of women assuming greater responsibility for themselves is in fact the preferred solution of contemporary culture. This is ironic, in that the women in question are already experiencing that they must assume too much responsibility both at home and at work, which, in the worst-case scenario, leads to burnout. A few months later, the article is quoted as a lead-in for the article "Good Girls Burn Out" ("Flinke jenter møter veggen") in *Stavanger Aftenblad* about the situation in Norway, where the claim is made that "Burnout is the latest public health issue. Young women are the most at risk."[101] Here the good girl syndrome, which until recently was virtually unknown, is recognized as a commonly known term: "Not long ago, burnout and the 'good girl syndrome' were terms most people had never heard of."[102] In the period of time starting in February 2004, at which time it was called "a type of diagnosis"[103] that *Aftenposten*'s interviewees used in reference to themselves, until September 2005, where it is declared to be "the latest public health issue", the status

[99] Ellen Kongsnes, "Blir syk av 'flink pike'-stempel" *Stavanger Aftenblad*, 22 September 2005, 38.

[100] Turid Børtnes, "Høytlønte kvinner mest syke" *Arbeidsmiljø*, 31 August 2005, n.p.

[101] Trine Lunde, "Flinke jenter møter veggen" *Stavanger Aftenblad*, 17 September 2005, 68.

[102] Ibid.

[103] Bugge, "Lider av 'flink pike'-syndrom" 6.

of the "good girl syndrome" has evolved from being an unknown commodity to acquiring scientific legitimacy.

In this period, several cases come to light in support of this and which indirectly help to consolidate the status of the "good girl syndrome" as an actual phenomenon. Student Bjørn Olaf Syvertsen answers in the university newspaper *Universitas* his own question of why boys perform more poorly in school with "Because they don't have the good girl syndrome."[104] NRK P2 broadcasts the radio documentary *This Is a Man's World*, which is introduced in the following manner:

> It is common knowledge that many young women suffer from the so-call 'good girl syndrome'. They feel the pressure of a requirement to excel at absolutely all times at work, while at the same time they fear they won't succeed to do precisely that. But what about the young men in working life? Which requirements must they live up to in their daily life and work?[105]

It is striking how the consolidation appears to occur through confirmation that the diagnosis is suitable for the female portion of the population but not for the male. In this way, the diagnosis is further verified by establishing to whom it *doesn't* apply.

This time period also appears to be a watershed moment in which the main focus of the public good girl conversation is still about the pressure young career women in their thirties with a husband and children are feeling, but parallel to this, a number of cases now emerge in which, for the first time, the focus is on teenage girls. An article in *Rogalands Avis* reports, "Eating disorders, loneliness and suicide attempts. A number of girls from the middle and upper class can't handle the pressure of our current society's ideal standard of excellence."[106] Chief Psychologist Rigmor Mogård at the Health Service at the University of Oslo explains that presumably well-functioning girls are now struggling more. Many of them have feelings of inadequacy which manifest in the form of stress-related complaints and moderate mental health ailments. Sociologist

---

[104] Bjørn Olaf Syvertsen, "'Flink pike'-syndromet" *Universitas*, 30 March 2006, n.p.

[105] Hege Dahl, "This is a man's world – en radiodokumentar om unge menn og krav på jobben" (NRK 2006), paragraph 3.

[106] Rogalands Avis, "Flinke jenter sliter" *Rogalands Avis*, 4 October 2004, n.p.

Karin Widerberg views this in the context of the "good girl syndrome" and the fact that young girls neither appear to escape the adult world's requirements to be clever and conscientious. In other words, the notion that well-integrated, intelligent girls are struggling more than previously has been in circulation for some time.

It appears that the "good girl syndrome" has become so incorporated in Norway that the term is now a given part of ordinary speech, an autonomous turn of phrase describing the expectation that women must please everyone. In 2005 the group Briskeby released a new album and in a promotional context the lead singer Lise Karlsnes stated: "We aren't suffering from any 'good girl 'syndrome about having to placate everybody."[107] The term pops up all the time as a derogatory adjective about overly ambitious subjects who are perfectionists. This is often found in music reviews of female artists—where the male reviewer usually thinks the musical expression is too polished. But not even Norway's current Prime Minister Erna Solberg has avoided such a label. In 2006 the Conservative Party scored poorly in the opinion polls and party veteran Gustav Heiberg Simonsen maintained that the time had come for new blood in the party leadership:

> We must have a leader who shows enthusiasm and inspiration. There's nobody who wants to recognize this. Erna is a 'good girl'. She is adept and correct, but the effect is too nit-picky and difficult. I think she should step down. Politics is about communication and we are failing to get our message across. We need someone who can fill people with enthusiasm.[108]

Further, "good girl" also appears to find expression in cases where the subject is perceived as overly controlled by external factors. In *Cosmopolitan*, Janne Kristiansen, a recruitment adviser at the University Hospital Helse Bergen, has the following advice for potential job hunters: "Be good at what you do, but don't be a good girl. Good girls who do everything right make me wonder whether they have any substance."[109]

---

[107] Dagsavisen, "Vi har god selvtillit" *Dagsavisen*, 4 October 2005, n.p.

[108] Marianne Johansen, "Høyre-veteran ber Erna gå av" *Dagbladet*, 4 April 2006, 10.

[109] Andreas Kokkvoll Tveit, "–Fjernt fra grasrota" *Klassekampen*, 21 September 2007, 5.

In an article about the Socialist Left Party (SV) in the government, the local government leader in Akershus Liv Heidi Brattås Remo remarks: "In the government, SV has become too much of a 'good girl'; too good to fight for a project, and not good enough at showing what we have achieved."[110] In both cases, the term "good girl" is understood as being the opposite of something genuine that stems from an inner motivation.

It should be added that there has been no shortage of opposing voices, although the statistics demonstrate that these have not been heard to any noteworthy extent. In 2011 *Dagens Næringsliv* columnist Eva Grinde explores the good girl syndrome and asks what is actually wrong with it when around 10,000 hours of practice are required to excel at anything; in this sense, being in possession of the qualities associated with a "good girl" would in fact be useful:

> Then 'good girl' qualities such as perfectionism, perseverance and conscientiousness come in handy. And there is nothing stipulating that these qualities cannot be accompanied by other qualities, which is the impression one often gets. Good girls can also be pioneers, courageous, creative and innovative, as exemplified by the success stories of women such as Pernille Sørensen, Sidsel Wold and Hadia Tajik. So, the question is: for whom in fact is the 'good girl syndrome' dangerous?[111]

Bergens Tidende journalist Ingrid Fredriksen also addresses the escalating use of the term "good girl syndrome": "So please, my fellow women: Let us not reduce ourselves to a group of losers. Just because we are good."[112] However, what best typifies the understanding of the term good girl in Norwegian public discourse of the 2010s is this article from *Aftenposten*'s youth forum *Si ;D* from 2011 signed "Good Girl (18)" (*Flink Pike*):

> When I have been pushing myself too hard for a long period of time, without stopping to check in on the state of my body and mind. I am a typical good girl. I want to get good grades at school, excel in my sport, work and

[110] Silje Midttun, "Raskt til topps" *Cosmopolitan*, 7 August 2006, n.p.

[111] Eva Grinde, "Ja til flinke piker!" *Dagens Næringsliv*, 16 May 2011, 22.

[112] Ingrid Fredriksen, "Ps" *Bergens Tidende*, 27 May 2011, 36.

> earn money, and have a rewarding social life along with it. This is why I have chronic headaches, a bad back and periods of heart palpitations and an ulcer induced by stress. On several occasions I have been asked to calm down or start setting priorities. The problem is that I can't give up any of these things and my brain functions in a way that makes me worry about everything that might happen. I can't just stop being good. It's a part of my personality. Unfortunately, this isn't just my problem. Young people should be offered a stress management course. I have no idea how to relax.[113]

There are several things that are striking about this article. It is permeated with a mentality of morbidity, in which being good and the requirement for perfection are the only explanations presented. At any rate, no other known diagnoses are mentioned, but a series of bodily symptoms are listed such as chronic headaches, a bad back, heart palpitations and an ulcer. The second striking omen is the young age of the author. Up to 2011, except for a few isolated, preliminary cases, the good girl label has predominantly been reserved for women in their early thirties who are suffering under the compound pressures of home and work. The solution presented by the author, incidentally, is also thought-provoking: a stress management course. The solution to the good girl syndrome is understood exclusively in health-related, therapeutic and individual terms. This *Si ;D* article is in many ways symptomatic of a large-scale shift in the "good girl" debate of the 2010s in Norway: the discussion moves away from a focus on young women in working life who have a husband and children to teenage girls and away from a political and systemic understanding related to working life and social welfare to an individualized framework, in which self-care and self-help prevail. The latter perception appears more and more to be the preferred solution also for the adult generation responsible. Jorunn Strand Askeland, communication consultant at Norwegian Church Aid, writes of the "good girl syndrome in the year 2012": "Good girls need to take a course in how to cope with the achievement society."[114]

In light of *the new openness* of the 2010s in Norway—which among other things includes the tendency for Norwegian celebrities to publicly

[113] "Flink pike (18)", "Flink pike-syndrom" *Aftenposten*, 18 September 2011, 23.

[114] Jorunn Strand Askeland, "Flink pike-syndromet anno 2012" *Vårt Land*, 13 January 2012, 29.

disrobe in the media by talking about their personal problems—it is neither surprising that the term "good girl" often appears as an explanation. Norwegian Progress Party MP Mette Hanekamhaug expresses in an interview with *Adresseavisen* her thoughts about why she was personally afflicted by anorexia: "Eating disorders often afflict people who hold themselves to a high standard. It is no longer enough to solely be a good girl; you have to be perfect; and this pertains to all areas of life. I have also been like this."[115] The deputy chairman of the Oslo Progress Party Aina Stenersen has also spoke openly to the media about her difficulties: "The good girl syndrome is very widespread in politics as it is elsewhere. For a long time, I was concerned about being perfect. The eating disorder shattered my idealized expectations and I struggled with that a lot."[116] In an article about television presenter Elin Tvedt's disappearance from the television screen, it was said that she: "struggled to be a good girl all the time. Because of this she was forced to take sick leave from her job on NRK's early morning programme *Frokost TV* in 2006."[117] In these cases the "good girl syndrome" leads to disablement of the afflicted individual.

A tendency that emerged during the 2010s was to attach the "good girl" label to well-documented medical and psychological ailments that are nonetheless without a clear cause. In an article about orthorexia—an excessive fixation with healthiness—in *Stavanger Aftenblad*, Monica Klungland Torstveit, associate professor in sports science at the University of Agder, states: "Typically found in a good girl/good boy endeavouring to excel in yet another field."[118] Physical therapist Gerd Søvli Wæraas writes in conjunction with an ongoing debate in *Adresseavisen* about the connection between fibromyalgia and the "good girl syndrome": "Otherwise I would like to rechristen the fibromyalgia diagnosis as the good girl syndrome. Women must learn to set boundaries at an early age, say no, listen to their bodies and learn to give a damn about being so

[115] Svanhild Naterstad, "Møter slagene" *Adresseavisen*, 31 December 2011, 27.

[116] Ingrid Hvidsten, "Bryter tabuet og forteller" *Dagsavisen*, 4 August 2012, 12.

[117] Jan Thomas Holmlund, "Elin Tvedt er tatt av skjermen" *Dagbladet* (2013), http://www.dagbladet.no/kjendis/elin-tvedt-er-tatt-av-skjermen/66756059, paragraph 21.

[118] Stavanger Aftenblad, "Når sunnhetsiveren tar overhånd" *Stavanger Aftenblad*, 2 December 2011, 30.

good."[119] And on World Mental Health Day *Troms Folkeblad* offered the following advice: "[T]alk to somebody a little bit about the so-called good girl syndrome, also known as CFS."[120]

The tendency to give the good girl phenomenon scientific legitimacy is now occurring on several fronts. Among other things, online tests got the wind in their sails in 2014, and what's more, with the approval of professionals. The website *ABC Nyheter* delivers the subject matter in the form of a checklist: "Do you suffer from the good girl syndrome?" Psychology specialist Sondre Liverød provides her own special list of questions typical of psychiatric diagnosis manuals: "If you can identify with more than one of these statements, it could be that you have a good girl syndrome."[121] The checklist reads as follows:

> I never accept being second best.
> I must be the best in most of what I do.
> I must always do my absolute best.
> I never manage to settle down properly
> I am very conscientious.
> I always meet my obligations.
> I often feel a constant pressure to achieve results and get things done.
> In relation to myself, I never get off easily.
> I don't make excuses for my mistakes but dislike myself when I don't perform to the very best of my abilities.
> I have so much to do that there is seldom time to relax.
> I am very competitive.
> Prosperity and status are important to me.
> My appearance must always be at its best.
> I deserve severe criticism when I make a mistake.
> I strive to keep everything perfectly organized.[122]

It has to be said about this checklist that it is rather inclusive—most people who have a trace of characteristics such as conscientiousness or

[119] Gerd Søvli Wæraas, "Fybriomyalgi/flink-pike-syndrom" *Adresseavisen*, 22 November 2011, 14.

[120] Troms Folkeblad, "Kom, vær med" *Troms Folkeblad*, 3 October 2012, 2.

[121] Marte Korsbrekke, "Sjekk om du lider av flink pike-syndromet" *ABC News* (2014), https://www.abcnyheter.no/livet/2014/01/14/191162/er-du-flink-pike

[122] Ibid.

ambition will be able to answer affirmatively to statements such as "I am very conscientious" or "I often feel a constant pressure to achieve results and get things done." And while the purpose of checklists in ICD or DSM classification systems is to help the examining party make a correct diagnosis, in these news articles there is a clear commercial interest in making the recognition factor as high as possible, so that the maximum number of readers will click on the article.

In 2015 the private psychologist centre HelpLink in Oslo also includes the good girl syndrome in its service repertoire and consistently refers to it as a "condition" for which they offer help on their website. HelpLink gives the following grounds for why they now also offer help for the good girl syndrome along with well-known disorders such as anxiety, depression and eating disorders:

> We receive many inquiries regarding the good girl syndrome (GGS). In recent years, the term has received increasing media attention. There are many who can identify with what they read and hear and are seeking more information. We therefore answer the most common questions about this condition.[123]

Accordingly, their reasoning is that the media writes about it, many identify with what is written and want to learn more, and therefore the psychologist group offers advice, guidance and treatment for this "condition". Under the heading "How can I tell if I am afflicted?" the following procedure is outlined:

> If you recognize yourself in the descriptions of GGS above and the complaints have been constant for a long period of time (six months or more) it can be a sign that you are afflicted. The most important thing however is not the name of the condition, but how you feel inside. If you are constantly tormented by a guilty conscience, uneasiness, worry, have an exaggerated fear of failure or of not measuring up, you have every reason to take this seriously. If you are unsure about why you are struggling, there's

[123] HelpLink Psykologsenter, "Spørsmål og svar om flink pike-syndrom" (2015), http://helplink.no/flink-pike-syndrom/

> nothing to be lost by having a conversation with a psychologist to receive clarification.[124]

The knowledge the psychology experts willingly and incessantly share in the media also appears to be absorbed by their target group. In *Bergens Tidende* eighteen-year-old Viktoria Merkesvik writes with insight about the "good girl syndrome" with an explicit basis in the above-mentioned Liverød to substantiate her critique of the school's focus on performance: "I'm not saying that the school society kills all young people, but a large number of us have our life spark extinguished or develop various disorders."[125]

In 2016 the TV2 series *Sykt perfekt* ("Pathologically Perfect") premiered and was introduced to viewers accordingly: "Never before have young Norwegian girls been so conscientious. Simultaneously, they have never struggled more with pressure, stress and mental health ailments. Meet seven brave girls who talk about how they are really feeling."[126] The series received a consistently positive response for providing an "appalling glimpse into vulnerable teenagers' desperate search for perfection" and the topic is also contextualized as related to being young in Norway, the land of prosperity, in 2016: "Their tearful accounts of never feeling that they are good enough are the dark side of the Norwegian gold medal."[127] In *Vårt Land* associate professor Margunn Serigstad Dahle views the series as an expression of the "Me generation" in the 2000s, in the context of which the self has been consciously and intentionally put front and centre and the individual is left to his or her own devices, for better or worse. According to Dahle's interpretation, the consequences of secularization and the loss of a relationship to God entail that many must now relentlessly administrate themselves to gain recognition: "You aren't given value; you must create it yourself – by performing to perfection."[128]

[124] Ibid.

[125] Viktoria Merkesvik, "Skolen – en besettelse" *Bergens Tidende*, 30 January 2016, 56.

[126] TV2, "Sykt perfekt trailer" (2016), https://www.tv2skole.no/ung/artikkel/67541, 00:10.

[127] Torstein Hvattum, "'Sykt perfekt' på TV 2: Modige jenter viser vei" *Aftenposten* (2016), https://www.aftenposten.no/kultur/i/63L3/Sykt-perfekt-pa-TV-2-Modige-jenter-viser-vei, paragraph 12.

[128] Margunn Serigstad Dahle, "'Sykt perfekt' speglar presset" *Vårt Land* (2016), https://www.vl.no/tro24/sykt-perfekt-speglar-presset-1.674304?paywall=true, paragraph 19.

However, a far less empathetic view of the series is voiced somewhat surprisingly on *Aftenposten*'s *Si ;D* pages, where Adelina Trolle Andersen speaks of being sick of hearing about the "good girl syndrome".

> You're not a victim because you feel you must spend several hours on social media comparing yourself with others. You're not a victim if you miss your best friend's birthday party because of football practice and a chiropractor's appointment. You are just self-centred.[129]

The article becomes one of *Aftenposten*'s most read pieces in 2016 and triggers a debate in which some of the TV series' participants also get involved. It appears that Andersen is not alone in feeling fed up, because while the newspaper searches from the second half of the 2000s show mainly a steady increase in the incidence, recent years show a slight downward trend: in 2005, the term *flink pike* appeared 76 times; in 2010 it appeared 304 times, leading to the top year so far of 2014 with 1229 hits, while for the subsequent year 2015 there were 628 hits, in 2016 426 hits and in 2017 333 hits.

Conclusion

The gender research website *Kilden kjønnsforskning.no* asked in 2016 an implicitly self-critical question: "Why are we so obsessed with good girls?" in the context of which gender researcher Harriet Bjerrum Nielsen recommended that we stop using the term, since to a very large extent it turns girls' achievements into an illness.[130] In the following months, a number of articles appear with the intention of reclaiming the expression "good girl" as a means of converting it into something positive one can say about oneself.[131] Although the "good girl syndrome" will not disappear

[129] Adelina Trolle Andersen, "Sykt perfekt? Nei, bare sykt selvopptatt" *Aftenposten*, 17 January 2016, 15.

[130] Eivor Mæland, "Slutt å bruk begrepet flink pike" *forskning.no* (2016), https://forskning.no/kjonn-og-samfunn/2016/02/hvorfor-er-vi-sa-besatt-av-flinke-piker

[131] Monica Sanden, "Ja, eg er flink! Eg har ikkje eit syndrom" *Bergens Tidende*, 9 April 2016; Inga Ragnhild Holst, "Hurra for flinke piker!", *KK*, 10 June 2016; Mari Helendatter Aarbakke, "Flink og ordinær", *Avisa Nordland* (2016), https://www.an.no/debatt/flink-og-ordinar/o/5-4-271583

overnight, it appears to be perceived by the most trend-conscious commentators as somewhat hackneyed. In the autumn of 2016, for example, psychology student Susanne Masvie made the observation in *Vårt Land* that the condition of "shame" (with the help of NRK's enormously popular television series for young people of the same name) has replaced the "good girl syndrome" as the latest disorder trend.[132] But even if the term should go out of style, it is not certain that this will result in the illness releasing its grip as easily. As Nietzsche commented in his time: "I am afraid we are not rid of God because we still have faith in grammar."[133] In the most recent example in the Norwegian media, appropriately on International Women's Day, 8 March 2018, eighteen-year-old schoolgirl Cecilie Gryte Fjelldal wrote insightfully in *VG*: "We young people no longer get sick from the 'good girl syndrome' but we are still carrying the virus."[134]

---

[132] Susanne Masvie, "Sunn og usunn skam" *Vårt Land*, 6 October 2016.

[133] Nietzsche, *Twilight of the idols/The anti-Christ.*

[134] Cecilie Gryte Fjelldal, "8 om 8. mars: Hadet 'generasjon prestasjon' – hei 'generasjon stress'" *VG* (2018), https://www.vg.no/nyheter/meninger/i/vmzdwj/8-om-8-mars-hadet-generasjon-prestasjon-hei-generasjon-stress, paragraph 2.

7

Self-Fulfilling Prophecies

"But just saying it could even make it happen" sings Kate Bush hauntingly on "Cloudbusting".[1] A number of examples can be found in the social sciences of different interactions between human ideas and behaviour. In psychology, there is the *Werther effect*. As the name indicates, it stems from the German author Johann Wolfgang Von Goethe's epistolary novel, comprising letters and diary entries, titled *The Sorrows of Young Werther* from 1774, which made him famous and allegedly triggered a wave of suicides on the part of young men suffering from broken hearts throughout Europe.[2] The Werther effect is the main reason why today's media is careful about reporting deaths as suicides and extremely reticent about giving descriptions of suicide methods, out of the fear of producing a rub-off effect. The Werther effect or the copycat effect, as it is also called, has been mentioned as raising cause for concern in recent years due to the potentially contagious effect of the media coverage of school shootings and terrorist actions.[3]

---

[1] Kate Bush, "Cloudbusting" in *Hounds of Love* (London: EMI, 1985).

[2] Johann Wolfgang Von Goethe. *The sorrows of young Werther* (London: Penguin, 1989).

[3] Nicholas Farnham and Marieke Liem, "'Can a copycat effect be observed in terrorist suicide attacks?'" *The International Centre for Counter-Terrorism – The Hague* 8, no. 4 (2017); Randy

O. J. Madsen, *Deconstructing Scandinavia's "Achievement Generation"*,
https://doi.org/10.1007/978-3-030-72555-6_7

Along the same spectrum of social ideas with the potential to trigger a specific type of behaviour, we also find *self-fulfilling prophecies*. Unlike the Werther effect, it is not the description of specific actions that is decisive here, but instead the very expectation of a type of behaviour on the part of influential individuals. A self-fulfilling prophecy in psychology can be defined as "a person's expectations that influence that person to change in a manner in keeping with the expectations".[4] This has been referred to as the *Pygmalion effect*, after a sculptor who fell in love with a statue he had carved, as also depicted in Ovid's *The Metamorphosis*. In modern psychology, the phenomenon has been given the updated epithet *The Rosenthal effect,* named after a study by Robert Rosenthal and Lenore Jacobson, where they demonstrated that a teacher who expects success from specific students unconsciously contributes to bringing this about.[5] The explanation can be that these students received more attention from the teacher and were challenged more than the students from whom the same level of progress was not expected.

Can a society then also evolve in response to an expectation, even at a macro level, such as by evolving in the direction of the achievement society? There is reason to believe so, according to Robert Merton, the inventor of the concept of self-fulfilling prophecies. Merton's explanation is based on his predecessor W. I. Thomas' famous theory: "If people define situations as real, they become real in their consequences."[6] A self-fulfilling prophecy is at the outset a false definition of a situation, which triggers a new form of behaviour, which in the end makes the initially false concept true. The unique validity of the self-fulfilling prophecy entails that its advocates tend to cite the development as evidence that they were right from the start. Merton gives the reader the example of the fictive Last National Bank, which bank director Cartwright Millingville

Borum et al., "What can be done about school shootings? A review of the evidence" *Educational Researcher* 39, no. 1 (2010).

[4] Store norske leksikon, "Selvoppfyllende profeti" *Store norske leksikon* (2017), https://snl.no/selvoppfyllende_profeti

[5] Robert Rosenthal and Lenore Jacobson, "Pygmalion in the classroom" *The Urban Review* 3, no. 1 (1968).

[6] Robert K. Merton, "The self-fulfilling prophecy" *The Antioch Review* 8, no. 2 (1948).

manages to the best of his abilities.[7] His bank has a certain amount of cash reserves, but most of its assets are tied up in speculative ventures. One day a large number of customers come to Millingville's bank at the same time. Other customers witness this and begin to grow worried. False rumours begin to circulate about how the bank is on the verge of bankruptcy and even more customers rush to the bank to withdraw their money. At the start of the day, the bank was not insolvent, but due to the rumours which caused customers in great numbers to withdraw their money at the same time, the bank was bankrupt by the end of the day. Merton adds that self-fulfilling prophecies are unique to human situations, while in the natural world they are impossible. Predictions about the arrival date of Halley's Comet will have no impact on its trajectory, while rumours about Millingville's bank influenced the actual outcome. The prophecy of a collapse brought about its fulfilment.

We saw in the last chapter how an abundance of contemporary diagnoses now exist which often depict the development in the Western world in a negative sense, according to various versions of alienation, disenchantment and anomie. If we are to take a term such as *reflexive modernization* seriously, this must necessarily also involve an openness to the possibility that contemporary diagnoses in themselves are reflexive, and we must actively anticipate that they can also have unintended consequences. In this context, sociologist Torben Hviid Nielsen has pointed out that diagnoses of contemporary society are not the same thing as descriptions of society, in that the former often focus on developmental features that can be of significance in the future and latent tendencies that can become manifest realities.[8] As an example, he mentions the *liberation* from traditional roles and traditions which influential diagnosticians of contemporary culture such as Anthony Giddens, Ulrich Beck and Zygmunt Bauman describe in detail as characteristic of late modernity and which is most relevant for the globe's wealthiest one-fifth, who control more than four-fifths of the assets. For the remaining four-fifths of the population, this liberation functions only in the form of an aspiration for a better life.

[7] Ibid.

[8] Nielsen, "De 'frisatte'. Om individualisering og identitet i nyere samtidsdiagnoser".

But Nielsen's admonitions about how to handle the diagnoses of contemporary society go beyond acknowledging the limitations of their representativeness. Giddens', Beck's and Bauman's diagnoses of our times all emphasize how the modern individual is reflexive in his or her options and life project of creating an identity, in contrast to former times when the transmission of knowledge about how things were to be done took place more or less automatically. Nielsen adds however: "if individuals understand their own life challenges in the terms of the diagnoses of contemporary society, the diagnoses can therefore – in a kind of double reflexivity – both become a self-imposed burden and assume the character of a self-fulfilling prophecy."[9] Ergo: If young people internalize many of the current diagnoses of our society as part of their own self-perception and framework of expectations for how life is—such as Bauman's hypothesis that identity has progressed from being something given to becoming a task—this can further intensify the responsibility the individual assumes for their own destiny. The diagnoses of contemporary society can therefore appear to be self-fulfilling. Nielsen provides an example using the urbanist Richard Florida's influential term the *creative class*, which Florida himself estimated comprised around one-fourth of the workforce in a number of European nations, while studies have shown that more than half the workforce of the EU nations now perceive themselves as creative workers.[10] In Sweden as many as 82 percent of wage-earners see themselves as belonging to the creative class. And as Nielsen fittingly comments: the distance between expectations and opportunities and self-understanding and reality represents an impending danger of further increasing the vulnerability of the liberated. *The double reflexivity* of the diagnoses of contemporary society is also fruitful as a gateway to the subject of this book—the living conditions and self-understanding of young people.

In this chapter, I will illustrate this by addressing how key terms such as "the achievement society", "the achievement generation" and "the good girl syndrome" addressed in the previous chapter became incorporated into Norwegian discourse.

---

[9] Ibid., 180.

[10] Ibid.

The Problem Without a Name

To endeavour to identify a single source that has contributed to the "good girl syndrome" becoming a self-fulfilling prophecy is probably futile. It is more likely a matter of myriad sources that have played a part in giving the concept its current manifestation. But if I were nonetheless to focus on a suitable case, there is perhaps no more obvious candidate than the book *Too Good for Her Own Good* from 1990 by the two American family therapists Claudia Bepko and Jo-Ann Krestan.[11] This book, which has been published in Norway in Norwegian translation, has previously also been singled out by Harriet Bjerrum Nielsen as one possible source behind the introduction of the term "good girl" (*flink pike*) in Norway.[12] But as illustrated in the last chapter, the term actually has a long history predating this book's publication and only a modest 3000 copies of the Norwegian translation were printed.[13] However, the possibility that this self-help book contributed to facilitating the emergence of a new understanding of "the good girl" remains. A rereading of the book twenty-five years after it was published raises suspicions of this.

Viewed from the vantage point of the current day, where the "good girl" in the context of Norway is often spoken of as a syndrome, it is interesting to note how Bepko and Krestan give their approach legitimacy already in the preface to the book by using their clinical experience from the field of substance abuse. They perceive this as an effective approach that is also valid for other problems: "We discovered that our work with alcoholism could be applied to and used in all families."[14] The strict social codes imposed on women can allegedly lead to a type of dependency in which the woman accepts a restricted gender role as a means of living up to the expectations of others:

[11] Claudia Bepko and Jo-Ann Krestan, *Too good for her own good! Searching for self and intimacy in important relationships* (New York: Harper and Row, 1990).

[12] Mæland, "Slutt å bruk begrepet flink pike".

[13] Anne-Berit Tuft, "Flink pike! Så god at du ikke har godt av det [private conversation]" (2018, 8 March).

[14] Bepko, Claudia, and Jo-Ann Krestan. *Flink pike! Så god at du ikke har godt av det?* (Oslo: Cappelen Damm, 1993), 7.

> In the process of talking about women's 'goodness,' we try to provide a broader context for thinking about behavior that is currently referred to as codependent. We hope we have provided a perspective that suggests that codependency may be a form of being too good, but that not all 'good' behavior is necessarily codependent. Rather, it's adaptive, it's behavior we've been taught 'works' if you're a woman.[15]

Here Bepko and Krestan establish a connection between exaggerated goodness and a medical explanation called "codependency syndrome", which one must assume many readers will uncritically accept, given the authors' professional expertise in the field of substance abuse and the seductive explanatory element that lies in combining a set of experiences into a syndrome under the spell of which the reader, like many other women, apparently finds herself. The reader is clearly expected to chime in affirmatively, "Yes, that's how I feel!" in response to this inviting medical explanation.

The historical starting point for Bepko and Krestan appears to be that the woman's role is at a crossroads, as the modern woman is tugged back and forth between the self-sacrificing housewife role of the past and the career woman of the future. In this context, Bepko and Krestan draw from Betty Friedan's influential book *The Feminine Mystique* from 1963, upon which they bestow the honour of having inspired the revolutionary upheaval that has occurred in the lives of women. In her day, Friedan brought to light women's longing for the freedom to pursue their own dreams, unfettered by the social norms dictating what a good woman and housewife were permitted to do. Friedan gave the consciousness of such subjugation currency by referring to it as precisely "the problem that has no name".[16] Herein lies the very key to the future of the nation and culture, Friedan wrote. "We can no longer ignore that voice within woman that says: 'I want something more than my husband and my children and my home.'"[17] Ten years later, Bepko and Krestan's project becomes both to show how women remain trapped by "the problem that has no name", even though many women now work outside the home, and to help

---

[15] Ibid., 8.

[16] Ibid., 14.

[17] Betty Friedan, *The feminine mystique* (London: Penguin, 2010), 20.

women articulate this overwhelming feeling of responsibility. The Norwegian edition reads, "In American society a new term was coined in the 1980s for this feeling of responsibility experienced by women – codependency. In Norwegian, we can call it the dependency syndrome. In reality, the dependency syndrome is another term for Friedan's feminine mystique."[18] Bepko and Krestan then provide the requisite theoretical foundation for what amounts to objectification through reference to their own experience with their clients:

> As therapists who have specialized in working with addiction for most of our careers, we've seen the concept of codependency reach and help many women who feel trapped and even harmed by their goodness, whether or not they've been affected by addiction.[19]

The shift from "the problem that has no name" to "codependency" is an illustrative example of Moscovici's concept of objectification, since something vague has been converted into something more concrete. It also demonstrates Moscovici's concept of anchoring, in that Bepko and Krestan situate the problem without a name in a clinical medicine framework. The question is merely whether their readers can achieve the desired liberating effect, or if it instead becomes, paradoxically, yet another form of subjugation. It would appear that Bepko and Krestan were at least farsighted enough to anticipate the danger of a potentially negative outcome, in that by way of introduction they inform the reader that their intention is *not* to categorize or pathologize:

> Finally, we've been concerned not to 'label' women's experience in any way. We've given names only to processes and to principles; we've named ideas about change. It's been our intention to convey respect for the conflicts we all encounter as women without resorting to a need to categorize or pathologize us for having them.[20]

---

[18] Bepko and Krestan, Norwegian edition. My translation.

[19] Bepko and Krestan, *Too good for her own good! Searching for self and intimacy in important relationships*, 15.

[20] Ibid., 8.

Based on what we know now, it is natural to wonder whether Bepko and Krestan's medical label became something of a self-fulfilling prophecy in the decades that followed, though not primarily for middle-aged women living in the bondage of requirements to please their husbands and children, but rather for the many teenage girls and some boys in puberty striving to satisfy both their own and other's high expectations and aspiring to perform optimally in school, at sports or in the gym and on social media. The physicist James Clerk Maxwell is purported to have said that what seems abstract to one generation becomes concrete for the next.[21] Maxwell's "law" appears to correspond astonishingly well with the "good girl syndrome". The syndrome arose in Norway as a common semantic point of reference for women in their thirties in the 2000s, women who were struggling with the notorious time pressure and balancing act of managing home and work, having a career and being a housewife. For their teenage daughters in the 2010s, on the other hand, this became an internalized disorder, with real physiological and psychological symptoms. But where Friedan encouraged women to seize the day by rejecting limiting, oppressive gender roles, the transmission of "the problem that has no name" to the young girls of today half a century later is paradoxically reduced to a good girl syndrome, which is rather an expression of a latent anxiety on the part of women, an inkling that breaking away from the archetypal activities of the past, such as home, husband and children, can still have brutal repercussions. It is as if society is still ambivalent about women's possibilities for self-realization, but this concern finds expression in a clinical self-diagnosis. The feminist motto "the personal is political" is transposed to "the personal is medical". The prescribed solutions are therefore exclusively individual and therapeutic—mindfulness and life and stress management. The good girl syndrome is a pertinent example of an observation made by the American psychologist Dana Becker: "Whereas the women's movement explained women's problems as arising from their oppression, psychology transforms them into mental phenomena."[22] Women have perhaps gained their freedom, but it has

[21] Moscovici, "The phenomenon of social representations".

[22] Dana Becker, *The myth of empowerment: women and the therapeutic culture in America* (New York: New York University Press, 2005), 137.

come at the price of an increased risk of physiological and psychological health problems. This paradoxical history of women's struggle for liberation via "the problem that has no name" illustrates how the governments of advanced liberal democracies in the second half of the twentieth century at all times strove to encourage the autonomous individual to manage his or her life by way of psychological and medical techniques, such as the monitoring and regulating of own stress levels. The British sociologist Nikolas Rose has commented on how late modern societies grant the freedom to choose, but only if one submits to subjectification in the form of constant psychological self-evaluation.[23] The good girl syndrome can thereby be understood as a logical outcome of this development whereby the many burdens of women's and girls' self-realizations are placed on their own shoulders. Potential moral accusations for renouncing the designated care-giving role of women of former times have perhaps fallen by the wayside, but only to be replaced by an internalized psychological stress.

When the Meritocracy Came to Norway

The search engine of the Norwegian National Library offers the option to conduct archive searches for books predating Atekst Retriever's database for Norwegian newspapers. The Norwegian term for the achievement society (*prestasjonssamfunnet*) would appear to stem from the Norwegian translation of British sociologist and Labour politician Michael Young's book *The Rise of the Meritocracy* from 1958. This sociological satire is a futuristic story set in the year 2034, at which time the politicians of Great Britain have found themselves obliged to employ human resources in a more efficient fashion due to global competition. For this reason, all citizens with an IQ over 130 are sorted out and placed in the leading positions of society. In the chapter with the suggestive title "From Seniority to Merit" the Norwegian translation reads as follows: "Before the achievement society was fully established, the merit principle may have been

[23] Nikolas Rose, *Inventing our selves: psychology, power and personhood* (Cambridge: Cambridge University Press, 1996).

necessary to uphold stability after the system based on succession was phased out."[24] In the English original however, the term "meritocracy" is used. A *meritocracy* is a form of rule in which the decision-makers are chosen because of their abilities and skills rather than because they win an election as in a democracy. In the Norwegian edition, the term meritocracy is translated as "achievement society", a term related to a meritocracy, but which signifies more exclusively the existence of expectations of performance excellence. It is possible that the Norwegian term for achievement society was used in the translation because Norway has not traditionally had an aristocracy like Great Britain and the assumption was that the term "meritocracy" would not hold the same relevance in Norway. The Norwegian edition contains a specially written epilogue, titled "Norway – on the path to an achievement society?" by psychologist Torild Skard, who was also a deputy member of the Norwegian Parliament. Skard begins by declaring that Young's predictions are overly pessimistic but she also recognizes two developmental features in the Norwegian society of the mid-1960s which do indeed foreshadow the emergence of the achievement society: the technological development which makes society more complex and the economic competition which makes productivity and efficiency dominant cultural values.[25]

There are several things that are remarkable about the incorporation of the term "achievement society" in the public discourse of Norway. Young's book is universally accredited with having introduced the term meritocracy into everyday speech, but ironically he was disappointed about how his concept of "elite rule" and "achievement society"—which he conceived of as something negative—appeared to become goals worthy of pursuit. A year before he died, Young wrote the comment "Down with Meritocracy" which appeared in *The Guardian*, in which he criticizes Great Britain's education system which only allows for the advancement of the members of a small class and he asks prominent Labour politicians led by the then Prime Minister Tony Blair to stop using the word meritocracy in a positive sense in their speeches: "Much that I predicted has

[24] Michael Young, *Intelligensen som overklasse* (Oslo: Pax, 1966).

[25] Torild Skard, "Norge – på vei mot prestasjonssamfunnet?" in *Intelligensen som overklasse*, ed. Michael Young (Oslo: Pax, 1966).

already come about. It is highly unlikely the prime minister has read the book, but he has caught on to the word without realizing the dangers of what he is advocating."[26] "The meritocracy" arose in other words as a prophetic warning about the future, a prediction which its creator later maintained had come true to a large extent.

In Norway, the use of the Norwegian term for "achievement society" initially follows a similar pattern. Besides Skard, one year later another Socialist People's Party politician, Dag Seierstad, criticized the achievement society, also referring to Young's vision of the future. It is nonetheless evident how also Seierstad does his own part to adapt "the achievement society" to conditions in Norway by toning down Young's more explicit focus on the theme of eugenics.

> Young's nightmare vision is probably not especially realistic but the achievement society that Norway is in fact becoming is not much more heartening. It is not based as unambiguously on intelligence as in Young's vision, but it is at least based on career performance and a sharp pair of elbows. It is among other things based on an insane terror of not managing to compete – on the international market, with classmates or with whatever else might be relevant.[27]

Several educators also followed suit in the years that followed. In Reidar Myhre's *Innføring i pedagogikk* ("Introduction to Educational Science") he discusses the potential dangers of the education society through direct reference to the achievement society, where he advocates a view of human life and a concept of universal edification that also encompasses something more than intelligence, efficiency and productivity.[28] And in the educational pamphlet "The Folk High School" (*Folkehøgskolen*) by Stein Fossgard, one of the sections is entitled "The human being and the achievement society" (*Mennesket og prestasjonssamfunnet*).[29] Fossgard

---

[26] Michael Young, "Down with meritocracy" in *The Guardian* (2001), https://www.theguardian.com/politics/2001/jun/29/comment, paragraph 4.

[27] Dag Seierstad, "Sosialismen og utdanningssamfunnet" in *Ny radikalisme i Norge. 34 skribenter i samfunnsdebatten*, ed. Torild Skard (Oslo: Gyldendal, 1967), 175.

[28] Reidar Myhre, *Innføring i pedagogikk* (Oslo: Fabritius & Sønners Forlag, 1969).

[29] Stein Fossgard, *Folkehøgskolen* (Oslo: Norsk Korrespondanseskole, 1972).

also discusses Young's dystopian futuristic story about the year 2034 and considers the similarity to the Norwegian society of his day. "There are many signs indicating that in Norway we are in the process of sliding into the achievement society."[30] Fossgard highlights the tendency of many people with high IQs to apply for desk jobs and how the staffs of the most important institutions of society are made up of experts, those with a high school diploma and higher education and not primarily labourers and farmers. For the time being, intelligence is still more or less evenly distributed throughout society, but there is a risk that this may change if the school system unilaterally focuses on the cultivation of theoretical abilities. Should this occur, "there's a big risk that we will slide slowly but surely into the achievement society".[31] I won't comment upon whether or not we today truly live in an achievement society, but reading Fossgard's analysis in retrospect it comes across as relatively visionary, in light of debates of current interest about the theorization of the school and professionalization of politics. In an interview with the journal *Minerva*, Statistics Norway adviser Øyvin Kleven was recently quoted as follows:

> Previously, people used to enter politics by way of trade unions, organizations, the church and local associations and often they only had primary or lower secondary school educations. Today there are fewer 'ordinary people' in politics. Instead we are at risk of a professionalization of democracy. This may be a cause for concern.[32]

Already in the 1980s, the "achievement society" appears to have become an accepted diagnosis of Norwegian society that is a cause of concern for an increasing number of people and not only from the Left. The prominent theologian and Conservative Party politician Inge Lønning writes: "It is not without reason that our type of society – the highly civilized, Western society of affluence – is occasionally referred to as 'the achievement society.'"[33] Lønning asks if we are headed for a more ruthless society

---

[30] Ibid., 74.

[31] Ibid.

[32] Kristian Meisingset, "–Vi risikerer en profesjonalisering av demokratiet" *Minerva* (2017), https://www.minervanett.no/vi-risikerer-en-profesjonalisering-av-demokratiet/, paragraph 50.

[33] Øyvind Dahl et al., *Etikk* (Oslo: Universitetsforlaget, 1983), 65.

in which human worth is converted into something socially quantifiable, as effect and function considerations are becoming increasingly dominant. The uneasiness about the achievement society and its effects can also come from the Right wing—for understood by Lønning as a threat against protection of the fundamental human worth of children and the elderly, the intrinsic value of whom is at risk of devaluation if people are increasingly assessed on the basis of their performance value.

Apparently, it does not take long before the psychological concern about what the achievement society is doing to us surfaces. One of the chapters in the pedagogical booklet "A Study Guide for Psychology" (*Studiehefte i psykologi*) by Thomas Blaasvær is titled "Today's lifestyle poses a threat to our nerves" and is written as a conversation between the author and psychologist Halvor Lyngestad, who describes the times as follows: "Our values are characterized by a cut-throat materialism [...] Within our social structure it's all about excelling – achieving something continuously, without any particular consideration for the 'soft values'."[34] In one of the subsequent paragraphs, with the heading "The Achievement Society" the following comment is made:

> Key words signifying problems in today's society, which in and of themselves can both trigger and bring about nervous disorders, are stress, the rat race and the productivity mentality. To be accepted today, you must achieve something at all times, produce unceasingly, accomplish something in one way or another.[35]

In short the idea of "the achievement society" as a growing threat to ordinary mental health is far from recent and has been with us since long before its crystallization as "the achievement generation".

[34] Thomas Blaasvær, *Studiehefte i psykologi* (Oslo: Bedriftsøkonomens forlag, 1984), 36.
[35] Ibid., 37.

Finally Somebody Who Understands Us

As illustrated above, the history of the third label, the "achievement generation", is not as lengthy as the other two concepts. In the last chapter, we saw that the Norwegian term for the "achievement generation" (*generasjon prestasjon*) was used for the first time in Norway by Charlotte Lunde as recently as in 2011 in reference to the smart drugs trend, to be later introduced as a general description of youth culture. The journalist Marit Bromark, who has written about children and young people's living conditions for several years and given lectures under the auspices of the Cultural Rucksack programme, was responsible for a number of these early texts about televised children's competitions, among other topics. In 2014, she also wrote the comment: "Had I been young today I would have quit on the spot", through which she aspires to give adults insight into the average Norwegian school day, filled with national standardized tests, vocabulary quizzes and several hours of homework after school.[36] The daily lives of students are replete with all manner of assessments ranging from beep tests in gym class to performance tests in music. Likewise, parents scarcely allow their children any room to breathe: "It's just that everything counts. Absolutely everything is the most important thing [...] And being clever does not help. Because even if you do well, it's never good enough."[37] As far as teachers are concerned, they insist that it's important for young people not to wear themselves out, but simultaneously drone on about how important the next assignment is, Bromark continues. On top of it all a fifteen-year-old is named the Norwegian national football team's saviour, an eighteen-year-old crowned Norway's greatest singing talent and teenage girls are continuously confronted with advertisements featuring photoshopped, bony models. "And we still wonder why our young people are so stressed?"[38] Bromark concludes rhetorically, which is reminiscent of Jens Bjørneboe's pointing a finger of blame at adults in his poem "The Brutality of Youth" ("*Om ungdommens*

[36] Marit Bromark, "Hadde jeg vært ungdom ville jeg sagt opp på flekken" *klikk.no* (2014), http://www.klikk.no/foreldre/kommentarer/hadde-jeg-vaert-ungdom-ville-jeg-sagt-opp-pa-flekken-2488929

[37] Ibid., paragraph 28.

[38] Ibid., paragraph 40.

råskap") from half a century before.[39] Bromark clearly struck a nerve. "Had I been young I would have quit on the spot" became one of the most popular social media posts of 2014—read by more than 300,000 Norwegians and shared 45,000 times on Facebook, also by the affected but amazingly resourceful young people themselves.[40]

In 2014 some upper secondary schoolchildren from Ålesund joined forces to start the youth initiative *Generasjon Prestasjon* ("Achievement Generation") under the direction of the non-profit organization "Young Entrepreneurship" (*Ungt Entreprenørskap*) in Møre and Romsdal's programme for schoolchildren and were quickly commissioned to hold lectures and organize workshops throughout all of Norway. In the *NRK Ytring* feature article "From achievement to depression" penned by Håkon Avseth from the *Generasjon Prestasjon* initiative, he tells readers about the origins of the organization:

> One autumn day in a grammar school in Ålesund we started the youth enterprise *Generasjon Prestasjon*. Some of us had read a feature article entitled 'Had I been young I would have quit on the spot'. The article was concise but comprehensible. The author put into words a lot of what we were thinking and offered a kind of helping hand that differed from what we were accustomed to, miles away from a know-it-all academic approach. What if we, as young people, who are smack in the middle of this, could talk about it?[41]

The students behind the initiative also stated that they were inspired by Ungdata after reading the newspaper article about the living conditions of young people today which made reference to the Ungdata studies.[42] Although first employed by the adult generation, young people now use

[39] Jens Bjørneboe, "Om ungdommens råskap" in *En sangfugl i en snare gikk – Jens Bjørneboe i utvalg*, ed. André Bjerke (Oslo: Bokklubbens Lyrikkvenner, 1981).

[40] Egmont Publishing, "500.000 tenåringsforeldre har ventet på dette" (2015), https://www.ntbinfo.no/pressemelding/500000-tenaringsforeldre-har-ventet-pa-dette?publisherId=7154035&releaseId=7302117

[41] Håkon Avseth, "Fra prestasjon til depresjon" *NRK Ytring* (2015), https://www.nrk.no/ytring/fra-prestasjon-til-depresjon-1.12369440, paragraph 6.

[42] Halvard Dyb, "Skoleelever startet bedrift inspirert av Ungdata" (2015), http://www.hioa.no/Aktuelle-saker/Skoleelever-startet-bedrift-inspirert-av-Ungdata

the term "achievement generation" in their own self-depictions. The consolidation appears to be a done deal. And not just in newspaper articles. The youth enterprise *Generasjon Prestasjon* was in existence for a mere two years and in that time they managed to travel throughout the country far and wide, distributing information, holding lectures and organizing motivational workshops to "reverse a dangerous mental health development".[43] The young people involved received a lot of attention from the media both locally and nationally and a number of commendations for their efforts on behalf of the mental well-being of young people.[44] And it appears that their efforts have had widespread penetration. Their video "Wake Up" (*Våkn opp*) with the catchy slogan: "We are the achievement generation in a world of depression, of too little communication and a focus only on the telephone" which was posted in 2016, has been viewed more than 300,000 times.[45]

Despite the best of intentions, the question arises as to whether initiatives such as this, through a national tour and social media campaigns in which they encourage lower secondary school students to speak about how they are feeling, may have in fact fuelled the development instead of slowing it down. Avseth's description of the problem on *NRK Ytring* is based on the following definition of performance pressure: "Our definition of performance pressure is when you perform to the extent that you are no longer doing it for yourself, but to satisfy the standards of others."[46] Based on this operational starting point, the youth enterprise *Generasjon Prestasjon* has mapped out the widespread scope of the phenomenon among young people:

> In 2014 we did our own survey on the experience of an overwhelming pressure stemming from school and work, appearance and clothing, and in social settings. Around 300 young people aged thirteen to nineteen took part and the results corresponded with our expectations. 87, 75, and 75

[43] Avseth, "Fra prestasjon til depresjon".

[44] Dyb, "Skoleelever startet bedrift inspirert av Ungdata".

[45] Generasjon Prestasjon, "Våkn opp – En reklamefilm for Generasjon Prestasjon" (2016 https://www.youtube.com/watch?v=Eg-0KPfLkrA&t=2s)

[46] Avseth, "Fra prestasjon til depresjon".

percent, respectively, felt an overwhelming pressure in relation to the categories mentioned.[47]

If we are to take these dramatic results seriously, they imply that the problem of pressure for young people is not large; it is enormous. Feeling that one is under an overwhelming pressure has become quite simply normal. The high figures, however, do not come as much of a surprise, given the broad definition of performance pressure on which the survey was based. In this context, the many methodological objections that could be raised are perhaps neither of interest. Instead, it is worthwhile to dwell upon the young people's own understanding of performance pressure. A possible source of inspiration for the youth enterprise *Generasjon Prestasjon*'s definition of performance pressure would appear to be psychologists Edward Deci and Richard Ryan's influential *self-determination theory*, where the emphasis is on how one of the benefits of an intrinsic motivation is protection from stress,[48] while extrinsic motivation is more associated with negative stress. Deci and Ryan encourage parents, coaches, leaders and educators who are interested in inspiring motivation and emotional engagement to take note of this lesson.

The incidence of being extrinsically controlled and feeling pressure from one's surroundings has not only risen to unprecedented levels for the achievement generation but also become pathogenic. Therefore, it has been made a requirement that all motivation be intrinsic, stemming from our authentic selves. In previous generations, individuals could decide for themselves what they were going to be to a far lesser extent than today—people were restricted by the need to enter the workforce much sooner than today—and that was the case without there being much talk about pressure whatsoever. The focus was on one's duties. As such, the entire idea of being under pressure must be viewed as a relatively new invention, conceived in step with individualization and in accordance with the Canadian philosopher Charles Taylor's idea of *the ethics of authenticity*—wherein the foremost source of a life of value is to

[47] Ibid., paragraph 13.

[48] Richard M. Ryan and Edward L. Deci, "Self-determination theory and the facilitation of intrinsic motivation, social development, and well-being" *American Psychologist* 55, no. 1 (2000).

be found in one's own private subjectivity.[49] For that reason it has now also become a widespread requirement among young people in Norway that all activities, including time at school, are to exist primarily for your own sake. This requirement should not surprise anyone but is simply the logical extension of the ideal of self-determination and autonomy. Paraphrasing Bjørneboe we must therefore ask: For the life of you, can you comprehend how they have become so exacting in their demands?

Proceed with Caution

The histories of the terms outlined above are all about different versions of self-fulfilling prophecies and illustrate the complexity of the relationship between phenomenon and concept. In principle, critical diagnoses of the contemporary age ironically can contribute to escalating the very phenomenon about which a warning is being issued. A conservative lesson that might perhaps be extracted from this would be that the authorities, media and other stakeholders should exercise greater caution in discussions of such diagnoses and not merely in relation to cases of suicide. If you consider the current news landscape, however, there is little indication that the media is practising any exemplary "proceed with caution" awareness in relation to the risk of self-fulfilling prophecies.

Students Provide a Causal Explanation

The headline on the front page of *Aftenposten* 10 July 2017 read, "School-related pressure is the cause of mental health complaints" and was illustrated with a photograph of three sixteen-year-old girls.[50] Upon reading the full article inside the newspaper, however, it turns out that the phrase school-related pressure is primarily based on young people's own perceptions of a cause and effect correlation, whereby the school day full of homework, tests and assessments is identified as the most important

[49] Charles Taylor, *The ethics of authenticity* (Cambridge, MA: Harvard University Press, 1991).
[50] Aftenposten, "Skolepress er årsak til psykiske plager" *Aftenposten*, 10 July 2017, 1.

source of the experience of more stress and pressure than previously. The backdrop for this perception, highlighted on *Aftenposten*'s front page, is recent research from NOVA presented in the report "Stress and Pressure in Young People" (*Stress og press blant ungdom*). The report presents the results of group interviews with twenty-nine tenth grade students in the Oslo school system, based on both Sletten and Bakken's knowledge report cited here (see Chap. 5), which highlights school-related stress and pressure related to body image and analyses from the Young in Oslo (*Ung i Oslo*) study of 2015.[51] The article serves as an illustration of how research today is often subsumed into a media cycle in which a selected message—over which the researchers' themselves have no further control—is consolidated and disseminated via the internet and social media. In the *Aftenposten* article in question, in order to understand the headline, it is necessary to read the subheading which is in a much smaller font. "School-related pressure is the cause of mental health complaints" is in fact the young people's own explanation for how things are connected. The main headline is presented with no quotation marks. It is also a matter of mental health complaints and not psychological disorders, although the article does inform readers about this. The facts of the article can be accordingly summarized as follows: students in the Oslo school system have answered youth researchers' questions in focus groups and questionnaires about whether they feel that the pressure they experience at school plays a part in causing mental health complaints. The not wholly surprising conclusion of the school being to blame is blown far out of proportion on the front page of Norway's largest newspaper, where it is presented as a new scientific discovery. It's not a given that the average reader will pick up on the nuances of the issue presented and there is a clear danger of the article being understood by *Aftenposten*'s 250,000 subscribers as meaning that the Norwegian school system in its furious pursuit for results is now causing psychological disorders in young people. But the article is wholly in keeping with the spirit of the times, of which perhaps *Aftenposten* is the foremost media representative in Norway, where the voices of youth to the greatest possible degree are to be heard.

---

[51] Ingunn Marie Eriksen et al., "Stress og press blant unge. Report no. 6/17" (Oslo: NOVA, 2017); Sletten and Bakken, "Psykiske helseplager blant ungdom – tidstrender og samfunnsmessige forklaringer. Notat no. 4/16".

Identifying with the Research

Tuesday, 22 August 2017, the newspaper *Klassekampen* printed a related feature article also typical of the times: "Girls make themselves sick with stress". The lead-in is striking: "Seven out of ten upper secondary schoolgirls experience school-related stress. Increasingly more are on medication."[52] The basis for the article is also here new findings from the Ungdata study where schoolchildren from the entire country have been asked about how they are doing and for the first time students have been asked to answer the question of whether they have experienced school-related stress. In the latter category it is clear that especially girls struggle to meet the expectations imposed on them. Sixty-nine percent of the girls asked in upper secondary school say that they often or very often feel stressed about their schoolwork. For boys, the figure is 33 percent. Simultaneously, 20 percent of the girls in lower secondary school and 28 percent of the girls in upper secondary school respond that they experience a high level of depressive symptoms. This is twice as many as the boys and the highest percentage since studies of this nature began in 2010. The expert *Klassekampen* uses as a source, Marit Uthus, associate professor at the Department of Teacher Education at NTNU, holds that we must now ask the question of whether school constitutes a risk to the mental health of young people, especially with respect to the testing that has become increasingly prevalent in the schools since the introduction of the National Curriculum for Knowledge Promotion (*Kunnskapsløftet*) in 2006. In the article, Uthus receives the support of Maria Glørstad, who is attending her second year at the upper secondary Cathedral School in Trondheim, and Alida Donaas, who just graduated from upper secondary school. Both state that they can "identify with the research" in which the school is singled out as the foremost cause of pressure and stress in young people: "There's an assessment hysteria. When we have tests all the time, how you perform on them becomes more important than any other

[52] Jo Røed Skårderud, "Jentene stresser seg syke" *Klassekampen*, 22 August 2017.

kind of learning."[53] Here one can sense how the idea of the achievement society influences the critique, based as it is on how an instrumental performance assessment gets in the way of actual learning. It is noteworthy that *Klassekampen*'s article reports that there is an assessment hysteria in the schools, which is even said to constitute a health risk for young people, without any reflection whatsoever about the fact that Norwegian young people are also being subjected to an assessment hysteria on another front, specifically, from youth researchers who are constantly inquiring about how they are actually feeling. This is strange, given that the girls in the interview even claim bluntly that they can "identify with the research".

Talking About It

A third example from the summer of 2017 is found in the newspaper *Bergens Tidende*, featuring a photo of six smiling and presumably healthy teenage girls, although the headline reads: "Girls experience more anxiety than boys. *BT* asked six schoolchildren to talk about what is causing them stress in daily life."[54] The article is based on a recently completed survey of 1719 students at eighteen different lower secondary schools in Hordaland done by Uni Research Health. The results showed that 22 percent of lower secondary school pupils are anxious. And the chance of developing anxiety symptoms is five times greater for girls. What should be done? One of the researchers behind the study, psychology specialist Solfrid Raknes, recommends "putting thoughts and feelings on the agenda for all children as early as from the age of three-four years, so that children can learn to notice when they are feeling afraid and tell adults".[55] Further, she recommends that parents tell their children about their own feelings of dread and how they have trained themselves to cope with such

[53] Ibid., 7.

[54] Bergens Tidende, "Jenter engster seg mer enn gutter. BT lot seks skoleelever fortelle om hva som stresser dem i hverdagen" *Bergens Tidende*, 28 June 2017, 1.

[55] Hilde Heian, "-Stadig flere unge sliter med angstsymptomer" ibid., 11.

feelings. None of the six girls *BT* spoke with has taken part in the survey, but they are familiar with the issue. One of the girls, Ida Aarestrup Haugland, informs the reporter that stress is a frequent topic of discussion among young people, too: "We talk a lot about the good girl syndrome. Many girls are expected to excel in many ways and on more levels than before. Everyone feels the stress of daily life."[56] She speaks of how she will call a good friend on the rare occasion she might feel stressed before an end of term examination. And even if girls are the hardest hit, she believes it is harder for boys to open up about it.

Overall, what is striking about the entire issue is how all the involved parties describe versions of *talking about it*. Experts recommend making thoughts and feelings a compulsory part of the curriculum starting from kindergarten and the psychologist also recommends that all parents be open with their children about their own anxieties. One of the girls apparently has a good working strategy which involves talking to a close friend, but she implies that "the silent" boys could benefit from learning how to talk about it. And in general, *BT* gives all involved parties an opportunity to talk about it—that is even underscored in the headline: "*BT* asked six schoolchildren to talk about what is causing them stress in daily life."[57] The assumption would appear to be that talking about it at all levels will provide a much needed catharsis in bringing the difficult pressure or shame

young people are feeling to the surface and out into the open and thereby offering purification. This therapeutic idea has apparently materialized in the Norwegian public discourse as part of the vision of the newfound openness which exclusively applauds celebrities, bloggers and others who come forward to bare their souls by talking about their mental health complaints. It has become the solution that everyone can support: "We are obliged to start talking about it", to cite a related article about eating disorders.[58] In many cases, this prevailing mentality is presumably correct. In clinical psychology, it has been well documented that

---

[56] Ibid.

[57] Bergens Tidende, "Jenter engster seg mer enn gutter. BT lot seks skoleelever fortelle om hva som stresser dem i hverdagen" ibid.

[58] Vilde Linnea Bredesen, "Jeg veide for mye for å få behandling. Beskjeden forverret tilstanden min" *Aftenposten* (2018), https://www.aftenposten.no/meninger/sid/i/RxrwaW/Jeg-veide-for-mye-

talking about it can be effective, in that the intensity of painful thoughts and emotions is often mitigated by putting the latter into words and sharing them with a trusted companion. But this can also be turned around by pointing out that we have not done anything but talk about it in recent years. One question that comes to mind is therefore whether the effect of society's eagerness to talk about it has been just as much to intensify as to mitigate, a phenomenon by the way which we will see in the next chapter is absolutely nothing new, but which it appears we have to a large extent forgotten about.

Conclusion

Combined, these three newspaper articles illustrate how research today becomes subsumed in media cycles, the course of which can have significance in terms of how we talk and think about young people's mental health. *Aftenposten*'s front-page story demonstrates how causal connections are inflated into universal truths based on the findings of a research report, where in reality what has been investigated is Oslo young people's basic narratives about their dissatisfaction with school. The *Klassekampen* article illustrates the lack of self-reflection about assessments, while the *BT* article shows contemporary culture's unilateral belief in the importance of talking about it. Combined, the articles demonstrate how the Norwegian media behaves as if the phenomenon we are dealing with is comparable to Halley's comet, while one should in fact have treated it as if it were Millingville's bank.

---

for-a-fa-behandling-Beskjeden-forverret-tilstanden-min%2D%2DVilde-Linnea-Bredesen, paragraph 19.

8

The Paradox of Health

Precisely thirty years ago the American physician Anthony Barsky marvelled over what he would later christen *the health paradox*.[1] Although the health of the US population objectively speaking had never been better, the same population reported in purely subjective terms that they were less satisfied with their own health. Based on objective parameters, people have never enjoyed better health than today, measured as life expectancy for men and women. In 2015, life expectancy in Norway was 84 years for women and 80 years for men, while in 1846 it was 50 years for women and 46 years for men.[2] Despite such formidable progress Barsky alleged that we feel subjectively sicker than before.[3] The threshold and tolerance for minor illnesses and isolated symptoms has decreased. There is greater willingness to assume the *role of the sick person*. People are quicker to seek medical help for isolated symptoms, and people suffering from acute and chronic illnesses spend more days in bed than previously. Barsky grouped the incongruence between objective and subjective health

[1] Barsky, "The paradox of health".

[2] Norwegian Institute of Public Health, "Forventet levealder i Norge", (2017), https://www.fhi.no/nettpub/hin/befolkning/levealder/

[3] Barsky, "The paradox of health".

O. J. Madsen, *Deconstructing Scandinavia's "Achievement Generation"*,
https://doi.org/10.1007/978-3-030-72555-6_8

conditions in the population into four categories of causes: (1) first, medical advances have lowered mortality from acute infectious diseases, resulting in a corresponding increase in the incidence of chronic and degenerative ailments. (2) Second, society's increased health awareness has led to more self-monitoring and greater awareness of physical symptoms and signs of illness in the average man and woman. (3) Third, the widespread commercialization of health and increased focus on health problems in the media has led to a cultural climate fraught with fear, insecurity and anxiety about illness. (4) And fourth, the progressive medicalization of daily life has engendered unrealistic expectations of a healing cure, due to which untreatable illnesses and unavoidable ailments are experienced as being worse than before. The final "prescription" Barsky then writes, based on these insights on the paradox of health, is that doctors should be more aware in the future of these contradictory consequences of medical advances, so that they do not unintentionally contribute to the growing dissatisfaction with the medical sciences and to undermining the feeling of health and well-being in the population.

Thirty years after Barsky's discovery, there are few indications that doctors, psychologists or society in general have attributed any particular importance to the paradox of health. Instead, the attitude is that everyone will improve their health, both objectively and subjectively speaking, through greater focus on and awareness of public health. The problem appears to be eternally defined as a lack of information or openness about health. Ergo, we can never have enough. Despite this lack of understanding about health's interactive nature, it is important to emphasize that taking the insights from Barsky seriously absolutely does not imply that we should stop treatment or preventive measures, but that the latter should be offered on the basis of thoroughly considered evaluations and a heightened awareness of the dilemmas inherent to an increased focus. More openness makes it quite simply easier to be sick, in both the positive and negative sense. The Norwegian public, with the exception of the random dissident,[4] appears, however, to have decided that the only thing

[4] See, for example, Per Are Løkke, "Å gå seg vill i åpenheten", *Morgenbladet* (2017), https://morgenbladet.no/ideer/2017/10/gar-seg-vill-i-apenheten?utm_content=buffer2c9f1&utm_medium=social&utm_source=facebook.com&utm_campaign=buffer

that matters is the positive effect. The Swedish idea historian Karin Johannisson once commented on how it is virtually taboo today to speak about cultural or interactive explanations for mental health disorders.[5] This "ban" became evident when *the new openness*, which entails a lower threshold for publicly sharing one's own psychological disorders, was under debate and author Linnea Myhre in the newspaper *Morgenbladet* under the fitting title "Openness for All" vehemently debunked the entire discussion:

> Psychological illness in the public sphere is not contagious – not in and of itself. Nobody chooses to have a psychological disorder and I doubt anyone can be bothered to pretend they have anxiety, bulimia or depression in the long run, neither for the sake of attention or with an eye to becoming a role model. There's nothing trendy about being sick.[6]

Myhre's depiction of the position of her opponents—purportedly claiming that psychological disorders are actively chosen by some, who are in fact simulating, motivated either by the need for attention or to jump on the bandwagon—is illustrative of how the understanding of contagion is underdeveloped in the public discourse. Mira Aaboen Sletten who works with mental health issues at Ungdata expresses a closely related view, going to great lengths to disprove the possibility that the influence of the media can play a part in the increase in reporting of mental health ailments: "At any rate it's strange if those who work with it locally don't see it if it is only a matter of young people who are especially sensitive or who are whiners."[7] With these kinds of mental models, all evidence that "infection" can actually occur becomes synonymous with monstrous accusations that mentally ill individuals have chosen the illness themselves or are just overly sensitive. And consequently, all inducements to further analysis and debate about the interactive nature of psychological

---

[5] Karin Johannisson, "Om begreppet kultursjukdom", *Läkartidningen* 105, nr. 44 (2008), 3131–32.

[6] Linnea Myhre, "Åpenhet for alle", (2017), https://morgenbladet.no/ideer/2017/11/myhre-apenhet-alle, paragraph 8.

[7] Arne Olav Hageberg, "Ein generasjon av stressa jenter", *Tidsskrift for Norsk psykologforening* 51, nr. 11 (2014), 963.

disorders are prematurely shut down because nobody wants to be viewed as inhuman, particularly in relation to those suffering from mental illness.

Cultural Oblivion

It is common knowledge that mental health disorders can be caused by genetic, biochemical and psychological or social factors and usually a combination of several such factors will be in evidence.[8] Although everything from the brain to social structures can be relevant to an understanding of psychological disorders, it still seems that we easily forget wholly fundamental insights from humanism and cultural psychology about what it means to be a human being when we speak about psychological disorders. This is possibly based on an erroneous conclusion that these disorders involve something unique and are thereby extraneous to the basic existential make-up of human beings, as if the fundamental logic of psychological disorders adheres exclusively to the laws of biological psychology and the medical and the natural sciences. These explanations are of course also relevant, but the type of true-false or nature-culture distinctions that we often employ in our understanding of psychological disorders are poorly suited for preserving their complexity, which involves everything from a synapse to society.[9]

In the book *Being Human* science historian Roger Smith poses the wholly fundamental question "What is human nature?"[10] But the answer to the question, Smith writes, is not to be found in nature but in culture. Human nature is not a thing waiting to be discovered but is instead always active in the work of understanding itself. In sum, humans are incomplete beings who can only complete themselves by way of culture. If there is nonetheless something such as biological universals that hold true for all human beings, it is not possible to describe this basic potential independently of its expression through specific forms of culture, Smith

[8] Malt, Retterstøl, and Dahl, *Lærebok i psykiatri (2nd edition)*.

[9] Ole Jacob Madsen, "Hinsides sant eller falskt: En undersøkelse av Ian Hackings teori om mentale lidelsers sosiale dynamikk", *Tidsskrift for Norsk psykologforening* 51, no. 9 (2014).

[10] Roger Smith, *Being human: historical knowledge and the creation of human nature* (New York: Columbia University Press, 2007).

emphasizes. The basic potential is encapsulated in the way we live; it never exists independently of lived life. Smith cites the anthropologist Clifford Geertz's statement about how "there is no such thing as a human nature independent of culture".[11] Based on this, some will perhaps categorize these theorists as radical social constructivists who deny human beings' biological nature. But they are not denying the significance of nature. Smith's basic point is simply that for the impulses of the body and the brain to be meaningful for us in any sense, we must carry out continuous interpretation, through which we put these signals into a semantic context, which we can then communicate about with our surroundings. And to do this we need culture in the form of language, images and mental models. Humans are quite simply interpretive animals, including when they are suffering.

If we relate this to Barsky, it simultaneously implies that if the culture in which we are living has a heightened focus on illness, this will make us more sensitive to signals sent by the body, more likely to interpret those signals according to illness categories and more inclined to seek professional help. And should one hear often that one is living under particularly difficult social conditions, conditions that are making many people sick, the immediate response would presumably tend to be the projection of problems and setbacks into such a potentially illness-inducing interpretive framework. This holds true especially for psychological modes of expression, as Nikolas Rose has previously pointed out: "When our culture provides us with life narratives couched in psychological terms, our lives really do become psychological in their design."[12]

Scientific Myths

This also entails that we must view psychological terms such as "stress", "anxiety" and "depression" both as collective terms for disorders that can be useful in a clinical treatment setting and as meaningful myths that

[11] Ibid., 35.

[12] Nikolas Rose, *Governing the soul: the shaping of the private self (2nd edition)* (London: Free Association Books, 1999), xviii.

human beings employ to understand their lives, with respect to both inner and outer influences. As implied above, however, we have an unfortunate tendency to think that the former precludes the latter. But even though myths have an archaic origin, this does not make them less true for human beings of today. Science does not repress the myths; it permeates them.

The American sociologist John Hewitt in the book *The Myth of Self-esteem* establishes a myth perspective for the term self-esteem, which since the early 1980s has experienced a phenomenal dissemination first in the USA and then in the rest of the Western world, to a large extent thanks to the way psychology and sociology have embraced it as a perspective.[13] The discourse about self-esteem is often buttressed by myth-like narratives about people who have cured themselves of all manner of addictions. *You Can Heal Your Life* is even the title of Louise Hay's popular self-help book, which, with 50 million sold copies, is one of the bestselling books in the world regardless of genre.[14] In such modern epic narratives, it is the belief in the infinite opportunities of the individual that is valued.

Every culture contains a set of beliefs about human nature, often called the folk psychology of a given culture. The US folk psychology has in recent decades been heavily influenced by the social sciences and by psychology in particular. What this implies is that Americans will tend to turn to psychological theories and research that can shed light on the meaning of human nature, our thoughts, feelings and actions. Hewitt gives an example of this through the story of an imagined bus accident that causes the tragic death of several students, in response to which the school administration calls in a crisis psychologist to offer the students therapy. Or when the US is faced with a drug epidemic, theories from psychology will be consulted in the search for a solution.

As a consequence of this world view, other myths such as *The Book of Job* from the Old Testament also become less credible, in contrast to myths that insist on the individual's possibilities for overcoming adversity and in the end emerging victorious over addiction, poverty or other

[13] John P. Hewitt, *The myth of self-esteem* (New York: St. Martin's Press, 1998).
[14] Louise Hay, *You can heal your life* (Carlsbad, CA: Hay House, 1984).

unfortunate circumstances. *The Book of Job* has meaning only in the presence of a folk psychology emphasizing human beings' submission to God. The function of myths is also to justify the social reality. The function of *The Book of Job* was to defend religious faith in meeting with adversity. Those who experienced adversity or distress were encouraged to accept their lot in life as God's will and submit instead of struggling against the circumstances. This type of belief system is naturally well suited for those who already benefit from the way society's resources are distributed. Psychological myths also justify the social reality by attributing the problems to the individual instead of the surrounding society. The belief that the individual can improve their lot in life by improving their self-esteem is a doctrine that celebrates the idea of the individual's infinite possibilities. On the one hand, the individual is attributed with formidable power to alter his or her fate, but, on the other hand, the myth of self-esteem entails that the individual is burdened with an enormous responsibility. It is the individual alone who is held responsible for his or her situation. The potential role the surrounding society can play is left out of this psychological mythology, Hewitt specifies.

British Resistance

The mythology Hewitt observed around him has also been demonstrated in other parts of the Western world and often goes by the name of *therapeutic cultures*, in which psychology serves as a unifying myth or system of meaning along the lines of a secular religion and where the diagnosis and illness categories play a not insignificant part, particularly in the lives of young people. In *Therapy Culture: Cultivating Vulnerability in an Uncertain Age*, British sociologist Frank Furedi explains the dialectic relation between the illness narratives communicated through the therapeutic culture and the impact of these on people.[15] Not only do the illness narratives provide a framework for how people are expected to feel and experience a problem, they also constitute an invitation to physical and

[15] Frank Furedi, *Therapy culture: cultivating vulnerability in an uncertain age* (London: Routledge, 2004).

psychological impotence, Furedi claims. As an example he mentions the growing problem of exhausted children in Great Britain and affiliated expert statements: "If you had asked eight-year-olds about stress 20 years ago, they would have looked blank, now they understand the concept and a significant number report experiencing it."[16] Here Furedi highlights how the fact that today's eight-year-olds understand stress in a manner unlike that of previous generations attests to the considerable influence psychology and the therapeutic ethos have had. With time, young people are beginning to give their experiences meaning through the psychological filter. They are thereby served a cultural recipe stipulating that difficult experiences are the source of an illness for which there is help to be found. In principle, people have no inner need to identify as sick, but the dominant cultural signals now offer a divine leadership that can give such burdens meaning. This continual analysis of human emotions as problematic leads sooner or later to the recycling of illness, Furedi warns. And as soon as painful responses become culturally validated as illnesses, they will eventually feel that way as well.

It can appear as if Furedi's warning to the authorities had a limited impact, in that one decade later, several others have pointed out the exact same problem. The British psychiatrist Anthony Daniels, who writes under the pseudonym Theodore Dalrymple, has commented on how reports from researchers on the incidence of psychological disorders in the population in and of themselves can contribute to producing the very phenomena in question. Dalrymple refers to the above-mentioned Werther effect and quotes the French seventeenth-century philosopher Blaise Pascal's statement about how man is a thinking reed, the most fragile in all of nature, but nonetheless full of self-awareness. On the basis of this insight, it is a mistake to treat the increasing prevalence of psychological disorders as a natural, straightforward fact, comparable to the incidence of hypothyroidism—an underactive thyroid gland—Dalrymple comments, since the risk of imitation must also be factored into the equation:

[16] Ibid., 112.

> No statement that a psychological disturbance has such and such a prevalence in such and such a population should be taken at face value, especially when it is a plea, as it often is, explicit or implicit as the case may be, for more resources to treat it, the supposed prevalence having risen shockingly in the last few years.[17]

As Dalrymple demonstrates, the problem is not merely that you will find what you are looking for, but that you will actually trigger what you are looking for. The British liberal thinker Claire Fox argues as well that the way adults discuss their worries infects their children, affecting how their offspring respond to problems in life. When children all the way down to the age of five report feeling "stressed", "anxious" or speak about "their well-being" do we believe they have learned this vocabulary on the playground? Fox asks rhetorically. Her explanation is that they have absorbed this from adults' therapeutic speech patterns and have been encouraged from an early age, by a host of professionals, to view themselves as emotionally vulnerable beings. But the constant flow of initiatives intended to help children handle stress, can quickly become self-fulfilling:

> So when the 'Preventing anxiety in Children through Education in Schools' programme holds lessons in cognitive behavioural therapy (CBT) for children in primary schools, I fear this will encourage children to be self-obsessive about their own interior emotional life, which they will inevitably verbalise as soon as one of the army of opinion poll surveyors asks them 'How do you feel?'[18]

How Does Infection Occur?

A culture can also be the carrier of infection, in addition to being a vital resource. But if one accepts the premise that human beings are *interactive types*,[19] who interact with classifications, research and public health mea-

---

[17] Theodore Dalrymple, *Admirable evasions: how psychology undermines morality* (New York: Encounter Books, 2015), 46.

[18] Claire Fox, *'I find that offensive!'* (London: Biteback, 2016), 77.

[19] Ian Hacking, *The social construction of what?* (Cambridge, MA: Harvard University Press, 1999).

sures, how does this occur? We already know that human phenomena such as terrorism, disablement, obesity and pain threshold are all potentially contagious when transmitted through the media, family association or social networks.[20] So why should psychological disorders be any different, however much they are not "in and of themselves" contagious, as Myhre reminds us. Strictly speaking, it is difficult to envision something being infectious in its own right. Even basic organisms such as bacteria and viruses need a drop of fluid, a door handle or a human being to transport them. Psychological disorders presuppose a certain degree of receptivity in the afflicted party. Here psychological disorders, on the one hand, and bacteria and viruses, on the other, go their separate ways with respect to infection, in that the latter exercise little of this unique form of consideration.

One of the most sophisticated approaches to the contagiousness of psychological disorders has been developed by the Canadian philosopher of science Ian Hacking through meticulous historical studies of the spread of dissociative fugue in France and parts of Italy, Germany and Russia in the late nineteenth century and multiple personality disorder in the USA in the late twentieth century.[21] Hacking, however, is not unaware of the rub-off effect in the regions of Scandinavia. In 2009, he was awarded the Holberg Prize by H.R.M. Crown Princess Mette-Marit in Håkonshallen in Bergen and surprised everyone with his knowledge of the Scandinavian cultural heritage when in his homage to human curiosity he paraphrased the Swedish soft-porn classic *I Am Curious (Yellow) (Jäg er nyficken – gul)* and *I Am Curious (Blue) (Jäg er nyficken – blå)*.[22] Hacking has otherwise worked with historical case material from Sweden of a completely differ-

[20] Nicholas A. Christakis and James H. Fowler "The spread of obesity in a large social network over 32 years", *New England Journal of Medicine* 357, no. 4 (2007); Gordon B. Dahl, Andreas Ravndal Kostøl, and Magne Mogstad, "Family welfare cultures", *The Quarterly Journal of Economics* 129, nr. 4 (2014); Michael Jetter, "The effect of media attention on terrorism", *Journal of Public Economics* 153 (2017); Solveig Engebretsen et al., "The peer effect on pain tolerance", *Scandinavian Journal of Pain* 18, no. 3 (2018).

[21] Ian Hacking, *Rewriting the soul: multiple personality and the sciences of memory* (Princeton, NJ: Princeton University Press, 1995); *Mad travelers: reflections on the reality of transient mental illnesses* (Cambridge, MA: Harvard University Press, 1998).

[22] "Deres Kongelige Høyhet Kronprinsesse Mette-Marit, statsråd, Deres Eksellense, Ludvig Holbergs minnefond og gjester", in *Prisseremoni Holbergs internasjonale minnepris og Nils Klim-prisen 25. november 2009*, ed. Holbergprisen (2009), 7.

ent nature and of greater relevance to the issue at hand. In the period between 2001 and 2007, there was an epidemic of *resignation syndrome* in children of asylum-seekers in Sweden. Initially the symptoms consisted of withdrawal from all types of social life and school refusal, but eventually the children also stopped interacting with their own families. And in the most serious cases, they stopped talking altogether, stopped moving and eating, so they had to be fed intravenously. Some of the children ended up in a mild coma. The afflicted children were all from Romani families, primarily from Kosovo and some from Serbia or former Soviet republics with a Muslim majority population such as Kazakhstan, Kirgizstan, Azerbaijan and Armenia. Usually it was the oldest child in the family who was afflicted and the victims were both girls and boys. Their families were seeking asylum in Sweden, but in half of the known cases the children fell ill before the application for asylum was submitted. Hacking, who by chance was a guest lecturer in Uppsala in the autumn of 2006, was consulted in conjunction with the epidemic due to his theory on *transitory mental disorders* and in 2010 he gave his final assessment after the controversy provoked by inflammatory issue had calmed down.[23]

Apparently, the epidemic was limited to Sweden. There is allegedly evidence of a similar disorder in Australia, but it was only in Sweden that it acquired epidemic proportions and only there was it publicized, becoming a source of national concern. When the issue became public knowledge in Sweden, not surprisingly clear positions for and against were generated, based on the above-mentioned true-false and nature-culture paradigms. There was a clear tendency for the Left to view the disorders afflicting the children as real, physical symptoms caused by the way the asylum process mistreated refugee families. The Right, on the other hand, had a predilection for viewing the children's illness as simulated or it was implied that their parents had drugged them, as a strategy to ensure being granted residency in Sweden. This division also found expression among the experts who were consulted. Child psychologist Marie Hessle was appointed national coordinator for children in the asylum-seeking process who were suffering from resignation syndrome and together with

[23] "Pathological withdrawal of refugee children seeking asylum in Sweden", *Studies in History and Philosophy of Biological and Biomedical Sciences* 41, no. 309–317 (2010).

head of research Nader Ahmadi they reached the conclusion that it was not a question of an actual syndrome, while an alternative report written by Dr. Göran Bodegård from the Karolinska Institute and the organization Save the Children emphasized that the cases must be considered from a medical trauma perspective. Hacking was invited to step into a minefield, to put it mildly. Hacking, who in previous works has overtly expressed his dislike of true-false questions and answers about psychological disorders, gives however, not surprisingly, a satisfactory explanation consistent with both alternatives.[24]

Hacking calls the conceptual model he establishes *the imitation and internalization model*, requesting a stronger emphasis on the latter, even though both processes are essential to an understanding of what could have taken place. The model is based on the term *learned helplessness* developed by the psychologist Martin Seligman in the 1960s, through studies of animals in which dogs were given electric shocks and it was observed that the dogs could respond with apathy and become incapable of avoiding shock-carrying stimuli also when this was possible.[25] Learned helplessness has since been explored further in the works of the paediatrician Bryan Lask, who describes young girls who won't eat, drink, walk, speak or take care of themselves, as if they are overcome by a feeling of hopelessness for a period of several months, which he called *pervasive refusal syndrome*. Hacking also credits psychiatry historian André LeBlanc for his idea, in that LeBlanc established connections between hypnosis, the placebo effect and the multiple personality disorder epidemic in the USA in the 1980s and submission to religious faith, which Pascal in his day recommended. Pascal's famous *wager argument* entailed accepting the existence of God in order to secure future salvation, even though one couldn't know for certain whether it was true: "If you win, you win everything, if you lose, you lose nothing. Do not hesitate then; wager that He does exist."[26] Hacking stresses that even though you can't just decide to believe, you can decide to behave in a manner which will eventually cause

[24] *Rewriting the soul: multiple personality and the sciences of memory*; *Mad travelers: reflections on the reality of transient mental illnesses*.

[25] Martin E. P. Seligman and Steven F. Maier, "Failure to escape traumatic shock", *Journal of Experimental Psychology* 74 (1967).

[26] Blaise Pascal, "Veddemålet", in *Pascal*, ed. Francois Mauriac (Oslo: Gyldendal, 1954), 92.

you to believe: by naively and slavishly imitating the practice of believers, taking the sacrament regularly and interacting with God-fearing people. Then you will in a purely psychological sense usually end up sincerely believing. What started as a performance ends up becoming a deeply rooted psychological state.[27] LeBlanc's studies of hypnotized subjects who typically report that they just follow instructions obediently and are wholly conscious, that at any time they can choose to defy the instructions to hold their arms at their sides, but in the end actually end up fully hypnotized, convinced LeBlanc of Pascal's foresight. The psychological anthropologist Tanya Luhrmann in a subsequent study of American Evangelical Christians, *When God Talks Back*, has also demonstrated that believing in God is something that must be learned, in the sense that Christians learn to be attentive to their own inner mental and emotional life to find proof of God's existence, which changes the experience of their inner lives and finally culminates with the believers experiencing a true, external, interactive and living spiritual presence.[28]

How did the children then end up with a pathological disability? Hacking's explanation is based on the fact that the above-mentioned Bodegård appeared on Swedish television during prime time programming when the first known cases occurred and he told television viewers that it was a matter of a life-threatening disease afflicting children seeking asylum.[29] Many of the asylum-seekers didn't speak Swedish, but due to strong informal networks between asylum-seekers in Sweden (allegedly all Romani people in Southwest Sweden know one another), information about the issue nonetheless became common knowledge among these groups through word of mouth. Hacking claims that imitation thereby occurred when the eldest child of the families in question took responsibility for the situation by copying the already known cases of resignation behaviour. He concedes that this can sound simple but reminds us that these Romani families were under extreme pressure in their situation and the children found a solution which through imitation and

[27] Hacking, "Pathological withdrawal of refugee children seeking asylum in Sweden", 316.

[28] Tanya M. Luhrmann, *When God talks back* (New York: Vintage Books, 2012).

[29] Hacking, "Pathological withdrawal of refugee children seeking asylum in Sweden".

internalization eventually became a painful reality over which they lost control as it evolved.

The national coordinator's report concluded with four critical questions to which Hacking held he could provide more or less valid answers:

1. Why did the problem manifest itself precisely at the beginning of the 2000s?
   Answer: A complete coincidence. The incidence of one or more children with long-term resignation syndrome was not possible to predict but neither was it surprising given the families' situation.
2. Why was there such a high incidence in Sweden after 2002?
   Answer: The snowball effect. The children began imitating and it became an accepted form of behaviour.
3. Why is the case unique to Sweden?
   Answer: It was a coincidence that the first cases occurred in Sweden; their dissemination occurred with the help of the media. Since neighbouring countries such as Norway and Denmark did not learn about the cases, there was nothing for others to copy.
4. Why did it afflict only children from a specific geographic region?
   Answer: Presumably because in this region there is a strong tradition of personal identity formation within the family and the children are expected to assume responsibility for the family at a relatively young age.[30]

By way of conclusion Hacking acknowledges that his explanation can perhaps seem unappealing for many of those who viewed the syndrome as real clinical cases, but he reminds us that the imitation and internalization model is still consistent with the trauma perspective. From the point of view of the authorities, who must act, it is possible to argue that both granting and denying a residence permit would remove the stressor for both the children and the families. But for the families who were granted residency, it nonetheless appears that several of the troublesome symptoms are still with them, in that internalization does not so easily release its grasp. Again and again it would seem that we need to be reminded of self-fulfilling prophecies' reality-producing consequences: "If people define situations as real, they become real in their consequences."

---

[30] Ibid.

The Illness Epidemic in Sweden

If we try to apply Hacking's imitation and internalization model to the public discourse on mental health and young people in Norway, the media attention is undoubtedly key, given the significant and repetitive exposure of recent years via social media, newspaper articles, television documentaries, films, research reports and workshops in the schools, feature articles, debates in the news and so on. At the same time, any pressure on Norwegian children to assume the role of a sick child, in the manner of the refugee children, is less apparent. But if we accept the premise that adolescence, as a transition from childhood to adulthood, is characterized by uncertainty and anxiety about working out one's identity, finding one's place and making a number of choices related to education, home, work, partner and children, then it's easy to understand that this transition can be experienced as a strain. Growing up in a country such as Norway in the 2010s also entails having every opportunity within reach. The institutional basis for having high personal ambitions is decidedly in place. And at the other end of the spectrum, the language for failure or experiencing adversity is permeated with a medical and psychological diagnostic mentality. It is therefore not so inconceivable that the available explanations in circulation in some cases can appear to be relevant categorizations in relation to life challenges, making it feasible that imitation and internalization will sometimes occur.

But Myhre is still right when he claims that infection does not happen all by itself. Hacking's model does not explain *why* some individuals become sick and others do not. As has been pointed out previously by others, even Hacking's model is lacking a participant.[31] So we must continue to abide by the individual vulnerability model in addition to Hacking's cultural approach to transitory mental disorders to even begin to approach the complexity of how psychological disorders can also be contagious. It is worthwhile recalling that Hacking in all his works detests either/or responses, including the question of whether certain illness epidemics are real or not: "What do *I* think?? Is it real or is it not? I am not

[31] Serife Tekin, "The missing self in Hacking's looping effects", in *Mental kinds and natural kinds*, eds. H. Kincaid and J. Sullivan (Cambridge, MA: MIT Press, 2014).

going to answer that question. I hope that no one who reads this book will end up wanting to ask exactly that question."[32] Hacking here highlights the point that to be able to even ask the question "Is it real N?" one must always include a noun, which in this case will be an *illness* or a *disorder*.[33] And even if we avoid the first category of errors, there's absolutely no guarantee that we will then receive a satisfactory answer: "A true or real disorder as opposed to *what*?", Hacking asks rhetorically.[34] To be able to answer we must know what a true or real psychological disorder is and that is far from straightforward.

What Hacking wants to show us instead is how a number of different psychological disorders arise and develop through an extremely complex interaction between human sciences such as medicine and psychology, and statistics and psychometrics and patients. The illness behaves in keeping with the classifications and the classifications change according to the behaviour of the illness. In this dynamic interaction, actors such as the media, the public authorities, interest organizations, technology and language are also involved. And in the midst of this fragmented landscape we find human patterns of disorders and illness experiences which to the greatest extent are real enough for the individuals in question, but the response pattern also fluctuates in step with scientific advances, technological innovations and the development of society. In other words, psychological disorders correspond with their own, unpredictable social dynamic beyond the realm of true or false, but at the same time with enough predictability to require us to factor in the researcher and research as always already being participants.

Reaping as We Sow

Hacking has also written about the interactive nature of research. When towards the end of the nineteenth century the authorities in Europe began taking an interest in suicide in the population, this led to an

[32] Hacking, *Rewriting the soul: multiple personality and the sciences of memory*, 16.

[33] Ibid., 11.

[34] Ibid.

increase in the number of suicide candidates who left a suicide note, as a final form of documentation for the state's statistic supervisors.[35] It was possibly motivated by a wish to be seen, even in the afterlife. This is not to say that people took their own lives so the state's statisticians would have figures for their reports; the personal motives were already in place, but the awareness of this investigatory practice had an impact on pre-suicide behaviour. And if we return to the recent youth research studies done in Norway, there are several methodological factors that merit further elucidation. A large segment of the surveys documenting the incidence of mental health complaints in young people is based on questionnaires. One of the most comprehensive and well known of these is presumably the Ungdata surveys of the Norwegian Social Research Institute NOVA at Oslo Metropolitan University, which are funded by the Norwegian Directorate of Health through an annual grant allocated via the government's fiscal budget. Since start-up in 2010, 665,000 lower secondary school students throughout Norway have been asked to indicate the degree to which they have experienced symptom descriptions such as "feeling that everything is hard work", "difficulties sleeping", "feelings of unhappiness, sadness or being depressed", "feelings of hopelessness about the future", "feeling stiff or tense" and "worrying about things a lot" by checking off "Not at all", "Very little", "Quite often" or "A great deal". The use of questionnaires for such purposes entails a number of well-documented challenges. In a scientific article in the *Canadian Medical Association Journal* from 2018, a warning is issued about the increasingly widespread use of self-reporting questionnaires to measure the prevalence of depression in the population as opposed to clinical interviews requiring greater resources, since the risk of overestimation is considerable.[36] Researchers refer to a number of studies in which both approaches have been used: in a study of medical school students using self-reporting questionnaires, 27 percent of the informants reported experiencing depression, while when clinical interviews were used, the result was only 9 percent. Similarly, in a study of patients who had under-

[35] "The looping effects of human kinds", in *Causal cognition: a multi-disciplinary debate*, eds. D. Sperber, D. Premack, and A. J. Premack (New York: Oxford University Press, 1995).

[36] Brett D. Thombs et al., "Addressing overestimation of the prevalence of depression based on self-report screening questionnaires", *Canadian Medical Association Journal* 190, no. 2 (2018).

gone obesity treatment surgery, self-reporting questionnaires showed that 19 percent reported struggling with depression, but when diagnostic interviews were employed, the incidence was found to be 7–8 percent.

"Are public opinion polls self-fulfilling prophecies?" David Rothschild and Neil Malhotra asked a couple of years ago.[37] The question stems from a study of the so-called bandwagon effect from psychology, which refers to the phenomenon of how human beings will do something simply because other people are doing it, regardless of what their own opinions might be, sometimes even flying in the face of these. The Polish social psychologist Solomon Asch demonstrated this phenomenon in his classic conformity study conducted in 1956, in which he disclosed how subjects of an experiment adapt with an uncanny swiftness to the majority's erroneous assessment of which line is the longest.[38] To find an answer to the question of whether public opinion polls can become self-fulfilling prophecies, Rothschild and Malhotra designed a trial in which they asked participants to state their support for three political proposals: reduce US troops in Afghanistan, free trade agreements and public funding of elections. The informants were first asked their opinion and, in the next round, were informed of the opinion of the majority and were subsequently again asked for their opinion.

Rothschild and Malhotra found three key social psychological mechanisms that can cause polls to produce conformity:

1. *Normative social influence.* People want to adapt to the preferences of the majority so they can feel that they are liked or are a member of the winning team,
2. *Informative social influence.* People believe others' interpretation of an unclear situation is more precise than their own and adapt to this.
3. *Cognitive dissonance.* People will change sides, joining the side they believe will win based on the opinion polls.[39]

---

[37] David Rothschild and Neil Malhotra, "Are public opinion polls self-fulfilling prophecies?", *Research & Politics* 1, no. 2 (2014).

[38] Solomon E. Asch, "Studies of independence and conformity: I. A minority of one against a unanimous majority", *Psychological Monographs: General and Applied* 70, no. 9 (1956).

[39] Rothschild and Malhotra, "Are public opinion polls self-fulfilling prophecies?".

The bandwagon effect is primarily used to explain voting behaviour, but it is not inconceivable that the processes in question can also be applicable to how informants in the Ungdata survey respond to questions about whether they worry too much or whether everything is hard work. Here it will not be the majority's opinion on political issues that will be the determining factor, but instead how they believe other young people whom they identify with will answer the same question. Rothschild and Malhotra find that the degree of influence is greatest in cases where informants have no strong prior opinions; in other words, when young people are confronted with Ungdata survey questions about which they have no clear conviction or ready response, they will tend to identify with what they believe will be the dominant response pattern. Gender roles can be an example of such a categorization that influences response patterns. The prevailing image that Ungdata has played a part in creating is one of girls who are struggling, unlike the boys, which can indicate a risk of over-reporting in girls and under-reporting in boys. When in the 2015 survey 56 percent of the tenth grade boys in the Oslo school system who were asked to specify the degree to which they have experienced "feelings of unhappiness, sadness or being depressed" replied "Not at all" and 30 percent "Very little", it is reasonable to conclude that for the most part they are fine. Simultaneously, there is cause to question whether this response pattern is in fact wholly in keeping with the fundamental existential condition of human beings, which entails that for everyone life entails feeling unhappy, sad or depressed from time to time.[40] Maybe the boys don't allow themselves to acknowledge that they sometimes have these feelings, or they don't want to report this in the surveys, which can stem from preconceived notions about the responses of other boys.

Compared with the attention the Norwegian public sphere gives to the results of these surveys, the silence surrounding the methodological challenges has been deafening, with a few notable exceptions. Health researchers Birgit Nordtug and Gunn Engelsrud have previously addressed how the political will to increase the investment in improved mental health

[40] Patrick Lie Andersen and Anders Bakken, "Ung i Oslo 2015. NOVA Rapport 8/15", (Oslo: NOVA, 2015).

among children and young people in Norway can be based on an uncritical application of research:

> In the Ungdata survey (which involves 63,000 young people), the questions about eating disorders include: 'I am concerned about losing weight.' 'I feel uncomfortable after I've eaten sweets.' 'I work out to lose weight.' Such surveys are not 'polls' about how many children and young people are struggling with eating disorders. To paraphrase Østerberg: The measurement of eating disorders is not identical to the field of inquiry eating disorders.[41]

Nordtug and Engelsrud base their analysis on sociologist Dag Østerberg's three types of understanding: identity, exteriority and interiority. The first two forms of understanding presuppose one another—the measurements and the field of inquiry are in a relation of mutual exteriority, which means that the incidence of psychological disorders will be the same whether it is measured or not.[42] When it comes to interiority however, it's a different story in that the different components are not independent; instead, they mutually influence one another. The psychological problems of young people are not an objective reality that can be mapped and measured without affecting it. It should also be mentioned in this context that the Labour Party's Tove Karoline Knutsen from the Standing Committee on Health and Care Services in a response concedes that she "struggles to understand the point" of Nordtug and Engelsrud's article, which indicates how little accustomed the public health policy sector in Norway is to addressing analyses of methodological challenges.[43]

University lecturer in the field of nursing Marthe Schille-Rognmo also addresses the problems of the methodological foundation in the Ungdata surveys in her master's thesis *Ungdata, Mental Health and Gender Differences*.[44] Here she examines whether the questionnaires affect girls and boys differently: Is it possible that the asking of questions, the practical implementation of the study and the expectations of gender-based

---

[41] Birgit Nordtug and Gunn Engelsrud, "Fra forskning til politikk", *Klassekampen*, 24 July 2015, 18.

[42] "Utvendig og innvendig forståelse", *Klassekampen*, 17 July 2015.

[43] Tove Karoline Knutsen, "Vi snakker forbi hverandre", ibid., 21 July 2015, 22.

[44] Marthe Schille-Rognmo, "Ungdata, mental health and gender differences" (Tromsø, 2017).

mental health differences all influence the presumed reliability of the results? As a theoretical point of departure, Schille-Rognmo stipulates that the Ungdata survey must be viewed as a component in a process of knowledge production, in the sense that reality is not simply being described as it is, but that those carrying out the survey are participating in its generation. In other words, there is a *recursive relationship* between knowledge and reality: something is recurring which contains itself and which corresponds with Østerberg's interiority.[45]

With respect to the methodological challenges, Schille-Rognmo stresses how the implementation of the Ungdata surveys takes place in the course of one 45-minute school period, during which the students fill out a digital questionnaire. The average, total time spent on the survey is 17.3 minutes. That breaks down to 0.12 minutes or 6.9 seconds per each of the 158 questions. This is of course efficient, but also contrasts greatly with the amount of time that would have been spent on clinical consultations. Another point Schille-Rognmo highlights is how almost all the questions that cover mental health have a negative implication and employ words such as "struggle", "problem", "unhappy", "sad", "depressed", "hopelessness", "stiff", "tense", "worried" and "lonely". And as she adds: when Ungdata asks about well-being, they do it in a manner that does not exactly lead to positive thoughts. The choice of words is not surprising in that the questions are modelled on the American diagnosis manual DSM-IV. A further problem that Schille-Rognmo underscores is how a question such as "Do you feel unhappy, sad or depressed?" equates largely what must be considered fundamental human emotions with psychological disorders. She emphasizes how the results of the Ungdata surveys are often presented by drawing attention to the stressed-out girls, with the boys playing supporting roles, which can also serve to consolidate different expectations on the part of boys and girls about who is struggling and thereby contribute to further exacerbating gender differences.[46] The more future respondents become familiar with the Ungdata surveys through new surveys, media coverage and political response, the greater the risk of this narrative accelerating and the more we risk

[45] Ibid.

[46] Ibid.

pushing the future generation's self-image and in particular that of young girls in the direction of the survey results. The increase of bodily ailments and depressive symptoms in young girls in the last two years' Ungdata surveys *may* be consistent with the impact of such a mechanism.

Professional Whistleblowing Systems

In the Norwegian Psychology Associations' journal (*Tidsskrift for Norsk psykologforening*) Anders Bakken, the leader of the Ungdata Centre, was recently asked to comment on Schille-Rognmo's critique.[47] Bakken insists on the accuracy of the image produced by Ungdata and points out that their surveys are used in more than 400 municipalities and they have received very little feedback claiming that the figures they are operating with do not correspond with the experiences of municipal healthcare workers. If, on the other hand, we had received more of this type of feedback, we would have exercised greater caution about drawing definitive conclusions, Bakken explains. As stated earlier, Sletten has previously offered a similar argument: "It is strange at any rate if those who are working with this locally don't see it."[48]

The arguments of both Bakken and Sletten are decidedly logical. Nevertheless, they rest on a premise that is far from given. It is not certain that healthcare workers will speak up, even when they perhaps should. The category of healthcare workers includes many occupational groups, but Sletten explicitly mentions community nurses throughout Norway. In the course of their one-hundred-year history, child health clinics have played a critical role in the work with infant mortality, vaccine programmes, prenatal care and public health. The child health clinics and school health services continue to perform an important function today but following on the heels of their gradual expansion, including incorporation of the population's mental health into their repertoire in the 2000s,

---

[47] Per Olav Solberg, "Mener Ungdata gir et nyansert bilde", *Tidsskrift for Norsk psykologforening* 55, no. 2 (2018).

[48] Arne Olav Hageberg, "Ein generasjon av stressa jenter", ibid. 51, no. 11 (2014), 963.

is the risk of over-involvement.[49] I have previously addressed this on the basis of an episode at a child health clinic, where I experienced that the service of a well-meaning support system, armed with a psychological perspective and with a normal distribution curve hanging above the desk, can become overly ambitious.[50] The community nurse was concerned about my one-year-old son who still couldn't walk. She found it appropriate to recommend a number of resource-intensive measures, when the lack of any objective basis in the first consultation should presumably have led her to close the case. In spite of the boy's otherwise wholly normal developmental history, physiology and mobility, she became worried about what it would do to his self-esteem when he saw other children his age who were able to walk. Now this experience, which I christened *child health clinicism*, is quite anecdotal, but it invites nonetheless the question of whether Norway's many community nurses have the requisite professional ballast to sound the alarm about potential pathologizing or if they are more likely to contribute to the same.

If we consult another profession that is in a unique position when it comes to questions of mental health and which is well on its way to making inroads into all the municipalities of Norway—the psychology profession—what is the status of the willingness there to sound the alarm about pathologizing? The dominant attitude in the psychology profession in Norway must in general be characterized as relatively inclusive. Most Norwegian psychologists these days appear to convene around Terent's adage "nothing human is alien to me" with a therapeutical twist: "no disorder is insignificant to me". In a panel debate where the question "Are we just becoming more and more 'psick'" was raised, psychologist Peder Kjøs expressed his view as follows:

> Is it an illness to think there's a great deal of pressure stemming from grades and all that? I would like to normalize this type of difficulty and call it life challenges. And I would like it to be something that gives you a kind of good reason to seek help. I could say that it's easy to say this when you're in

[49] Ole Jacob Madsen, "Psykologiens innflytelse i velferdsstaten", in *Forvaltning av makt og moral i velferdsstaten: Fra sosialt arbeid til "arbeid med deg selv"?*, eds. Randi Kroken and Ole Jacob Madsen (Oslo: Gyldendal Akademisk, 2016).

[50] "Helsestasjonismen", *Morgenbladet*, 29 July 2016.

private practice. But it's what I think. You know, the whole business of first-world problems and luxury problems and all that, which are the kinds of questions one gets, especially if one is in private practice and has an office in an affluent neighbourhood such as Homansbyen, the way I do. So, I don't think so, that people have this. And when these parents send their young daughters to a psychologist, I don't think this is a matter of luxury problems and nonsense and foolishness. I really don't think so. I have yet to meet a client who I thought would have been better off spending their money on a new jumper.[51]

A similarly liberal view was expressed by the Chief Adviser of the Norwegian psychology association Andreas Høstmælingen in a debate about pathologizing in the *Tidsskrift for Norsk psykologforening*:

When we create diagnostic terms for disorders that are completely common in life, clearly we are pathologizing normality. But this need not be solely negative. It's also an expression of a culture that recognizes that normal life is difficult.[52]

In the *Morgenbladet* feature article of last year entitled "A catalyst for greater inequality" ("*En katalysator for økte forskjeller*") psychologist Simon Thorsell Næs wrote a timely, critical commentary on the development of the quickly growing market of private psychology services, the accessibility of which would appear to accommodate the most resourceful and well-to-do clients:

Through different channels the private actors claim that 'everyone' can benefit from talking with a psychologist, whether it's a matter of stress, performance anxiety, the wish for improved self-esteem or healthier relationships. In this way they contribute to targeting specific individuals and universal challenges as candidates for psychological treatment.[53]

---

[51] Psykologisk Salong, *Psykologisk Salong*, podcast audio, Blir vi bare psykere og psykere? 2018, https://podtail.com/no/podcast/psykologisk-salong/psykologisk-salong-2-blir-vi-bare-psykere-og-psyke/, 57:00.

[52] Andreas Høstmælingen, "Et forsvar for sykeliggjøring", *Tidsskrift for Norsk psykologforening* 54, no. 6 (2017), 571.

[53] Simon Thorsell Næs, "En katalysator for økte forskjeller", *Morgenbladet* (2017), https://morgenbladet.no/ideer/2017/11/en-katalysator-okte-forskjeller, paragraph 9.

But even with a basis in this commendable class perspective, Næs also champions the same fundamental view that everyone should be included, when in the next sentence he hastens to add: "When an increasing number of Norwegians seek out services to help them with the above-mentioned problems at an early stage, there is most likely a wholly real, personally experienced need behind it."[54] There is correspondingly reason to believe that every young person who contacts a community nurse or psychologist is experiencing a real, personally experienced need. And the willingness of health professionals to question this need will be correspondingly non-existent.

What Bakken and Sletten leave out of their logical reasoning is how professions are informed by profession-based thought. A well-known bias is often called *déformation professionnelle*: if you only have a hammer, you see nails everywhere. All professions possess a latent drive to expand their own mandate, which can be motivated by everything from idealism to self-interest. This can ideally be counteracted by a strongly developed ethical awareness of necessary prioritizing or humility about the limitations of the profession, but it is difficult to detect this in the current practice of the psychology profession. Instead, what is confirmed is the validity of the American linguist Noam Chomsky's apt observation: "One waits in vain for psychologists to state the limits of their knowledge."[55] This does not necessarily mean that the portrait Ungdata has produced of how Norwegian young people *actually* are doing must be wrong, but as a safeguard, I would propose that the evidence supports the belief that "one waits in vain" if one expects corrective interventions from the psychology profession, in the event we were to pathologize large portions of the young population.

[54] Ibid., paragraph 9.

[55] Noam Chomsky, "Psychology and ideology", in *The Chomsky reader*, ed. James Peck (New York: Pantheon, 1987), 182.

Double Reflexivity

The idea that it is possible to address the health of young people in a manner similar to that of an oceanographer who can take regular samples to measure the water temperature or the CO_2 concentration of the water surface, without the ocean noticing this, is not without its consequences. Because young people, parents, teachers, community nurses, politicians and journalists must necessarily take the research into account, both with regard to the actual questionnaires the young people are asked to fill out and the dissemination and attention devoted to the results in reports, campaigns, the media and the public sphere. The above-mentioned NOVA report "The experience of stress and pressure in youth" (*Stress og press blant ungdom*), which was commissioned by the Directorate of Health and the Ministry of Children and Equality, investigated what might lie behind the increase in self-reported mental health ailments in girls in recent years.[56] In the report one finds that 53 percent of the girls and 26 percent of the boys in the tenth grade in Oslo schools report experiencing mental health ailments "quite often" or "a great deal". The young people themselves appear to attribute these symptoms to stress and particularly stress caused by school. The report has employed focus group interviews with youth and investigated how the young people personally understand and experience stress and pressure. With respect to coping strategies for stress, the researchers in the report emphasized how the young people's solutions consistently ranged from withdrawal, such as taking a break, to emotional strategies, such as enlisting support and understanding, or that which they characterize as more extroverted strategies, such as working harder, becoming more efficient or tougher, or learning better stress management methods. A common feature is nonetheless that the young people believe that they must personally change the situation. This is also the NOVA researchers' thought-provoking conclusion: "None of these strategies entailed changing the source of stress or reducing the external pressure. Protesting against or removing the source of stress does not appear to be an option the young people consider."[57]

[56] Eriksen et al., "Stress og press blant unge. Rapport nr 6/17".

[57] Ibid., 59.

This is of course essential if we recall how neoliberalism's view of human life is to a large degree based on individualization and not least personal accountability, whereby the individual is expected to manage him or herself. This appears to have become the dominant social landscape for Norwegian youth as well.

An even more alarming question, however, is whether with this state-financed knowledge production, using the analytical terms "stress" and "pressure" which researchers invite young people to apply to their lives, can be reasonably expected to arrive at any other conclusions? Can it be that the terms instead spread and legitimize an individualistic and neoliberal mentality under the guise of science? The NOVA report dedicates an entire chapter to stress.[58] Here you can read about Hungarian endocrinologist Hans Selye's ground-breaking studies of animals where he identified three physiological reactions to threats or troublesome events: the alarm reaction, the stage of resistance and, finally, the stage of exhaustion. Selye held that especially the last type of reaction is harmful to health because it is associated with high blood pressure, cardiovascular disease and other adaptive difficulties. The report also adds that the previous research on stress which Selye represented tended to emphasize negative events in people's lives, whereas today's studies of stress are more geared towards a constant strain in people's daily lives, not least the pressure of requirements and expectations.

Rather than approaching stress as a universal, physiological phenomenon according to which the reaction to running into a bear in the woods would be the same for a cave man as for modern man and woman, Dana Becker is interested in how the contents of "stress" as a concept have changed significantly since Selye introduced it as an object of scientific study in *Nature* in 1936.[59] In Middle English of the period between 1150 and 1500 "stress" referred to "hardship or force exerted on a person for the purpose of compulsion", indicating that stress was the will of another being imposed on the individual, in contrast to today where we understand it as being integrated in the self. And all the way up to more mod-

[58] Ibid.

[59] Dana Becker, *One nation under stress: the trouble with stress as an idea* (New York: Oxford University Press, 2013).

ern times, "stress" was a name for "what was hard and had to be endured", which in turn required strength and bravery.[60] In the 1949 edition of the Merriam-Webster dictionary, "stress" is defined wholly without reference to human beings, as "the action of external forces; especially to overstrain".[61] An image that was used to illustrate stress was of a ship being tossed about by the stress of bad weather. Stress was something temporary, like a storm, whereas today, stress has become a constant in Western contemporary culture. And although we refer to stress as both an external force, outside a person, and an internal state, it is increasingly the internal state that appears to be accentuated, Becker concludes. An article in the national daily *VG* entitled "Stress-test yourself" illustrates her point.[62] Here an established term regarding "dangerous obesity" is revised as "dangerous stress". It is illustrated by the picture of a young, beautiful woman, but the blush of her rosy cheeks has spread upward to her temples and become glowing stressors. It is therefore important to separate the stress—the interior danger—from life. The next step is then to hold different stressed groups in society accountable, a move that Becker calls *stressism*.[63] The concept of stress draws in the outside—in a way that leads to our ending up with the belief that we must change ourselves so we can adapt to the living conditions of society, rather than changing those conditions. "The chameleon nature of the concept of stress makes it possible to obscure or conceal social problems by individualizing them in way that mostly disadvantages those who have the least to gain from the status quo, among them women and the poor",[64] Becker points out. As such, the concept of stress carries out what Becker and the cultural historian Mary Poovey characterize as the task of *ideological work*—to absorb contradictions and pave the way for the acceptance of simple, dominant conceptions as common sense. The *VG* article's underlying logic is that stress-testing is important to be able to recognize our own inherent stress and keep it at bay so as to stay healthy. When conceived in this way, it is

---

[60] Ibid.

[61] Ibid.

[62] Eliese Laustsen, "Stresstest deg selv", *VG*, 22 May 2013.

[63] Becker, *One nation under stress: the trouble with stress as an idea.*

[64] Ibid.

difficult to thematically address the underlying causes of stress, since the problems are presented as being individual lifestyle problems. This is otherwise in keeping with the liberalist individualism's view of illness, in which the individual is primarily understood as sick, rather than relating it to the illness-producing features in the development of society. And some groups will very likely be perceived as more stressed than others. It is hardly a coincidence that "Stress-test yourself" is illustrated with the picture of a young woman, since Becker shows how stress literally exploded in parallel with the feminist backlash of the 1980s, during which working mothers were warned of the price of wanting to "have it all". Becker documents how the message that women must learn to de-stress became more popular during this period, and stress mastery became an essential part of daily self-care, whereby solutions emerged from designated industries including everything from yoga and mindfulness courses and self-help literature to stress-alleviating medications. Meanwhile, the structural inequality between American men and women and the development of welfare benefits in the USA remained for the most part unmodified.

Becker's point is not to make stress relative by saying that people *shouldn't* have experienced specific events as stressful, or to cast doubt on people's experiences of stressful events, but to show how the concept of stress leads to specific behaviour. When the NOVA researchers express surprise or concern about how protesting against or removing the source of the stress sufferers are experiencing in their bodies does not even appear to be an option for the Oslo students participating in their surveys, then it's both commendable and alarming at the same time—commendable, because such findings can perhaps help us address the issue of young people's experiences of stress and pressure from another angle, so we do not prescribe individual remedies such as school courses in stress and life mastery. Hopefully this is what the authors have in mind when on the final page of the report they conclude by saying: "More knowledge about the meaning of 'stress discourses' or how we speak about stress and mental health ailments in different contexts and whether this influences what the young people report is also needed."[65] But at the same time it is alarm-

[65] Eriksen et al., "Stress og press blant unge. Rapport no. 6/17", 103.

ing, because the conclusion demonstrates how little they appear to have reflected upon how they have personally taken part in inviting young people to discuss their lives in terms of concepts such as stress and pressure, which exclusively encourages thinking and talking about oneself in an individualized and personally accountable manner. It is difficult to predict the types of effects commissioned reports of this nature can have. But a less than unlikely scenario can be that they lead to a greater focus on stress and pressure as problems in the schools, and the implementation of measures such as life and stress mastery courses in the schools, which further consolidate the idea that stress is something the individual must handle by learning strategies. This is presumably something the most resourceful students will manage and take advantage of, in contradistinction to those with fewer resources, who will thereby be even more likely to blame only themselves for their misfortune.

Conclusion

Most social scientists, in the course of their education, will hear about *reflexivity*, since the social sciences' field of inquiry is other people and human-made phenomena. But as the sociologist Per Otnes has pointed out: "But why is this requirement so easy to write about and so correspondingly difficult to practice?"[66] The reasons Otnes proposes are the lack of a methodological procedure for how this critical activity shall be carried out, uncomfortable self-realizations, or that reflexivity is viewed as irrelevant to the subject in question. In the context of youth research, one could perhaps add factors such as a lack of interest on all sides, from the commissioning body in the Ministry to the media and the public sphere, since reflexive moderation is not as easily applied in the ecosystem of modern research as are alarming figures or statistics. A more prosaic explanation less based on a critique of power can quite simply be a shortage of time: When shall we do this work that does not necessarily produce any tangible results?

[66] Per Otnes, "Innledning", *Sosiologisk Årbok*, no. 2 (2001), iii.

To practise what one preaches, we can also ask here how it is possible to prevent contemporary diagnoses such as “the achievement society” from becoming self-fulfilling prophecies? If we consult the authors, Merton pointed out that self-fulfilling prophecies do not occur automatically but can only occur when fear is transformed into a reality, which can happen primarily in the absence of an intended institutional control. It is a large leap from the American federal authorities’ fluctuating control over the banking system to the actual social development of the current era. But the emergence of several of the self-fulfilling prophecies is occurring in a historically unparalleled period of individual liberation, under the guise of maximizing the individual’s freedom and autonomy. Becker also comments on how the concept of stress appears more and more to camouflage the individual’s feelings of uncertainty and fear. It is undeniably ironic how the concept of stress thrives under liberal individualism, which promises an abundance of freedom, but which can lead to a lack of freedom in the manner of greater anxiety about “the dangerous stress”. Women’s freedom of choice in particular appears to encounter a medicated curtailment, also in Norway as in the case of the “good girl syndrome”, where women blame themselves and their oversized ambitions for subjecting themselves to a kind of stress that is hazardous to health.

Sociologist John Thompson has previously analysed how ideology can perform by way of different modalities, such as illness metaphors.[67] An example he gives is how former Prime Minister Margaret Thatcher described a change in the perception of Great Britain from “the English illness” to “England has the cure”. By implementing illness and health metaphors, Thatcher succeeded in clouding the actual social and economic circumstances that brought us to where we are. What is achieved by combining “good girl” with “syndrome”? And who benefits from this use of illness metaphors? Applied to the materials we have before us, it will entail that the labels both the surrounding society and young people themselves use, such as “achievement generation” and “good girl syndrome”, function as an ideology that entrenches a specific understanding of the relation between individuals and their life conditions. Accordingly, these terms can do some ideological work, serving individual interests

[67] John B. Thompson, *Ideology and modern culture* (London: Polity Press, 1990).

which are not necessarily always those of the young people themselves. The descriptions of the problems appear most of all to engender the proposal of solutions involving individual stress and life mastery coping strategies, which inevitably make the individual even more accountable. And now that “the problem that has no name” finally has a name, it has suddenly become difficult to conceive of other possible names.

9

Conclusion

Not only are you young, you are young and simultaneously confronted with images of how you as a young person should be.

—Thomas Ziehe. (Ziehe, "Ungdom och modernitet", 53)

A RECURRING THEME OF THIS BOOK has been how Norwegian youth are doing, objectively speaking, and how they experience their lives, subjectively speaking. A concluding report on the status quo from an event on Norway's National Day fully demonstrates the discrepancy: on 17 May 2014 two teenagers, Stine Smedsland and Thea Ågedal Mjåland, gave a speech in Byremo, a small town in the northern part of Audnedal municipality in the county of Agder, nest to a monument erected in memory of those who had been killed during the Second World War. In 2011, Audnedal topped the list of the best-places-to-live municipalities in Norway.[1] Although the two young women reside in the best municipality in the fifth best country in the world, as evidenced by the rankings, and were about to dedicate this moment to the young people who gave their

[1] Ole Petter Pedersen, "Kommunebarometeret", *Kommunal Rapport*, 14 April 2011.

O. J. Madsen, *Deconstructing Scandinavia's "Achievement Generation"*,
https://doi.org/10.1007/978-3-030-72555-6_9

lives for the society with abundant benefits that we all enjoy, Smedsland and Mjåland find it appropriate to question how their peers are *actually* doing:

> Young people today are under pressure to succeed from all sides. There are requirements to excel at school, there are requirements for clothing and appearance, and it's also important to be popular both on social media and in real life. We live in one of the best countries in the world. You would think we would have a better chance to succeed than ever before but how are we really? We take part in well-being surveys at school that show the same results as elsewhere in Norway: many young people are struggling in their daily lives and feel stressed about measuring up.[2]

Young people personally experience pressure from all sides to succeed—to be clever, attractive, popular—both virtually and in real life—and simultaneously they admit that the conditions to ensure their success have never been better, although well-being surveys from the schools demonstrate that this is not the case, that many of their peers struggle in their daily lives with stress related to feelings of inadequacy. This apparent paradox is nonetheless not contrary to logic: after concluding their public schooling, members of previous generations went to work to guarantee themselves and their family a necessary income; there was no time for teenagers to think about what they should become or who they wanted to be. What existed in the way of external sources of strain were primarily *the duty to perform*. But now that the development of society has taken giant steps through *freedom from* poverty, hunger and unemployment and a substantial increase in prosperity has occurred, new opportunities emerge and with these also new pitfalls. As Pascal Bruckner says, pointedly: "We are probably the first society in history to make people unhappy about *not* feeling happy."[3] But as Neil Young has countered: "Though my problems are meaningless, that don't make them go away."[4] With the ideal of success comes inexorably not only the reality of failure, but also the awareness that failure is a possibility, which clearly can cause worries,

---

[2] Stine Smedsland and Thea Ågedal Mjåland, "17. mai i Grindheim 2014", in *Avis frå Byremoelevar*, eds. Janne Åvesland, Ingrid Stulien, and Elise Hobbesland (2014), 65.

[3] Bruckner, *Perpetual euphoria: on the duty to be happy*.

[4] Neil Young, "On the beach", in *On the beach* (New York: Reprise, 1974).

anxiety and stress. It is otherwise striking how young people themselves will cite the research results, which provides us with the truth about how young people are really doing, a truth that is disturbing. Of course it is—the ideal of success constitutes a goal that is both exalted and elusive. It is up to young people themselves to come up with the meaning of success. In addition to this come the unintended consequences of increased interest in and consciousness-raising about how youth are actually doing: more introspection, more registration of diffuse bodily and mental ailments, increased reporting of these and greater awareness about the problem when the results are headlined in the media, which in turn feeds the next generation of young informants with information about how difficult adolescence is, especially for girls. If they do not feel pressured and stressed to begin with, then public opinion makes it a point to remind them of it constantly. Beyond this, there is a steady stream of research reports which also truly give cause for concern about some areas of young people's lives, which the media is happy to publicize, in contrast to the big picture which shows that most young people growing up in Norway today actually are doing quite well. At least for the time being.

Summing Up the Book

The individual chapters of the book have provided different perspectives on how youth are actually doing. In Chap. 2, "The Pathologies of Modernity", and Chap. 3, "The Pathologies of Late Modernity", I explored the critique that has surrounded modernity since the time of its inception, in which a somewhat gloomy picture is painted of young people's possibilities for living a good life in late modernity. In Chap. 4, "Young, Privileged and Sick", I investigated how some of these contemporary norms and ideals can come to prevail in Scandinavian young people's lives and illness narratives in purely subjective terms. In Chap. 5, "Youth Under Pressure", I've compiled the existing research and statistics on internalized and externalized behaviour ranging from suicide to sexual debut, which in purely objective terms indicates that young people today are doing relatively well, although there are some indications that especially young girls are experiencing a substantial amount of psychological ailments in the form of pressure-induced ailments, worries and stress. In Chap. 6, "Social Representations", I investigated the media development of leading depictions of the current age and youth, such as "the achievement society", "the achievement generation" and "the good girl syndrome". In Chap. 7, "Self-Fulfilling Prophecies", I addressed the issue of how these concepts can paradoxically contribute to reinforcing the developmental features, not least youth research which in recent years has received considerable attention in the public sphere. In Chap. 8, "The Paradox of Health", I discuss how humans are interactive beings who always interact with their scientific classifications, including persons suffering from psychological illnesses.

It is common knowledge that people tend to emphasize findings that confirm their already existing beliefs and that they are correspondingly sceptical of opinions that run counter to these. Readers who position themselves politically on the Left will therefore possibly be most enthusiastic about Chaps. 2–4 and less enthusiastic about Chaps. 6–8, while Right wing readers will possibly prefer Chaps. 6–8, but be more ambivalent about Chaps. 2–4. The reader's sympathies and antipathies are what they are. One ambition of the book has simply been to explore the question of how young people *are* doing from perspectives that can shed light on established truisms, although none of the individual chapters in and of themselves necessarily offer an exhaustive explanation. Hopefully all the perspectives have something to offer, but that depends on whom, what and which aspect you are seeking to illuminate.

Neither can I avoid a number of areas of uncertainty attached to the book's analyses. It is possible, for example, to cite the last chapters as proof of the fact that young people's mental health issues are to a large extent media-driven and therefore also exaggerated. But whether I have succeeded in documenting that infection has occurred on a broad scale in Norway by way of the media remains an unanswered question. One can remark that the terms "achievement generation" and "good girl syndrome" have had significant exposure in the media for several years now, but it is only in the measurements of recent years that we see a clear increase in self-reported ailments in the Ungdata survey. If the media-contagion explanation is correct, why didn't it kick in previously? It is also possible to question whether young people absorb much of what is found in the media. A current study of the media habits of youth discloses that a number of young people don't read traditional news sources at all.[5] And for those who still do, their minds cannot be viewed as a kind of tabula rasa that uncritically absorbs everything written there. Further, there are clearly objective sources of stress and pressure in everything from the school, specific requirements for the body and physical appearance, social media, the labour market and economic disparities. And as I will address below, it is doubtful that the term "achievement generation" provides a representative image of how most young people are doing. The concept says first and foremost something about society's preferred representation of young people (also one of the main topics of this book) more than about young people in and of themselves. The book is therefore best read as an investigation of how we speak about the current challenges facing young people.

The Answer Is Served

One of the main problems with trying to get to the bottom of how we are actually doing is the propensity to believe that the answers to complex social factors are only satisfactory if they can be reduced to either-or answers, upon which we must choose which of the two alternatives is most worthy of our endorsement. Instead, we should endeavour to think that opposites can be simultaneously true. In the anthology *This Idea Must Die*, the point is made that in order to make new scientific advances possible, existing, limiting scientific ideas must first be buried.[6] Editor John Brockman has therefore invited 175 of the world's leading scientists to perform their own personal coup de grace on an idea standing in the way of progress. The psychologist Eldar Shafir's contribution opens with the description of an inventive drink *Hot and Iced Tea* by the British celebrity chef Heston Blumenthal, who is known for his molecular

[5] Hallvard Moe and Hilde Sakariassen, "Bruksmønstre for digitale nyheter", (Bergen: University of Bergen, 2018).

[6] John Brockman, ed., *This idea must die* (New York: Harper Perennial, 2015).

gastronomy.[7] The drink is a syrupy brew prepared in a glass with a partition running down the middle; the glass is then filled with half hot tea and half iced tea. Due to the gel-like consistency of the liquid, when the partition is removed, the two types of tea remain separated long enough to allow dinner guests to enjoy a perfect hot and iced tea simultaneously. And as Shafir emphasizes: as you imbibe Blumenthal's drink, there is no point in arguing about whether it is hot or cold. It is both. Opposites need *not* be mutually exclusive. And that is how things are to a great extent both in the world and in the sciences—and especially the social and behavioural sciences—he points out. This is the case even though we will tend to think about this differently. For example, when it comes to joy and sadness, we think of them as being mutually exclusive. But recent research findings on emotions indicate that positive and negative affects should not be viewed as opposite poles on a continuum, but rather feelings that can be experienced at the same time, Shafir writes. If asked right after having seen specific films or having completed a final exam, it was people who tend to feel a fundamental sense of both bliss and sadness. The same holds for whether people will be good or evil in a given situation, in that we now know that contextual nuances determine on which side people will land. Shafir refers to a classic study in which theology students were instructed to give a sermon about the Good Samaritan. Half of the candidates were convinced that they had plenty of time before the sermon, while the other half were told that they were late. On the way to the sermon, each of the theology students came across an injured man in need of assistance. The majority of those who had plenty of time stopped to help but only 10 percent from the group who believed they were late stopped. Just like in the example of the tea drink, the pastors-to-be were both caring and indifferent; small random events turned them in one direction rather than the other, Shafir reasons. With regard to the issue of children in general, we also have a propensity to seek the type of answers through which one scenario will categorically exclude the other: "Young people have never been better off!" or "Young people have never suffered so much!" But with the hot and cold tea in mind, it's possible to

[7] Eldar Shafir, "Opposites can't both be right", in *This idea must idea*, ed. John Brockman (New York: Harper Perennial, 2015).

chime in that the human being of today is to be pitied, given the unique challenge we are facing *and* to remember that it has always been held that mankind is to be pitied. In sum we can therefore conclude: "Hasn't it always been difficult to be young?" Of course. "Are we more attentive to how young people are doing today than previously?" Undoubtedly. "Do the youth of today experience a type of performance pressure that is unique?" Definitely. "Doesn't every generation believe that the next will be the last?" Of course. "But can all these hypotheses be true simultaneously?" Actually, yes.

The Unbearable Distortion of the Media Society

To accept the inherent complexity of things, however, is not the same as accepting that the images created of young people are true in the sense of being representative. Forty years ago, the journal *Samtiden* published the article "The media's distortion of society" (Det media-vridde samfunn) written by sociologist and later Labour Party Cabinet Minister Gudmund Hernes.[8] Hernes asks fundamental questions about the impact media distortion has on the development of society. While discussing the media's influence on politics, Hernes writes: "Because *the way* information is presented affects not only *what* we understand, but also our understanding of *how* issues are addressed and resolved and *which* issues *should* be addressed."[9] The filtering of information by the media would also appear to be in force today, exemplified by images of youth, such as "the good girl syndrome" and "the achievement generation".

[8] Gudmund Hernes, "Det mediavridde samfunn", i *Forhandlingsøkonomi og blandingsadministrasjon*, ed. Gudmund Hernes (Oslo: Universitetsforlaget, 1978).
[9] Ibid., 189.

Media Templates

As illustrated in previous chapters here, articles about young people who are struggling, depicted as "the achievement generation" and frequently personified as "good girls", were prevalent in the Norwegian media in the mid-2010s. Such personalized stories fulfil several of the criteria Hernes holds to be necessary to make an impact on a society distorted by the media and suffering from an attention deficit. For example, this is achieved through use of *specific examples* whereby the presentation of unique circumstances serves to undermine any analysis of the universal. But the many news items also appear to refer to one another. Media Studies scholar Jenny Kitzinger has coined the term *media templates* inspired by newspaper articles about child abuse.[10] The term stems from the much-discussed media incident from Cleveland, England, in 1987, at which time over the course of a six-month period, 121 children were removed from their homes by the child welfare authorities due to suspicions of sexual abuse. A subsequent investigation nonetheless concluded that most of the allegations of sexual abuse were unfounded. A total of 94 of the 121 children were returned to their homes. Subsequent incidents in other locations, such as the Orkney Islands, were then referred to in the British media as "yet another Cleveland". Application of the Cleveland template required the existence of a fixed set of stereotypes, prejudices and interpretations. The Cleveland case had established a template, according to which any new cases of families whose children were removed by the child welfare authorities were understood as further examples of the original story. This recollection occurred on the production side, in terms of how the journalists did preparatory work, wrote and angled the story, and in the story's reception. Using focus groups, Kitzinger demonstrates how the public used its knowledge of the original cases to understand the subsequent cases. Another well-known example is media stories about heart transplants from the 1980s, which typically follow the process from the desperation of the person waiting for an organ, the fear that time is running out, the operation that provides the

[10] Jenny Kitzinger, "Media templates: patterns of association and the (re)construction of meaning over time", *Media, Culture & Society* 22, no. 1 (2000).

opportunity to escape death and the press conference afterwards which becomes an arena for hope. Today a heart transplant needs additional appeal to qualify as news—one example would be a dying Palestinian who donates his heart to save an Israeli.[11] Kitzinger also shows how some templates can be *reversed* when their currency is weakened: the stories about the child welfare authorities' infringement of the rights of wholly ordinary families eventually became old news, but a reversal involving a father from Cleveland, who was actually a condemned child abuser, would revitalize the interest.[12]

It is possible to demonstrate the existence of similar media templates in the many articles about struggling youth in Norway. In 2013, *Aftenposten*'s front page bore the following headline: "Good girls work themselves sick" ("*Flinke piker sliter seg syke*").[13] The headline is accompanied by a photograph of eighteen-year-old Lisa Jakobsen, who was named student of the year and in her own words had "thousands" of irons in the fire, until she finally became ill from all the stress. In the interview, Jakobsen admits that she both lives under and suffers from a relentless drive for perfection.[14] Three years later, the same newspaper published a follow-up article where again we meet Lisa as a twenty-one-year-old and it turns out she is doing relatively well. Immediately the story reverses the media template we usually associate with the typical, alarming achievement generation headline and the reader is reassured: "For the majority everything will be fine."[15] Journalist Miriam Lund Knapstad also asks self-critically on behalf of the media: "Have we focused too much on the achievement generation?"[16] But such reversals still appear to be in the minority; the alarmist articles about the younger generation continue to dominate the news cycle.

---

[11] Clive Seale, "Health and media: an overview", *Sociology of Health & Illness* 25, no. 6 (2003).

[12] Kitzinger, "Media templates: patterns of association and the (re)construction of meaning over time".

[13] Knapstad, "Sykt flinke".

[14] Ibid.

[15] "På videregående var de slitne, stressa og 'sykt flinke'", ibid., 22 October 2016, 35.

[16] Ibid., 37.

Media Favouritism

Another known source of error that is relevant to the achievement generation is the media's inherent propensity to focus on the reporting of negative events rather than positive. The famous psychologist Steven Pinker wrote a comment in *The Guardian* in which he sums up the problem concisely: "Whether or not the world is really getting worse, the nature of news will interact with the nature of cognition to make us think that it is."[17] Applied to the subject under investigation, this can be transposed as follows: "Whether or not young people are really worse off than before, the nature of news will interact with the nature of cognition to make us think that they are." Why is this true? Pinker refers to a well-known mental defect which the Nobel Prize winners Amos Tversky and Daniel Kahneman call the *Availability heuristic*: people estimate the probability of an event or the frequency of a phenomenon based on how easily it comes to mind.[18] Every time a memory approaches the top of the result list in the brain's search engine for reasons other than frequency, either because it's recent, powerful, violent, unique or upsetting, people will overestimate its probability, he reasons.[19] Applied to the subject at hand, it means that because we often hear about the achievement generation and the good girl syndrome in the media, the tendency will be to overestimate the importance of such phenomena as a cause of psychological complaints and disorders. And because we often read about young people who are struggling, we will overestimate the prevalence of psychological complaints and disorders in this group. Again, this will potentially trigger additional measures, studies and attention targeting the mental health of young people, in that the basic philosophy holds that it is important to talk about it. This in turn nourishes an illness-based mentality which young people will employ as a cultural reservoir when they are interpreting and positioning themselves. As such, given the availability heuristic,

---

[17] Steven Pinker, "The media exaggerates negative news. This distortion has consequences", (2018), https://www.theguardian.com/commentisfree/2018/feb/17/steven-pinker-media-negative-news, paragraph 4.

[18] Ibid.

[19] Ibid.

the media's favouring of negative features can paradoxically contribute to compounding the mental health problems of young people.

Skewed Reporting

A number of factors can cause skewed reporting. The phenomenon *disease prestige* means what it says—that some illnesses are held in higher esteem than others.[20] The hierarchies between the illnesses associated with the highest prestige, according to Dag Album and Eivind Engebretsen, are based upon the nature of the illness itself, the typical form of treatment, the average patient and the existing research on the illness. Illnesses in the upper regions of the body, such as the brain, heart and blood, appear to enjoy a higher prestige than those located lower in the body, not to mention those without any connection to a specific organ. Accordingly, brain tumours, heart attacks and leukaemia are highly ranked, while psychological disorders are correspondingly low. Album and Engebretsen's studies are limited to the evaluations of doctors, but there is reason to believe that the media also reflects specific types of disease prestige. Here the criteria for prestige will presumably be contingent upon which disorders generate the greatest interest and greatest number of clicks on the part of readers.

In one of the first in-depth articles about the achievement generation in the Norwegian national media in *VG Helg* in 2014, the leader of the Ungdata study Anders Bakken was asked whether "Norwegian girls have become so good that it's making them sick?" to which he replied: "Previously it was drugs and a problematic family life that made children depressed. Now privileged young people are also struggling."[21] It is of interest that the latter claim appeared to become particularly popular in the media in the subsequent period and it's interesting to speculate about why. Of course, it can be explained by news value. We are used to thinking about psychological disorders in connection with drug/alcohol abuse or a troubled family life and as affecting those with fewer resources. But

[20] Dag Album and Eivind Engebretsen, "Sykdomsprestisje", *Praktiske Grunde*, no. 1–2 (2013).

[21] Kreutz-Hansen, Hole, and Johannessen, "Generasjon prestasjon", paragraph 11.

now also resourceful young people are being affected, which tells us something universally valid about our society. At the same time, we must assume that the perception of privileged young people who are also struggling becomes popular because it is basically a more welcome media template—the message of being privileged but mentally ill is quite simply better click-bait than being underprivileged and mentally ill.

There are also indications that Bakken felt his statement received far too much attention. In the following year in connection with the release of the Ungdata report for 2015, Bakken specifies in an article in the press that ambitious girls are not the ones who are struggling the most: "The young people who are struggling the most with psychological ailments, are less happy at school, they do less homework, play truant more and to a lesser extent than the others are planning to pursue higher education."[22] He even admits that it would now be expedient to nuance this image somewhat: "There are also well-integrated and ambitious youth who are struggling, but it is pertinent to ask whether this group has perhaps received a bit too much attention from the media in recent years."[23] It is seldom that researchers publicly disavow media reports on their own research in this manner, so here Bakken deserves credit for doing so. And Mira Aaboen Sletten has meritoriously challenged the media narrative about good girls and shown that subjective health ailments are most prevalent in young people from families with a low socio-economic status.[24]

These disavowals illustrate how research today is often filtered via the media through specific images of youth in which some aspects have a tendency to be highlighted, while other aspects—which in reality can be more representative—are kept in the background. This can be problematic for several reasons: public opinion can be misled to believe that one group is struggling more than is actually the case, which in turn can have consequences for the priorities established for future research funding or treatment schemes. The images can also have repercussions for those who are struggling, so we cannot just think about this as a media template, but

---

[22] Høgskolen i Oslo og Akershus, "Ikke de mest ambisiøse jentene som sliter mest", (2015), https://www.ntbinfo.no/pressemelding/ikke-de-mest-ambisiose-jentene-som-sliter-mest?publisherId=15678779&releaseId=15768335, paragraph 5.

[23] Ibid., paragraph 8.

[24] Sletten, "Psykiske plager blant ungdom: sosiale forskjeller og historien om de flinke pikene".

also as an *illness template* with which young people are expected to conform. A question that arises in response to the many articles about performance pressure experienced by today's youth is whether the articles in and of themselves constitute a pressure under which the interview objects confirm the image produced of a generation of young people under pressure. In the *VG+* article, we hear about twenty-three-year-old Therese Wilhelmsen who is struggling with panic attacks, where the interviewee first points out that she "has always been a nervous person" and that both her father and grandfather died in the course of the same year, but finally, the discussion returns to the usual explanations: "But performance anxiety has also been a triggering factor for the panic attacks. I've always felt that I've been the worst and the ugliest in my class. I felt I had to work, work, work to become as good as the others."[25] Here one wonders whether she's felt an underlying pressure to confirm the preferred explanations for her disability. And if what we are dealing with here is a sub-species of what Thomas Ziehe has noted previously, young people today are forced to become reflexive due to a constant confrontation with contemporary images of how they as young people should be.[26]

The Reality 2.0

French-Moroccan sociologist Eva Illouz commented a decade ago on how the media today plays a critical part in collecting, legitimizing and disseminating a psychological view of the world and becomes a platform for a therapeutic self by acting as an intermediary between professional experts and the public, the latter in their role as clients.[27] In other words, it is not only a matter of the media twisting the truth of scientific psychology, although that is also a problem, but that the distorted image of society created by the media in the final analysis takes part in determining the direction of psychology's development, since it continuously feeds us

[25] Kingsrød-Olsen and Storrøsten, "Slik tok Therese og Jannicke kontroll over panikkangsten", paragraph 21–23.

[26] Ziehe, "Ungdom och modernitet".

[27] Eva Illouz, *Saving the modern soul: therapy, emotions, and the culture of self-help* (Berkeley, CA: University of California Press, 2008).

with specific skewed perceptions of illness, which sooner or later become realities for the young people, the adults around them and the professionals themselves.

The Generation Label

Using labels to characterize generations is a peculiar exercise. Social anthropologist Kirsten Danielsen has clarified what we are in fact talking about when we speak of generations:

> When we speak about generations it implies – in the narrow sense of the word (the generational unit) – that the generation has an awareness of itself; a feeling of belonging to 'our times' is required. A generation characterizes itself as being different from those who come before and after them.[28]

From this, we can conclude that even though it is highly doubtful that the "achievement generation" is an adequate characterization of all Norwegian youth born in the 2000s, the term is nonetheless something many young people will relate to as a point of reference connected to the contemporary age. Simultaneously, we should be aware that also the contemporary age is being written by the victors. Generalizations about cohorts have an unfortunate tendency to collapse under more scrupulous inspection.[29] As an example, take one of the most incorporated descriptions of a generation, the so-called 1968 Generation, which triggers associations of student protests, radical counter-movements, long hair, drugs and rebellious rock and roll. But from a purely demographic standpoint, most Norwegians who were young in the late 1960s were absolutely not rebellious students, but rather ordinary workers who to a large degree resembled their parents' generation. Social anthropologist Runar Døving has pointed out how this "generation" was in fact made up of a small, influential minority:

---

[28] Kirsten Danielsen, "I vår tid. Tre artikler om generasjon, modernitet og livshistorier", (Oslo: Norsk Gerontologisk Institutt, 1994), 12.

[29] Michael Hobbes, "Generation screwed", (2017), https://highline.huffingtonpost.com/articles/en/poor-millennials/

> The generation of '68 was not a generation but rather a clique. A group of political people in the spirit of the times who indeed had (and have) great influence on society, but most of those who were born in the 1940s were interested in earning a good salary, in social welfare benefits, a fifth week of holiday, in their children's welfare and parents' health – like everyone else.[30]

Døving's point is precisely that the entire generation concept is an elite phenomenon which is often used about and by small, yet dominant groups in society. Applied to "the achievement generation", the elite element can encompass resourceful youth who are both privileged and capable of getting their unique challenges on the agenda in social media, national newspapers and other forums. There is, on the other hand, a large, silent majority who do not necessarily correspond with this categorization, but who have fewer resources for the communication of their needs and suffering.

Wanted: "The Stagnation Generation"

So why doesn't the media write more about those who are most afflicted with mental health ailments, who often have bad relationships with their parents, fewer friends, those who are more frequently bullied and are less happy in their local community than those with good mental health? And those who have more experience with crime and drug and alcohol abuse? In a panel discussion under the direction of the "Psychology Saloon" (*Psykologisk salong*), researcher Leila Torgersen from The Norwegian Institute of Public Health proposed the following explanation:

> We are middle class people. Newspaper journalists are from the middle class. We are very interested in these good girls who are doing so well in school. What's important to keep in mind is that there are still more children experiencing mental health problems from families with low levels of education. The focus is on our children.[31]

[30] Døving, "Generasjon A", paragraph 16.

[31] Psykologisk Salong, *Psykologisk Salong*, 45:24.

Could it be true that this group receives more attention because the news producers and treatment professions are more familiar with the members through their own children? Articles about "the others", on the other hand, to a large extent would require moving outside of one's own select circle and into other parts of the country, outside of the communities in which most of the leading national media outlets operate. If we again consult Goodhart's much discussed value gap between the world views of the modern "anywheres" and more traditional "somewheres",[32] there are a number of indications that the achievement generation represents a typical "anywhere" issue that is not necessarily experienced as being equally relevant outside of central Oslo and the upper-middle class throughout Norway. While working on this book I spoke with a teacher in Moss secondary school, who, in response to a question regarding the achievement generation, replied that he hadn't noticed signs of it to any remarkable extent in his students; on the contrary, the problem was that the majority did not seem to be especially motivated.

The author Maria Kjos Fonn has also stated that we seldom hear from the young people who fall between the cracks or are excluded: "The achievement generation" and "the feelings generation" do not adequately capture the reality encountered by many *millennials*. There is also a "stagnation generation" among us—but where are they in the image produced by the media and relevant literature?[33] Fonn does find a few glimpses in fictional narratives, such as when NRK's popular television series for young people *Skam* ("Shame"), in a rare low-key episode, shows Vilde caring for her debt-ridden, depressed, bedridden mother or in Jan Kristoffer Dale's short story collection *Arbeidsnever* ("Working Man Hands") where he "depicts a group of millennials who are young but not promising. The shame over a lack of education and employment, low income and loneliness runs deeper than the television series named after the feeling in question."[34]

The Swedish author Therese Bohman has explored media representation in further depth by addressing how the very description "good girl

[32] Goodhart, *The road to somewhere.*

[33] Maria Kjos Fonn, "En mur av muligheter", *Samtiden* 127, no. 3 (2017), 52.

[34] Ibid., 53.

syndrome" is based on a specific class affiliation.[35] Popular feminism would convince girls that the solution to the good girl syndrome is for young girls and adult women to stop being so clever. To say to hell with it, quite simply. That may appear to be sound advice, but as Bohman points out, such advice often stems from a privileged class background which the adviser personally does not bother to reflect upon:

> Rejecting the good girl is a middle-class norm. [...] Violation of norms seems paradoxically to be a kind of middle-class tradition – much like the tradition of rebelling against tradition. But for those in need of a safety net to fall back on, a norm of norm-violation can be a curse, and culminate in running one's existence into the ground – the kind of ground which is never a real risk for the person encouraging violation of norms.[36]

The advice to become a rebellious Pippi Longstocking instead of her proper, boring best friend Annika can have costly repercussions for people from the working class, for whom cleverness at school is the only means of moving up and ahead, Bohman points out. For many it remains true that goodness first and foremost creates opportunities rather than limitations. An upwardly mobile class journey is founded on goodness and has potentially revolutionary implications for the good girl's future. Certain revolts take place in silence, Bohman concludes.

Left-Wing Media?

The way the Norwegian media has embraced the term "achievement generation" also reflects the dominant perception of reality in the segment of Norway holding the power of definition. In the USA, the leading generation-labels such as "millennials" and more overtly critical characterizations such as "the Me generation" and "generation snowflake" speak to different societal concerns and perceptions than those found in Norway. A constantly recurring point of contention is whether it makes

[35] Therese Bohman, "Til duktighetens försvar", in *Klassresan*, eds. Tobias Krantz and Karin Rebas (Stockholm: Bertil Ohlin Förlag, 2015).
[36] Ibid., 71.

any difference that Norwegian journalists vote to the Left of the average Norwegian. A counter-argument is often made regarding the growth of the far-right Progress Party in recent decades, about which historian Martin Eide has claimed: "Essentially no Norwegian journalist would vote for them, but the development in journalism towards a tendency to focus on individuals, strong feelings and melodramatic elements has of course produced a kind of media coverage and publicity that has been advantageous for them."[37] But as media studies researcher Kjersti Thorbjørnsrud has stated, nobody is neutral in terms of values and that includes Left-wing journalists who "influence the perception of what is given".[38] Applied to the theme of this book, it's conceivable that in recent years, Norwegian journalists have accepted the achievement generation diagnosis as a given because their basic political views entail an underlying acceptance of a "that's how capitalism is" mentality, in which increased competition and performance pressure have huge human costs.

The descriptions of generations can also encompass and promote political interests and perceptions of reality. A term such as "generation snowflake" has the effect of confirming the identity of the Right wing as a group that puts the importance of freedom of expression above all else, unlike the young generation of rights-conscious, identity politics warriors. "The achievement generation" has the effect of confirming the identity of the Left-wing as a group opposing capitalism's competitiveness and devoted to their conviction that the social structures are the cause, and above all, not the young people personally. In both cases, the foremost function of the image of a generation the labels represent is to confirm the truth of a group's world view: either freedom of expression is under threat because the West has lost its self-confidence and forgotten to protect its universal values or human worth is endangered by capitalism, which can be seen popping up constantly in our institutions, such as in the school's performance requirements. The conservatives see the Left-wing's tendency to blame society as a sign of decline at a time when the national sentiment is weakened and young people are primarily

---

[37] Glenn Slydal Johansen, "Forskere uenige om venstrevridde journalister", (2015), https://journalisten.no/2015/05/forskere-delt-om-venstrevridde-journalister

[38] Ibid., 7.

dedicated to criticizing the society of which they are a part.[39] The Left, on the other hand, has its demonized image of the Right as white, privileged individuals who don't particularly care about those more disadvantaged than themselves.

What Must Be Done?

As stated in the introduction to this chapter, the question of how young people are actually doing is encumbered by considerable uncertainty and is also an illustrative example of what Hacking calls "moving targets"—the objects of social scientific research change constantly because our investigations interact with and change them.[40] Despite this uncertainty, I have collated some potential measures below which may not be able to be implemented in a practical sense, but which identify neglected and problematic aspects of the existing practice.

A Good Enough Society

As Freud reflected in his day, a condition for ensuring that people, young and old alike, will thrive, is for the culture to foster a system that does not oblige individuals to live beyond their psychological means. On the basis of this, some historical eras and forms of society can be viewed as more or less successful, and those that are less expedient can be defined as neurotic civilizations. Ryan LaMothe has stipulated that to be able to make such diagnoses of a contemporary society, we must necessarily have a clear idea of what characterizes *a good enough society*.[41] The source of inspiration here is the British paediatrician Donald Winnicott's well-known concept of "a good enough mother", which has since been updated to the more gender-neutral "a good enough parent"—for which the basic formula for

[39] Thomas Sowell, "Mascots of the anointed", in *The Thomas Sowell reader*, ed. Thomas Sowell (New York: Basic Books, 2011).

[40] Ian Hacking, "Making up people", *London Review of Books* 28, no. 16 (2006).

[41] LaMothe, "The travails and tragedies of a market civilization: a psychology of faith perspective".

mental health is to refrain from seeking perfection, both in oneself and one's child. The following questions come to mind as an expansion of the idea of a "good enough" civilization: "What kind of civilization would promote and contribute to mental health? What type of civilization contributes to social well-being? Does well-being include all citizens?"[42] And we might add to this the question of why some people struggle with mental health ailments and disorders in specific cultures, while others are spared. The answer seems roughly to be forms of society in which social, political and economic stressors do not overburden the individual's psychological means. The Ungdata surveys in a wealthy welfare state such as Norway also confirm that children from poor families struggle the most. Youth who experience that their family is financially disadvantaged, consistently report far more psychological ailments than youth from well-to-do homes.

Different Medicine

As explained in the preceding chapters, we are presumably dealing with at least two different groups of young people who are afflicted with psychological disorders: a growing group of more privileged young people who are struggling with new risks, particularly associated with the requirements of the new individualism, on the one hand, and on the other, the more traditional, disadvantaged group for whom key terms are nonaffluent, family problems, abuse, drug/alcohol abuse, bullying and school absenteeism, and who continue to represent the majority of the cases. For these different groups, it is reasonable to assume that different social medicines should be prescribed. As the physician Ingebjørn Bleidvin put it in *Bergens Tidende*: "The first group goes around feeling things too much and expecting too much from life. The other group feels things too little and should expect much more from life."[43] Bleidvin specifies that it's a matter of striking a difficult balance between removing the

[42] Ibid., 156.

[43] Ingebjørn Bleidvin, "Det me ikkje snakkar om", *Bergens Tidende* (2017), https://www.bt.no/btmeninger/kommentar/i/OR23E/Det-me-ikkje-snakkar-om, para. 9.

stigma of mental illness so the latter group will find it easier to seek help, while the former group must take care not to exaggerate their focus on what they are feeling by constantly checking the balance of their happiness account so that even the smallest of setbacks in the group's self-realization project constitutes the basis for declaring themselves ill. The tendency towards polarization in this generation's idea of illness also entails a danger that well-intended, general measures will never reach the largest group and can prove superfluous, or even, paradoxically, further compound the problems of the other, smaller group.

The Disadvantaged Among Us

An underlying consequence of the distorted interest in the most resourceful group as opposed to the disadvantaged group is how the latter has greater difficulties in being heard even though they are known to have the greatest need. In a discussion in the journal *Syn og Segn,* psychology specialist Arnhild Lauveng remarks on the danger of our giving too much help to those who need it the least, and here she mentions specifically the example of youth who are struggling with performance pressure: "Why should a child with sick parents, who has lived in poverty, with parents who are psychologically ill and possibly addicts, be delivered into the hands of untrained healthcare professionals in an institution, while youth with resourceful parents and a good social network are given therapy sessions with specialists?"[44] Næs, also cited above, has addressed the problem of how low-threshold mental health services are often filled to capacity by resourceful individuals with higher education who in principle are least vulnerable to mental illness.[45] As an example, the Norwegian Institute of Public Health's evaluation of a low-threshold mental health scheme (*Rask psykisk helsehjelp*) revealed that among those who solicited help from the service, 45 percent had higher education, while the average in the population at large is 30 percent. Persons with a low level of education and low incomes tend to postpone seeking help and their ailments therefore

[44] Eskil Skjeldal, "-Det ville nok vore lurt å gje meg aktiv dødshjelp", *Syn og Segn* 124, no. 2 (2018).
[45] Næs, "En katalysator for økte forskjeller".

become compounded and more destructive. And because of late intervention, they derive fewer benefits from the treatment in municipal services and must often be referred to national-level specialist services. The threshold for receiving help there is high, however, for both children and adults. And in this manner, the system reinforces already existing differences. Næs also points out that the growing market of private psychologist practices, for those who can afford it, has no admission criteria and you can get an appointment the same day; stress, performance anxiety, self-esteem and healthier relationships are on the menu,[46] along with the "good girl syndrome". The time for the psychology profession to review its essentially amiable "everyone is included" and "no disorder is insignificant for me" motto, seems overdue, and in all likelihood we must contend with, to a greater extent, and address social ethics dilemmas pertaining to the use of resources and prioritizing, a task which the medical profession has up until now proven best equipped to carry out.

We Need to Talk About It

We have seen throughout this book how the strategy of talking about it consistently appears to be the supposed social medicine accorded the greatest credence. In accordance with the ideal of achieving a mental hygienic catharsis through verbalization of the inner, emotional life, increasingly more young people are requesting life and stress mastery as a part of the Norwegian school system's curriculum to prepare the young for a long working life. The adults among us have also requested this. In 2015, a number of key actors, among them the Norwegian Psychological Association, the Norwegian Psychiatric Association, Norwegian Council for Mental Health, Mental Health Youth, the School Student Union of Norway and the Norwegian Association of Secondary School Teachers joined forces in the campaign "The Book We are Missing" (*Boken som mangler*) to bring psychology into the schools:

[46] Ibid.

> For generations, the school has taught classes about students' physiological health. Physical activity and nutrition have been central themes on the curriculum. The purpose of all instruction is to give children tools so they can manage in life. But the ABCs of their thoughts, feelings and actions are not in their book bags. THIS IS NOT ONLY A SHAME – IT IS INCOMPREHENSIBLE.[47]

The campaign would prove successful. As a part of the curriculum renewal of the Knowledge Promotion Programme (*Kunnskapsløftet*), it has now been decided that *public health and coping strategies* will be one of the three interdisciplinary subjects of priority, along with *democracy and citizenship* and *sustainable development* starting in the autumn of 2020.[48] The school is to help train students' competencies in the realm of social and emotional skills. It still remains to be seen what the nature of these subjects will be in practice, but in light of the above issue, one must question whether a life-mastery class in which students are to develop their social and emotional skills will help the largest disadvantaged group of young people. How is it expected that this group will derive benefits from such instruction and develop competencies, if part of the problem is that they are not present, either mentally or physically? While for the other, more privileged group, "the achievement generation", one must consider whether a life-mastery class from official quarters will only serve to consolidate the already existing perception of being personally responsible for dealing with the stress and pressure in their lives.

The Ludvigsen report, one of the key supporting documents for the white paper on renewal of the Knowledge Promotion scheme, states in its recommendation that students of the future must strengthen their ability to learn how to learn through psychological strategies such as *metacognition and self-regulation*.[49] The question, however, is whether there is a risk of the students to an even larger degree than previously being thereby

[47] Norwegian Psychological Association et al., "Boken som mangler", (2015 https://www.psykologforeningen.no/foreningen/nyheter-og-kommentarer/aktuelt/krever-psykologi-i-skolen#opprop), 2.

[48] Stortingsmelding, "Meld. St. 28. Fag – Fordypning – Forståelse. En fornyelse av Kunnskapsløftet", (Oslo: Kunnskapsdepartementet, 2016).

[49] NOU, "NOU 2015: 8 Fremtidens skole: Fornyelse av. fag og kompetanser", (Oslo: Kunnskapsdepartementet, 2015).

held responsible for their own learning. The experiences from other countries, such as Canada, can suggest this, where psychologist Jack Martin and social worker Ann-Marie McLellan offer the following status report:

> In the absence of any clear and convincing distinction between self-regulation and teacher or psychologist regulation of student conduct and learning, all that has changed is a redirection of responsibility for the maintenance of appropriate levels of student conduct from psychoeducators to students themselves.[50]

In Norway, psychologists Ida Brandtzæg, Stig Torsteinson and Guro Øiestad and authors of the book "Seeing the Pupil From the Inside-out" (*Se eleven innenfra*), which in principle welcomes psychology into the school, have posed a timely question about whether the belief in improving students' mental health knowledge and competencies through the curriculum renewal of the Knowledge Promotion scheme can have the effect of undermining the relationships between teachers and students.[51] The life-mastery initiative in the school system has been chiselled out within the parameters of individualization and accountability, which have been specifically pinpointed as social variables that create problems for many students. It is doubtful that the planned training will equip the students to change them.

Life Sucks

If there is one book that is lacking in the school system, is it necessarily "The ABCs of thoughts, feelings and actions"? One question is whether the achievement generation would actually be better served with a reality-check about existence, *The Tragedy Reader*, rather than "a gym class for

---

[50] Jack Martin and Ann-Marie McLellan, *The education of selves: how psychology transformed students* (New York: Oxford University Press, 2013), 154.

[51] Ida Brandtzæg, Stig Torsteinson, and Guro Øiestad, "Folkehelse og livsmestring i skolen", *Tidsskrift for Norsk psykologforening* 54, no. 8 (2017).

thoughts and feelings".[52] Here there is an abundant canon of texts to choose from that could serve to remind young people of life's tragic realities, such as German philosopher Arthur Schopenhauer's radically dark vision: "Life swings like a pendulum backward and forward between pain and boredom."[53] When the goal of existence is no longer to do your duty, but to enjoy life as much as possible, which indeed also becomes a duty, even the most minor setback acquires the nature of something scandalous. In such a cultural climate, it is not surprising that tragic insights on the meaninglessness of life are not much in demand. Kaja Melsom has even suggested that the tragedies should be given a renaissance: "To counteract today's freedom ideal, we need modern tragedies that warn us against believing that as long as we just listen to ourselves and make the 'right' choices, we will be rewarded with a long and happy life."[54] Svend Brinkmann has taken inspiration from the Ancient Stoics and recommends instead of attentiveness to how you are actually feeling, to try thinking about something or someone that/who really means something in your life, such as your children and to imagine how it would feel if they were to be lost.[55] Young people who don't have children can replace the child with a mobile phone. The mental exercise will hopefully engender more gratitude for what we have, whether this be a beloved child or an iPhone.

Existentialism, Where Did You Go in the Midst of All the Chaos?

The fact that it should even be necessary to give this type of advice today can indicate that something has been lost. This raises the question of whether existentialism's language for being, with its emphasis on death, alienation, meaninglessness and freedom, has been lost. In the

[52] Tor Levin Hofgaard, "Psykologi må bli pensum!", *NRK Ytring* (2015), http://www.nrk.no/ytring/psykologi-ma-bli-pensum_-1.12499881

[53] Arthur Schopenhauer, *Verden som vilje og forestilling* (Oslo: Solum, 2000), 177.

[54] Melsom, *Den fordømte friheten*, 149.

[55] Brinkmann, *Stand firm: resisting the self-improvement craze.*

achievement society, existentialism's *being* becomes secondary knowledge,[56] and the current, always online, 24/7-satiety does not leave much room for the pursuit of existential contemplation. One of existentialism's progenitors, Nietzsche, predicted precisely such a development, even though the Internet had not been yet invented, when in the late nineteenth century, he foresaw how the modern human being would replace a device such as "God" with the earthly ideal of happiness and health whereby everything becomes small. Here it is ignorant apathy that prevails rather than raw anxiety about the basic conditions of existence.

When I was doing my psychology studies in the early 2000s, excerpts from the American psychiatrist Irvin Yalom's great work *Existential Psychotherapy* were still on the syllabus, but they are not any longer. It is apparently less important for the psychologists of tomorrow to learn the basic questions about existence.[57] Instead, the diagnostic language of illness, heavily informed by health sciences such as psychology and medicine, is increasingly prevalent. A number of others have commented, among them the Norwegian philosopher Lars Fredrik Svendsen, on how common colloquialisms such as "a cold", "headache", "tired" and "fed up" appear to have been replaced by medical and psychological labels such as "influenza", "migraine", "burn-out" and "depressed".[58] The Swedish philosopher Fredrik Svenaeus has also noted how little we value the significance of illness and suffering today in his book *Homo Patologicus*:

> We abandon the question of why we are suffering and replace it with the cultivation of different diagnoses. This tendency does not represent any scientific advancement; it is instead a kind of abuse, or at least an exaggerated use of medical terminology in our desperate attempt to give suffering a rational explanation and meaning.[59]

---

[56] Emil Valdimarsson, "Kig op, drop selviscenesættelsen, og forpligt dig til noget større", *Politiken*, 21 July 2018.

[57] Irvin David Yalom, *Existential psychotherapy* (New York: Basic Books, 1980).

[58] Gunnar Ringheim, "Vår tåleevne er svekket", *Dagbladet*, 21 November 2009.

[59] Fredrik Svenaeus, *Homo patologicus: medicinska diagnoser i vår tid* (Hägersten: TankeKraft, 2013), 57.

Svenaeus illustrates this through the example of waking up at the devil's hour with the cold sweats: had this been the 1950s, we would have viewed it as *existential anxiety*, while today we will tend to view it as *a panic attack*. The former interpretation invites contemplation over one's life, while the latter is treated by a visit to the doctor. Another of the founders of existentialism, the Danish philosopher Søren Kierkegaard, in his work *The Concept of Anxiety*, described precisely this feeling of anxiety as a serving spirit that haunts us to remind us of freedom's possibility: "Then the assaults of anxiety, even though they be terrifying, will not be such that he flees from them. For him, anxiety becomes a serving spirit that against its will leads him where he wishes to go."[60] The view of anxiety as a "serving spirit" is far-fetched for us today. Existentialism can be criticized for overly romanticizing negative feelings, leading to the unnecessary cultivation of disorders. But it does contain the space and a language for life's darker aspects, which our current therapeutic culture has largely banished. An illustrative example is the underlying view of emotions informing the popular psychoeducational self-help kits for *Psychological First Aid* which are used in Norwegian kindergartens and schools, child health clinics and treatment institutions to teach children and young people to assume control over their own lives.[61] Positive thoughts are here represented by the good-natured figure Green and negative thoughts are represented by the grim and devilish Red. The message is hard to misinterpret: painful thoughts and feelings are something to be kept out of life in the interests of mental hygiene.

To the Root of the Problem

But if this is a real problem today, the responsibility for its reintroduction can naturally not be left on the shoulders of young people alone. And the proposal for *The Tragedy Reader* can, like life-mastery courses in the schools, be accused of insufficiently diverging from the framework of

[60] Søren Kierkegaard, *Begrepet angst* (Oslo: Oktober, 2001), 203.

[61] Solfrid Raknes, *Psykologisk førstehjelp barn* (Oslo: Gyldendal Akademisk, 2010); *Psykologisk førstehjelp ungdom* (Oslo: Gyldendal Akademisk, 2010).

individualization and accountability. This would require a more radical approach. The Latin American liberation psychologist Ignacio Martín-Baró operated with an idea about *consciousness-raising* according to which no intervention in the life of an individual could be considered successful unless the person was thereby equipped to change some of the objective life conditions under which he or she is living.[62] Changing somebody's feelings or thoughts in reaction to a situation is not enough, and neither is life and stress mastery, or tragedy studies. On the other hand, interventions that enabled young people to challenge the existing representations of youth created by the media, such as "the achievement generation" and "the good girl syndrome", would be a place to start. Initially this could entail raising the consciousness of youth in terms of how these categorizations are not neutral in any sense, but have their unique creation story, which has brought us to where we are today, a situation in which few are able to see any solution other than having the school teach students strategies for coping with stress and pressure. This in turn could inspire young people to employ alternative representations of themselves and their generation, which could ideally lead to new visions to challenge the entire mentality underpinning self-optimization and accountability through extreme regulation of own body, psyche and life. This would clearly be in the spirit of Nietzsche and Dufour, in that rather than passively conforming to the prevailing religious and political ideologies, individuals will become capable of creating new "Gods", utopias and concepts.

Silence Is Golden

Another point that is rarely spoken about by the enlightened culture of confession is whether the well-intended concern of parents, healthcare workers, politicians and other official figures can paradoxically become a suffocating over-protectiveness. In a refreshing manoeuvre, the psychoanalytically oriented psychologist Per Are Løkke put a pin in young people and instead directed his focus on the parents involved:

---

[62] Ignacio Martín-Baró, "The role of the psychologist", in *Writings for a liberation psychology*, ed. Ignacio Martín-Baró, Adrianne Aron, and Shawn Corne (Boston: Harvard University Press, 1995).

> The idea about 'being close' is a key term for the new parenthood. Parents want to abolish the traditional, role-based distance to their children. But this heated investment in their children also has unfortunate side-effects. The parents seek to create an illusory closeness with their children, the consequence of which becomes that the capacity to tolerate life experiences connected to psychological pain, separation and loneliness is undermined.[63]

Løkke also bases his insights on Winnicott, who in his time specified that neither parents nor society for that matter should be too quick to intervene in young people's struggles with separation issues or psychological conflicts. If the adult generation prematurely provides ready responses in the form of diagnoses or manuals, young people are deprived of the building blocks required to personally create the basis for individuation and creativity. Many will instinctively object to this old-fashioned, laissez faire attitude to the problems of youth, but rather than being based on cold indifference, the argument derives from an analytical insight: if parents become *too* involved in the normal development of young people, the latter risk formation of what Winnicott called a *false self*—the development of a "successful mask" primarily designed to please and reassure adults. Løkke explains how Winnicott's understanding of adolescence was contingent upon a transaction phase in which one was to adapt to a new, interior landscape, from biological maturation through the body's sexual and aggressive impulses, to the need to stand up to one's parents and even *not* be understood. The spirit of our times appears to be a monomaniac focus on the diametrically opposed solution:

> We see that Winnicott's advice, to 'wait', 'have confidence', 'give them time and space' and 'not interrupt' has been discarded on the junkpile of history. Today it is on the contrary a matter of intervening and controlling as quickly as possible. Professional expertise has moved away from old and more complicated models that required a subjective assessment of whether it is right to wait or get involved in each individual case. Today it is always best to intervene as early and as quickly as possible.[64]

[63] Per Are Løkke, "Å hakke seg ut av egget", *Tidsskrift for Norsk psykologforening* 53, no. 3 (2016), 202.
[64] Ibid., 204.

Of course, there will be young people requiring timely help from adults and in need of psychological or medical treatment; Løkke also acknowledges this and cites a critique of Winnicott about how at times he put too much faith in the resilience of youth. But at this juncture, when it is not possible to intervene too soon, it becomes appropriate to ask whether the time has not come to recuperate Winnicott's view from the junkpile as a necessary counterweight.

An adult approach to handling the dilemma, of course, is not to close our eyes to the problems, but neither can we close our eyes to the reality that the eyes that see are unable to observe from the outside, the way an astronomer can observe Halley's Comet without having an impact on its appearance. Maybe we can learn something from its return after all; the last time it was in the Earth's vicinity was in 1986 and is not expected back again until 2061. The idea of a new survey and subsequent media coverage about the living conditions of young people every seventy-fifth year is taking things a bit too far, but a certain waiting period between each time we carry out soul-searching on a national scale, in which all young people are asked: "How are you really doing?" is probably not a bad idea. Naturally, it is in the interest of research to acquire data on a regular and timely basis, but perhaps we could at least be more restrictive about not publicizing the data in the media quite so often, in that young girls' psychological disorders in particular have a tendency to be blown out of proportion. And it is likely that the young people will thereby acquire more time and space to develop visions beyond that of purely self-accusatory notions about how they must learn better coping strategies for stress. And then one could direct the resources that have been freed up towards more targeted measures for the disadvantaged group.

Nothing New Under the Sun: The Youth of the Past

> What has been will be again, what has been done will be done again; there is nothing new under the sun. (Ecclesiastes 1:9)[65]

[65] Bibelselskapet, *Bibelen. Det gamle og det nye testamentet* (Oslo: Bibelselskapet, 2011), 742.

Discussing the well-being of young people can trigger associations of air bubbles trapped behind wallpaper. If you flatten the bubbles in one place, they will unavoidably pop up somewhere else on the wall. When I grew up in the 1990s, the worries about young people were especially about *peer pressure to smoke and drink*. Now that young people are becoming more respectable, spending less time out with their friends and generally proving less inclined to indulge in drugs and alcohol than before, the adult concern nonetheless does not seem to be disappearing, but is instead displaced onto anxieties about the pressure school or social media are imposing on the minds of their children. The sum of worries appears to be just as constant as the sum of burdens, a point that finds expression in headlines such as "The mobile phone is young people's new drug of choice".[66]

To worry about the younger, coming generation is also an activity as old as civilization itself. A much-cited quote about the young that is often attributed to Socrates can be found in Norwegian newspapers dating as far back as 1948:

> The children of our time love luxury, they have bad manners, they despise authority, show no respect for the elderly, they waste time instead of learning anything useful. Children are now the tyrants of the home, rather than its servants. They no longer stand up when adults enter the room. They contradict their parents, interrupt the conversations of adults, slurp their food, sit with their legs crossed and tyrannize their teachers.[67]

This quote has since then appeared more than sixty times in Norwegian newspapers, but remarkably enough, only once in the 1970s, the decade which the American author Tom Wolfe in his day christened *The Me Decade* to capture the introverted dwelling upon the self that was becoming increasingly popular among young people.[68] It is tempting to speculate about whether the adult generation's eagerness to apply an apologetic attitude to the youthful excesses of the time was at an all-time low during

---

[66] Tybring-Gjedde, "Mobiltelefonen er ungdommens nye rusmiddel".

[67] Lillehammer Tilskuer, "Lørdagskroken", *Lillehammer Tilskuer*, 31 July 1948, 6.

[68] Tom Wolfe, "The 'me' decade and the third great awakening", *New York Magazine*, 23 August 1976.

that decade. It is not at all certain the Socrates said this, however, in that there are no direct written sources. Some have cited Aristophanes' comedy *The Clouds* from 423 BC as a possible origin, where Socrates is ridiculed and embodied by one of the characters, who says: "In my day, children were seen but not heard."[69]

Despite the apparently universal nature of adults' complaints about young people, there would appear to be an important difference today. The annual Ungdata reports, by comparison, do not depict an image of rebellion in any sense, but rather a well-adjusted, active and home-loving generation of Norwegian youth, most of whom are content and very satisfied, although a significant percentage experience worries in their daily lives. In particular, there are many girls who find school to be stressful—mental health ailments are on the increase and not just for girls, but in the surveys of recent years, for boys as well. Generational diagnoses such as the "CV Generation" and "Generation Perfection" indicate that the worries of today are not in any sense about morality, 2500 years after Aristophanes, but about the psyche. A hypothesis that can explain the "achievement generation" can therefore be that we are dealing with an apparently unceasing complaint on the part of the parental generation about youth, but in contrast to previous eras, this dissatisfaction is now not primarily moral indignation, but rather a therapeutic concern. This hypothesis is compatible with historical studies of shifts in values in the twentieth century up to the present day, which show that intolerance is receding, while fear is on the rise.[70] In short, we are perhaps less morally judgemental of others' alternative lifestyles, but also generally more worried about just everything.

I have previously described a *therapeutic turn* in Western contemporary culture in which psychology assumes the role of the religion of our times, in keeping with the liberal, secular individualism and where morality doesn't have much currency, while mental and physical health become the standard against which everything else is measured.[71] The adult

[69] Aristofanes, *Skyene* (Oslo: Aschehoug, 1977), 71.

[70] Alberto Acerbi et al., "The expression of emotions in 20th century books", *PLOS ONE* 8, no. 3 (2013).

[71] Madsen, *The therapeutic turn. How psychology altered Western culture.*

generation's dismay over the moral decline of the coming generation thereby appears to be increasingly replaced by worries about something being hazardous to the health. "*What does it do to us*?" becomes the fundamental question we continually ask about all new social changes, even climate change.[72] And as I have demonstrated in the preceding chapters, we often allow our personal scapegoats to colour our perception of what is the most hazardous to young people's health, whether this be capitalism, the Conservative party government's result-oriented education policy or the digital see-and-be-seen platforms such as Instagram, Snapchat and Facebook.

Don't Speak: The Young People of Today

Maybe there is another underappreciated difference between then and now, as society and the adult generation become more morally tolerant but emotionally speaking more worried about how we think about young people? The NRK series *Lisenskontrolløren* ("The Viewing License Controller"), which serves up cultural history from the Norwegian Broadcasting Corporation's abundant archives, can help to illustrate this point. An episode on the subject of young people is introduced by a clip from the time of colour television's infancy in the 1970s, where an older woman is asked the question: "What do you think about the young people of today?" to which she replies with a smile: "They don't do anything. They're living the good life."[73] Host Njål Engesæth then cuts to an interview in black and white, with the young people themselves, presumably from the 1960s, who understand the current state of affairs somewhat differently: "The way things are now I am not happy at all."[74] The implication is that adults have always failed to understand youth and youth have always complained about how it is to be young. Engesæth effectively illustrates how a series of recurring themes in the social debate about

[72] "'Hva gjør det med oss?'", *Tidsskrift for Norsk psykologforening* 51, nr. 11 (2014).

[73] Njål Engesæth, "Lisenskontrolløren: Ungdom", (Oslo: NRK, 2017 https://tv.nrk.no/serie/lisenskontrolloeren/sesong/4/episode/3/avspiller), 0:03.

[74] Ibid., 0:14.

young people in the year 2020, such as that there are too many performances, testing and theoretical requirements in the schools, have been issues of concern for several decades. But there is an important difference all the same. Today it is unusual to come across adults who respond that young people do not do anything and are living the good life. The prevailing opinion, on the contrary, is that young people do far too much and are subjected to more requirements and greater pressure than previously, as expressed by Norway's King Harald in his New Year's address, cited in the introduction to this book. The explanation for this shift can be that when adults no longer regard young people with a strict, moral gaze, but rather with therapeutic, empathetic concern, there is less distance in the assessments of how they are doing than before. "The generation gap that disappeared" is youth researchers Tormod Øia and Viggo Vestel's description of the change in the relationship between young people and adults of today, which they hold leads to a new, more positive and dialogic relationship.[75] The sociologist Willy Pedersen has even speculated about whether the field of youth research attracts "adult children", who thereby receive a much welcome opportunity for contact with something childish.[76] Adults cease to serve as a contrast to youth's eternal complaining—and instead become equal allies who agree that young people are having a difficult time. But a consequence of this equalizing of the generations can be that young people instead become more insecure and worried, which in turn makes adults even more uneasy about how they will manage. In this sense, we are perhaps dealing with a mutually reinforcing effect of alarming observations, which people previously recovered from with greater facility. Adults of previous generations were quicker to respond with moral indignation about young people and thereby more inclined to declare that young people had a life that was too easy. Therapeutic assessments of how young people are doing, on the other hand, will tend to lead to conclusions that they are struggling. Ironically, moral prejudices about young people's lifestyle are therefore perhaps healthier therapeutically speaking than the widespread, well-

[75] Tormod Øia and Viggo Vestel, "Generasjonskløfta som forsvant", *Tidsskrift for Ungdomsforskning* 14, no. 1 (2014).

[76] Willy Pedersen, *Ungdom er bare et ord* (Oslo: Universitetsforlaget, 1994).

intentioned concern for young people of our day, where they shall preferably be *both* seen and heard on all channels.

Now and then one sees signs that young people also long for the moral authority their parents formerly represented. A couple of years ago, the twenty-two-year-old Westerdal student Johanna Holt Kleive related an episode from when she was thirteen and wanted to rebel against her parents so she painted skulls on her bedroom closet. The response of her mother, however, was far more understanding than condemning: "How nice that you found a form of self-expression, sweetie."[77] Kleive hits the nail on the head when she concludes with the following appeal: "I want the previous generation to call me a spoiled brat."[78]

A key element of the adult-child relationship has traditionally been the passing down of a moral code from one generation to the next. One of the most important components of the adult role has been to raise children with a set of religious or ethical rules for how they should live. However, many signs indicate that we have become squeamish about morality in the current cultural climate, since the distinction between *morality* and being *moralistic* is in the process of breaking down. Nobody today wants to be moralistic. This is not to say that today's parents refrain from involvement with their children, the opposite is rather the case, but the particular aspect of child-rearing that pertained to passing on a moral core from one generation to the next appears to be changing.[79] Authority is no longer a given and has thereby been usurped by something else. And an obvious candidate is the anti-authoritative therapeutic gaze, which with an empathetic expression asks: "How are you doing, really?" and "Do you want to talk about it?"

[77] Johanna Holt Kleive, "Forbanna på følelses-tv", *Dagens Næringsliv* (2016), http://www.dn.no/etterBors/2016/04/20/1130/Psykisk-helse/forbanna-p-flelsestv, paragraph 4.

[78] Ibid., paragraph 11.

[79] Foros and Vetlesen, *Angsten for oppdragelsen. Et samfunnsetisk perspektiv på dannelse (2nd edition).*

Generation Screwed: The Young People of the Future

Labels for youth such as "the achievement generation" also disclose something about contemporary culture, such as that there is a plethora of opportunities for young people that will enable them to evolve and grow as they wish in the name of self-realization and that they are living in the land and era of opportunity. It is very likely that this will change and is already in the process of doing so for many young people if one looks to countries less privileged than Norway. The news site *Huffington Post* published an article with the suggestive headline "Generation Screwed", which reflects the fact that the millennium generation of the USA, the generation born between 1982 and 2004, is probably facing the most serious economic recession since the Great Depression of the 1930s.[80] It is only half as likely that young Americans today will own their own home, compared to 1975, while student loans have increased on the average by 300 percent. A thirty-five-year-old journalist Michael Hobbes starts by explaining that, like many others of his generation, he has waited a decade for adult life to commence. But it is increasingly difficult when the rent consumes half of your income, you have not had a permanent job in years and savings are running out. Hobbes describes an economic situation in which many young people must live with their parents, postpone getting married and buying a home and wait longer to have children than any previous generation. Simultaneously, they are forced to hear from the older generation in the USA that the problem is simply that they are far too sensitive, lazy or spoiled. But as Hobbes specifies, the defining experience for the millennium generation is not helicopter parents or *Pokémon Go* but rather uncertainty about the future.[81] In Norway, we have been privileged enough that young people have been spared such recessions but that can change in the future. An OECD report from 2018 highlights that the labour market for fifteen- to twenty-nine-year-olds in Norway is still the most favourable of all the OECD nations, but the employment rate among young people has decreased significantly in

[80] Hobbes, "Generation screwed".

[81] Ibid.

Norway in recent years, and the number of new jobs on offer has not kept up with population growth, predominantly due to increased immigration from Central and Eastern Europe.[82]

There is one topic which has not yet been discussed, but which constitutes a highly legitimate cause for youthful despondency: human created climate change. Here the young people of today have an objective reason to fear the future, given the prognoses from the UN climate panel and the world's leading climate scientists. The most recent prognoses establish that there is now only a 5 percent chance of meeting the UN's climate targets, which means that the climate changes will become uncontrolled and inhospitable conditions such as extreme heat in some regions will be the outcome.[83] In the book entitled tellingly "How do we answer?" (*Hvad skal vi svare?)*, Arne Johan Vetlesen and the Danish sociologist Rasmus Willig point out how the relation between generations up until now has been defined by the idea that every generation shall leave its house to the next generation in slightly better condition than when they personally assumed ownership.[84] In the age of globalization, the house is now represented by the entire globe, but there are many indications that the coming generation must be prepared to inherit an earth that ecologically speaking will be in worse condition than when it was inherited by the previous generation.

Climate has only to a very limited extent been addressed in the context of diagnoses of young people's current living conditions, but as a part of the 2017 election in Norway, psychologist and acting member of parliament for the Green Party, Per Espen Stoknes argued that environmental policy is also the right social medicine for the coming generation: "It is pretty meaningless to offer young people individualistic psychotherapy and medication as long as the society they are growing up in destroys precisely what they need the most: a feeling of security about the future [...] Then 'the achievement generation' can become 'the quality of life generation'."[85] Stoknes here enacts a longed-for revision of the usual

[82] OECD, "Investing in youth Norway", (Paris: OECD Publishing, 2018).

[83] Adrian E. Raftery et al., "Less than 2 °C warming by 2100 unlikely", *Nature Climate Change* 7 (2017).

[84] Arne Johan Vetlesen and Rasmus Willig, *Hvad skal vi svare?* (Copenhagen: Hans Reitzel, 2017).

[85] Per Espen Stoknes, "Feil medisin!", *Klassekampen*, 24 August 2017, 23.

discussion about the achievement generation, where the achievement society's mainstays of competition and growth are now challenged by the necessity to live more sustainably. At the same time, it is alarming if the reorientation only becomes a pretext for further assessments of quality of life and mental health on a national scale. The Green Party has even proposed a new national survey every year which will ask the population: "How are you doing?":

> Norwegian youth are living in the richest country in the world, they have more things than ever before, yet a record number are taking migraine medication, have psychological problems and don't see the point of living, says Green Party MP Per Espen Stoknes, who is also a psychologist. He maintains that this clearly illustrates that it is possible to better facilitate an experience of having a meaningful life in Norway.[86]

Although the climate crisis is the most important issue of our times, there is cause for scepticism if the proposal leads to more national soul-searching, measurements and media attention on how young people are *really* doing. But hopefully the measure will not lead to the climate issue being made subordinate to issues of quality of life and mental health, but instead be a step towards realization of a more ecologically sustainable society, where the vision of a good enough society is based on values other than a unilateral cultivation of the growth of the Gross National Product (GNP).

Conclusion: Overloading "Young People"

Thirty years ago, the German youth researcher Thomas Ziehe gave a lecture at the Nordic Summer University in Stockholm in which he speculated about how what he called the *youth discourse*, in other words, how we speak and think about young people, will evolve in the time ahead, which in the current context seems quite appropriate.[87] Ziehe noted as far

---

[86] Solveig Ruud, "Hvordan har du det? Det vil fire partier på Stortinget nå ha svar på", *Aftenposten* (2018), https://www.aftenposten.no/norge/politikk/i/RxrpEO/Hvordan-har-du-det-Det-vil-fire-partier-pa-Stortinget-na-ha-svar-pa, paragraph 3–4.

[87] Ziehe, "Ungdom och modernitet", 53.

back as in the 1980s an increasing projection overload for the category "youth" which he predicted would only escalate. The explanation Ziehe proposes is that the youth discourse has become a metaphor for debates about current cultural and social problems related to lifestyle, modernization and the future. Speaking about young people is therefore also to carry out a kind of futurology or research on the future. If we seriously consider Ziehe's claim, it entails that in all the discussions about the achievement generation there is more at stake than just how the young people are doing; it is also about how we are all doing and where we are headed as a society. Young people and our understanding of youth is quite simply a seismograph for the state of the world. Given this ambiguity, we should keep in mind that we have been discussing both how young people are doing and how we are *all* doing. And the advice for how we can best meet these challenges will not necessarily be the same.

In terms of the former, an almost compulsory element would be to remind ourselves that being young has always been difficult. In the above-mentioned unusually self-critical article in *Aftenposten*, where the reader sees that the three girls who represented the achievement generation three years before are now thriving and the article's author asks in retrospect whether the media has given this group too much attention, "Norway's national psychologist"[88] Peder Kjøs assures us: "It's very common to go through a period between the ages of fifteen and twenty when things are experienced as difficult and a struggle. Maybe we shouldn't dramatize things so much."[89] In short: It gets better.

If on the other hand we use "youth" as a prism for discussing some basic human conditions, in other words life in late modernity, it is not certain that this advice will hold water. A key scene from Trier's portrait of the contemporary age *Oslo August 31* (discussed in Chap. 1) can illustrate this. In a scene, Anders' best friend asks him how he is doing and Anders acts out his friend's false reassurances: "It will get better, it will all work out", upon which he states in disillusionment: "It won't you know."[90]

[88] Hege Lyngved Odinsen, "Åpen om sønnens psykiske problemer", *VG+* (2016), http://pluss.vg.no/2016/08/06/2495/2396_23673654, paragraph 2.

[89] Knapstad, "På videregående var. de slitne, stressa og 'sykt flinke'", 36.

[90] Trier, "Oslo, August 31st", 20:52.

For him, as a thinking, sensible human being who doesn't live in the world's (second) happiest country, the only expiatory solution is to allow his life to come to an end along with the film. In short: It *doesn't* get better.

However, it is not in fact irresolute thirty-year-old men who primarily are feeling *the fatigue of the self* in meeting with the twenty-first century's mandate to administrate and optimize one's self; it is instead teenage girls. The most common explanation we hear for why young girls in particular report increasingly more mental health ailments is the story of the fifteen-year-old girl who spends too much time on Instagram, Snapchat and other social media, whereby the effect of social comparisons and dissatisfaction with her own body, appearance and personal success rate produces unhappiness. This is sometimes presented in combination with explanations based on personality psychology, such as how girls are on average more conscientious than boys and are therefore more sensitive to requirements or that in a purely biological sense, they have a more limited window of possibility to have children and therefore less time to get their lives on track. Such explanations, however, have a tendency to focus on social media as a scapegoat rather than viewing screen-based activity as a catalysing medium for something larger. A more radical explanation may be that the young girls growing up today are the first generation to be confronted with a neoliberal culture exceeding national parameters, in which self-management, self-adjustment and self-staging are key ingredients. Globalization's tentacles inexorably find their way into their bedrooms by way of broadband cables and fibre optics. Up to now, teenage boys have been shielded from this pressure due to more liberal gender role requirements, but it would appear they are now also feeling the weight of it. And the ideal of well-trained and thin bodies does not end at the border of the skin, but also fully involves the psyche.

In the contemporary anthropology study *Transnational Popular Psychology and the Global Self-Help Industry*, researchers investigate how political processes of change are reconfigured as invitations to transform the self, using popular psychology and self-help as global remedies.[91] Here they launch the concept of *the thin self*—a desocialized, depoliticized

[91] Daniel Nehring et al., *Transnational popular psychology and the global self-help industry* (London: Palgrave, 2016).

and atomized self which by way of self-help and popular psychology is invited to undergo personal change and achieve goals, cultivated under a neoliberal global order permeated by the dawning instability of traditional institutions and ways of life: "The thin self is confronted with a daily life full of stress, anxiety and uncertainty about the future and the prescribed solutions never have any impact on the root political, social and economic causes of such feelings."[92] Instead, "the thin self" must look within to find new methods for adapting to the expectations for success in late capitalist culture. We are presumably seeing the contours of something similar in Norway, whereby the problems that emerge in the aftermath of the global trend are first registered in the lives of online teenage girls, not unlike the canaries sent into the mines to warn workers of dangerous gases. And for that reason, the public discourse about how young people is really doing will most likely continue with unabated strength in the foreseeable future: because what we are in fact talking about is how all of us are *really* doing.

It may appear that we are now witnessing the fulfilment of Ziehe's prediction, that in the future, the problems of young people and adults will be interwoven to a greater extent: the young, and in particular girls, are forced to both become adults earlier and acquire the discipline that will cultivate their future selves, while society continues to discuss problems that pertain to all of us as if they solely pertained to youth. A clear example of this is the concern about young people's use of social media, which also applies to adults to a great extent. Or the half-hearted admission heard all the time from adults about their lack of interest in environmental and climate change issues, quickly followed by the reassurance: "But my children, they are very interested!" It is as if discussing by way of young people becomes a welcome filter which neatly holds our anxiety at bay. This confusion constitutes a problem for the young people themselves, as Ziehe noted, if a disparity arises between society's preoccupation with the myth of youth and the adults' lack of interest in the actual lives of youth. In this sense, "the achievement generation" can be understood as a widespread adult fantasy about a life dedicated exclusively to self-realization, while the interest in less privileged groups whose situation is

[92] Ibid.

far more representative of young people on the whole is lukewarm at best. And this naturally is also a problem for adults, if we constantly overload the discourse about youth without confronting the problems of our times in any other way except by empathetic, but profoundly empty "how are you *really* doing?" gestures. One thing, at least, is certain: the problems will simply continue to grow if we do not start addressing them in an adult fashion.

References

A-magasinet. "Gåten Martin [The riddle Martin]." *A-magasinet*, 12 February 2016, 1.

Aarbakke, Mari Helendatter. "Flink og ordinær [Good and ordinary]." *Avisa Nordland* (2016, 4 March). https://www.an.no/debatt/flink-og-ordinar/o/5-4-271583.

Aass, Hans Petter. "Kommisjonens 38 punkter [The commission's 38 points]." *VG*, 30 January 1999, 4.

Acerbi, Alberto, Vasileios Lampos, Philip Garnett, and R. Alexander Bentley. "The expression of emotions in 20th century books." *PLOS ONE* 8, nr. 3 (2013): e59030.

Adorno, Theodor W. and Max Horkheimer. *Dialectic of enlightenment: philosophical fragments.* Stanford, CA: Stanford University Press, 2002.

Aftenposten. "[Annonse] [Ad]." *Aftenposten*, 6 November 1907, 4.

———. "Skolepress er årsak til psykiske plager [School pressure the reason for mental health complaints]." *Aftenposten*, 10 July 2017, 1.

Ahlström, Kristofer. "Jag är inte narcissist, men [I am not a narcissist, but]." *Dagens Nyheter*, 16 April 2017, 12–15.

Ainsworth, Susan, and Cynthia Hardy. "The enterprising self: an unsuitable job for an older worker." *Organization* 15, nr. 3 (2008): 389–405.

O. J. Madsen, *Deconstructing Scandinavia's "Achievement Generation"*,
https://doi.org/10.1007/978-3-030-72555-6

Album, Dag, and Eivind Engebretsen. "Sykdomsprestisje [Disease prestige]." *Praktiske Grunde*, nr. 1–2 (2013): 85–92.

American Foundation for Suicide Prevention, "Suicide statistics" (2020), https://afsp.org/suicide-statistics/.

Amundsen, Bård. "Kriminaliteten nesten halvert blant ungdom – mer enn dob-let blant eldre [Crime almost halved among youth]." *forskning.no* (2017, 12 July). https://forskning.no/samfunn-barn-og-ungdom-kriminalitet-samfunnskunnskap/2017/07/kriminaliteten-nesten-halvert-blant.

Andersen, Adelina Trolle. "Sykt perfekt? Nei, bare sykt selvopptatt [Sickly perfect? No, just morbidly self-centered]." *Aftenposten*, 17 January 2016, 15.

Andersen, Patrick Lie, and Anders Bakken. "Ung i Oslo 2015. NOVA Rapport 8/15 [Young in Oslo 2015]." Oslo: NOVA, 2015.

Antonioni, Michelangelo. *Blow-up*. Beverly Hills, CA: Metro-Goldwyn-Mayer, 1966.

Apotekforeningen. "Bruken av paracetamol og NSAID i Norge 2003–2014 [The use of paracetamol and NSAID in Norway 2003–2014]." (2015). https://www.apotek.no/Files/Filer_2014/Nyheter/150213%20Faktanotat%20paracetamol%20og%20NSAID.pdf.

———. "En undersøkelse om ungdommers forhold til paracetamol [An investigation of youth's relation to paracetamol]." 2015.

———. "Unges bruk av antidepressiva fortsetter å øke [Young people's use of antidepressants continues to increase]." *Apotekforeningen* (2017). https://www.apotek.no/Default.aspx?ID=8444.

Aristofanes, *Skyene* [The clouds]. Oslo: Aschehoug, 1977.

Arnett, Jeffrey Jensen. "The evidence for generation we and against generation me." *Emerging Adulthood* 1, nr. 1 (2013): 5–10.

Asch, Solomon E. "Studies of independence and conformity: I. A minority of one against a unanimous majority." *Psychological Monographs: General and Applied* 70, nr. 9 (1956): 1–70.

Askeland, Jorunn Strand. "Flink pike-syndromet anno 2012 [The good girl syndrome in the year of 2012]." *Vårt Land*, 13 January 2012, 29.

Avseth, Håkon. "Fra prestasjon til depresjon [From achievement to depression]." *NRK Ytring* (2015, 21 May). https://www.nrk.no/ytring/fra-prestasjon-til-depresjon-1.12369440.

Baehr, Peter. "The 'iron cage' and the 'shell as hard as steel'." *History and Theory* 40, nr. 2 (2001): 153–69.

Bakken, Anders. "Ung i Oslo 2018. NOVA Rapport 6/18 [Young in Oslo 2018]." Oslo: NOVA, 2018.

———. "Ungdata. Nasjonale resultater 2017, NOVA Rapport 10/17 [Ungdata. National results 2017]." Oslo: NOVA, 2017.

———. "Ungdata. Nasjonale resultater 2018, NOVA Rapport 8/18 [Ungdata. National results 2018]." Oslo: NOVA, 2018.

Bakken, Bente. "Hvordan unngå 'flink pike'-syndromet [How to avoid the good girl syndrome]." *Dagsavisen*, 18 October 2004, 18.

Barker, Mike. *The handmaid's tale: faithful episode 5*. Los Angeles: Hulu, 2017.

Barsky, Anthony J. "The paradox of health." *New England Journal of Medicine* 318 (1988): 414–18.

Baudelaire, Charles-Pierre. *The painter of modern life*. London: Penguin Classics, 2010.

Baudrillard, Jean. *The consumer society: myths and structures*. London: Sage, 2003.

Bauman, Zygmunt. *Liquid modernity*. Cambridge: Polity, 2000.

———. *Postmodernity and its discontents*. Cambridge: Polity, 1997.

Beck, Ulrich. *Risk society: towards a new modernity*. London: Sage, 1992.

Beck, Ulrich, and Elisabeth Beck-Gernsheim. *Individualization: institutionalized individualism and its social and political consequences*. London: Sage, 2002.

Becker, Dana. *The myth of empowerment: women and the therapeutic culture in America*. New York: New York University Press, 2005.

———. *One nation under stress: the trouble with stress as an idea*. New York: Oxford University Press, 2013.

Bepko, Claudia, and Jo-Ann Krestan. *Flink pike! Så god at du ikke har godt av det?* Oslo: Cappelen Damm, 1993.

———. *Too good for her own good: searching for self and intimacy in important relationships*. New York: Harper, 1990.

Berardi, Franco. *The soul at work*. Los Angeles: Semiotext(e), 2009.

Bergens Tidende. "Jenter engster seg mer enn gutter. BT lot seks skoleelever fortelle om hva som stresser dem i hverdagen [Girls worry more than boys]." *Bergens Tidende*, 28 June 2017, 1.

Bergland, Camilla. "Eksperter: Slik kan foreldrene takle 'det tause opprøret' [Experts: This is how parents can handle 'the silent rebellion']." *VG* (2014, 23 September). https://www.vg.no/nyheter/innenriks/skole-og-utdanning/eksperter-slik-kan-foreldre-takle-det-tause-opproeret/a/23301970/.

Beverfjord, Alexandra. "Under overflaten [Under the surface]." *Adresseavisen*, 16 February 2001, 11.

Bibelselskapet. *Bibelen* [The Bible]. *Det gamle og det nye testamentet*. Oslo: Bibelselskapet, 2011.

Binkley, Samuel. *Happiness as enterprise: an essay on neoliberal life*. Albany: Suny Press, 2014.

Bjørneboe, Jens. "Om ungdommens råskap [On the youth's brutality]." In *En sangfugl i en snare gikk – Jens Bjørneboe i utvalg*, edited by André Bjerke, 59. Oslo: Bokklubbens Lyrikkvenner, 1981.

Blaasvær, Thomas. *Studiehefte i psykologi* [Study guide in psychology]. Oslo: Bedriftsøkonomens forlag, 1984.

Bleidvin, Ingebjørn. "Det me ikkje snakkar om [What we don't talk about]." *Bergens Tidende* (2017, 3 November). https://www.bt.no/btmeninger/kommentar/i/OR23E/Det-me-ikkje-snakkar-om.

Bly, Robert. "Foreword: Mitscherlich and his uncomfortable thoughts." In *The society without the father*, xii-xxi. New York: Harper Perennial, 1993.

———. *The sibling society*. New York: Penguin, 1997.

Bohman, Therese. "Til duktighetens försvar [Defending capability]." In *Klassresan*, edited by Tobias Krantz and Karin Rebas, 66–72. Stockholm: Bertil Ohlin Förlag, 2015.

Bor, William, Angela J Dean, Jacob Najman, and Reza Hayatbakhsh. "Are child and adolescent mental health problems increasing in the 21st century? A systematic review." *Australian & New Zealand Journal of Psychiatry* 48, nr. 7 (2014): 606–16.

Borge, Arne. "–Kierkegaard var ingen selvhjelpsguru! [Kierkegaard was no self-help guru!]" *Vårt Land*, 13 May 2017, 32–34.

Bornäs, Hanna. "'Att inskolas som vuxen' – medikaliseringen av unga vuxnas psykiska lidande i Sverge [Socialized into maturity]." In *Snart er vi alle pasienter. Medikalisering i Norden*, edited by Hilde Bondevik, Ole Jacob Madsen and Kari Nyheim Solbrække, 155–89. Oslo: Scandinavian Academic Press, 2017.

Borud, Håkon. "Å være flink er ingen sykdom [Being good is no disease]." *Aftenposten* (2015, 21 September). https://www.aftenposten.no/meninger/kommentar/i/2XA4/A-vare-flink-er-ingen-sykdom.

Borum, Randy, Dewey G. Cornell, William Modzeleski, and Shane R. Jimerson. "What can be done about school shootings? A review of the evidence." *Educational Researcher* 39, nr. 1 (2010): 27–37.

Brandtzæg, Ida, Stig Torsteinson, and Guro Øiestad. "Folkehelse og livsmestring i skolen [Public health and life-coping in school]." *Tidsskrift for Norsk psykologforening* 54, nr. 8 (2017): 766–67.

Brandtzæg, Petter Bae. "Social networking sites: Their users and social implications – a longitudinal study." *Journal of Computer-Mediated Communication* 17, nr. 4 (2012): 467–88.

Bratt, Nina. "Minimisser i rampelyset [Mini misses in the limelight]." *Aftenposten*, 3 November 1984, 23.

Braun, Virginia, and Victoria Clarke. "Using thematic analysis in psychology." *Qualitative Research in Psychology* 3, nr. 2 (2006): 77–101.

Bredesen, Vilde Linnea. "Jeg veide for mye for å få behandling. Beskjeden forverret tilstanden min [I weighed too much to get treatment]." *Aftenposten* (2018, 14 February). https://www.aftenposten.no/meninger/sid/i/RxrwaW/Jeg-veide-for-mye-for-a-fa-behandling-Beskjeden-forverret-tilstanden-min%2D%2DVilde-Linnea-Bredesen.

Breivik, Anders Behring. *2083 – A European declaration of independence.* London: Andrew Berwick, 2011.

Brinkmann, Svend. *The joy of missing out: the art of self–restraint in an age of excess.* London: Polity, 2019.

———. *Stand firm: resisting the self-improvement craze.* London: Polity, 2017.

———. *Standpoints: 10 old ideas in a new world.* London: Polity, 2018.

Brockman, John, red. *This idea must die.* New York: Harper Perennial, 2015.

Bromark, Marit. "Hadde jeg vært ungdom ville jeg sagt opp på flekken [If I was young I would quit on the spot]." *klikk.no* (2014, 4 December). http://www.klikk.no/foreldre/kommentarer/hadde-jeg-vaert-ungdom-ville-jeg-sagt-opp-pa-flekken-2488929.

———. "Prestasjonsbarna: – I dag er det ingen arena for det vanlige, bare for det som er best [The achievement children]." *foreldre.no* (2014, 24 May). http://www.klikk.no/foreldre/barn/prestasjonsbarna-1447809.ece.

Bruckner, Pascal. *Perpetual euphoria: on the duty to be happy.* Princeton, NJ: Princeton University Press, 2000.

Brundtland, Gro Harlem. "Statsministerens nyttårstale [The prime minister's New Year's speech]." NRK TV, 1992 https://tv.nrk.no/serie/statsministerens-nyttaarstale/FAKN70000191/01-01-1992.

Buer, Liz. "Kvinnfolk: Itj så lætt-skræmt [Women: Not so easily scared]." *Dagbladet*, 19 October 1997, 3.

Bugge, Mette. "Lider av 'flink pike'-syndrom [Suffering from good girl syndrome]." *Aftenposten*, 6 February 2004, 6.

Bush, Kate. "Cloudbusting." In *Hounds of Love.* London: EMI, 1985.

Byklum, Kari, and Christine Gulbrandsen. "–Jeg kjenner meg ikke igjen i ungdomspresset [I don't recognize myself in the youth pressure]." *Fædrelandsvennen*

(2016, 18 March). https://www.fvn.no/familieogoppvekst/%2D%2DJeg-kjenner-meg-ikke-igjen-i-ungdomspresset-8883b.html.

Børtnes, Turid. "Høytlønte kvinner mest syke [Highly paid women most sick]." *Arbeidsmiljø*, 31 August 2005, n. p.

Carr, Michelle. "Dream deprived: A modern epidemic?" *Psychology Today* (2017, 22 August). https://www.psychologytoday.com/blog/dream-factory/201708/dream-deprived-modern-epidemic#_=_.

Castellacci, Fulvio, and Vegard Tveito. "Internet use and well-being: A survey and a theoretical framework." *Research Policy* 47, nr. 1 (2018): 308–25.

Cederström, Carl, and André Spicer. *Desperately seeking self-improvement: a year inside the optimization movement.* New York: OR Books, 2017.

———. *The wellness syndrome*. London: Polity, 2015.

Center for selvmordsforskning. "Statistik [Statistics]." (2020, 6 November). http://statistik.selvmordsforskning.dk/.

Chomsky, Noam. "Psychology and ideology." In *The Chomsky reader*, edited by James Peck, 157–82. New York: Pantheon, 1987.

Christakis, Nicholas A., and James H. Fowler "The spread of obesity in a large social network over 32 years." *New England Journal of Medicine* 357, nr. 4 (2007): 370–79.

Christie, Agatha. "4.50 fra Paddington [4.50 from Paddington]." *VG*, 30 August 1971, 13.

Collishaw, Stephan. "Annual research review: Secular trends in child and adolescent mental health." *Journal of Child Psychology and Psychiatry* 56, nr. 3 (2015): 370–93.

Crary, Jonathan. *24/7: late capitalism and the ends of sleep*. London: Verso, 2014.

Crawford, Robert. "Healthism and the medicalization of everyday life." *International Journal of Health Services* 10, nr. 3 (1980): 365–88.

Dagsavisen. "-Vi har god selvtillit [-We have good self-confidence]." *Dagsavisen*, 4 October 2005.

Dahl, Gordon B., Andreas Ravndal Kostøl, and Magne Mogstad. "Family welfare cultures." *The Quarterly Journal of Economics* 129, nr. 4 (2014): 1711–52.

Dahl, Hege. *This is a man's world – en radiodokumentar om unge menn og krav på jobben*. NRK2006. Radio.

Dahl, Øyvind, Geir Lahnstein, Tove Lindemann, Inge Lønning, Åse Madsen, Helge Seip, Anfinn Stigen, and Liv Wergeland Sørbye. *Etikk* [Ethics]. Oslo: Universitetsforlaget, 1983.

Dahle, Margunn Serigstad. "'Sykt perfekt' speglar presset ['Sickly perfect' mirrors the pressure]." *Vårt Land* (2016, 13 January). https://www.vl.no/tro24/sykt-perfekt-speglar-presset-1.674304?paywall=true.

Dalrymple, Theodore. *Admirable evasions: how psychology undermines morality.* New York: Encounter Books, 2015.

Danielsen, Kirsten. "I vår tid. Tre artikler om generasjon, modernitet og livshistorier [In our time]." Oslo: Norsk Gerontologisk Institutt, 1994.

Davies, William. *The happiness industry*. London: Verso, 2015.

Debord, Guy. *The society of the spectacle.* New York: Zone Books, 1995.

Dostoyevsky, Fjodor. *Notes from the underground* (1864). https://www.planetebook.com/free-ebooks/notes-from-the-underground.pdf.

Duckert, Hege. "Smerte uten hjerte [Pain without heart]." *Dagbladet*, 8 July 2000, 13.

Dufour, Dany-Robert. *The art of shrinking heads: on the new servitude of the liberated in the age of total capitalism*. Cambridge: Polity Press, 2008.

Durkheim, Émile. *The division of labor in society*. New York: Free Press, 1997.

———. Émile. *On suicide*. London: Penguin Books, 2006.

Dyb, Halvard. "Skoleelever startet bedrift inspirert av Ungdata [Pupils started a company inspired by Ungdata]." (2015, 23 April). http://www.hioa.no/Aktuelle-saker/Skoleelever-startet-bedrift-inspirert-av-Ungdata.

Døving, Runar. "Generasjon A [Generation A]." (2016). https://kristiania.no/artikkel/media/generasjon-a.

Egmont Publishing. "500.000 tenåringsforeldre har ventet på dette [500.000 parents to teenagers have been waiting for this]." (2015, 6 February). https://www.ntbinfo.no/pressemelding/500000-tenaringsforeldre-har-ventet-pa-dette?publisherId=7154035&releaseId=7302117.

Ehrenberg, Alain. *The weariness of the self: diagnosing the history of depression in the contemporary age*. Montreal: McGill-Queen's University Press, 2010.

Eikefjord, Eirin. "Prestasjonspikene [The achievement girls]." *Bergens Tidende* (2014, 23 September). https://www.bt.no/btmeninger/kommentar/i/852gx/Prestasjonspikene.

Ellingsen, Christian Lycke. "Selvmord hos unge [Suicid among young] [personal communication]." 2018, 23 January.

Elliott, Anthony, and Charles Lemert. *The new individualism: the emotional costs of globalization (revised edition.)*. New York: Routledge, 2009.

Elster, Jon. *Making sense of Marx*. Cambridge: Cambridge University Press, 1985.

Engebretsen, Solveig, Arnoldo Frigessi, Kenth Engø-Monsen, Anne-Sofie Furberg, Audun Stubhaug, Freiesleben de Blasio Birgitte, and Sivert Nielsen

Christopher. "The peer effect on pain tolerance." *Scandinavian Journal of Pain* 18, nr. 3 (2018): 467–77.

Engen, Runa Victoria, and Tormod Strand. "Politiet om 150 tenåringer: – Vi greier ikke å stoppe dem [The police on 150 teens: - We can't manage to stop them]." (2018, 30 April). https://www.nrk.no/norge/politiet-om-150-tenaringer_-_-vi-greier-ikke-a-stoppe-dem-1.14029325.

Enger, Cecilie. "Eneste høne i kurven [The only hen in the basket]." *Dagens Næringsliv*, 13 February 1999, 32.

Engesæth, Njål. *Lisenskontrolløren: Ungdom* [The license inspector: Youths]. Oslo: NRK, 2017 https://tv.nrk.no/serie/lisenskontrolloeren/sesong/4/episode/3/avspiller.

Engstad, Carl Christian. "–Ungdommene trives [-The youth enjoy oneself]." *Lillesands-Posten*, 29 July 2016, 7.

Eriksen, Edvin M. "Generasjon prestasjon [Generation achievement]." *Harstad Tidende*, 27 September 2014, 22.

Eriksen, Espen. "Kirsti på medaljeplass? [Kirsti get into the medals?]" *VG*, 8 April 1967, 15.

Eriksen, Ingunn Marie, Mira Aaboen Sletten, Anders Bakken, and Tilmann von Soest. "Stress og press blant unge. Rapport nr 6/17 [Stress and pressure among youths]." Oslo: NOVA, 2017.

Erikson, Erik H. *Childhood and society*. New York: Pelican, 1950.

Espe, Torunn. "Kvifor vert nokon sjuk av å vere flink? Ei undersøking av flink pike-syndrom sett i lys av sosial representasjonsteori og identitetsprosessteori." ['How can anybody become ill by being good?]" University of Oslo, 2015.

F5. "Generasjon prestasjon [Generation achievement]." In *MGP Jr.* 2017. Oslo: NRK, 2017.

Fardal, Signy. "Blått blikk i gul sofa [Blue gaze in yellow sofa]." *Dagens Næringsliv*, 5 September 1992, 16.

Farnham, Nicholas, and Marieke Liem. "'Can a copycat effect be observed in terrorist suicide attacks?'" *The International Centre for Counter-Terrorism – The Hague* 8, nr. 4 (2017): 1–34.

Ffytche, Matt. "Psychoanalytic sociology and the traumas of history: Alexander Mitscherlich between the disciplines." *History of the Human Sciences* 30, nr. 5 (2017): 3–29.

Fisher, Mark. *Capitalist realism*. Winchester: Zero Books, 2009.

Fjelldal, Cecilie Gryte. "8 om 8. mars: Hadet 'generasjon prestasjon' – hei 'generasjon stress' [8 on March 8]." *VG* (2018, 8 March). https://www.vg.no/nyheter/meninger/i/vmzdwj/8-om-8-mars-hadet-generasjon-prestasjon-hei-generasjon-stress.

Flaubert, Gustave. *Madame Bovary*. London: Penguin, 2003.
"Flink pike (18)". "Flink pike-syndrom [Good girl syndrome]." *Aftenposten*, 18 September 2011, 23.
"Flink pike". "'Flink pike'-syndromet [The good girl syndrome]." *Adresseavisen*, 20 January 2014, 15.
Fonn, Maria Kjos. "En mur av muligheter [A wall of posibilites]." *Samtiden* 127, nr. 3 (2017): 50–53.
Foros, Per Bjørn, and Arne Johan Vetlesen. *Angsten for oppdragelsen. Et samfunnsetisk perspektiv på dannelse* [Child-rearing anxiety] *(2nd edition.)*. Oslo: Universitetsforlaget, 2015.
Fossgard, Stein. *Folkehøgskolen* [Folk university college] Oslo: Norsk Korrespondanseskole, 1972.
Fox, Claire. *'I find that offensive!'*. London: Biteback, 2016.
Fredriksen, Ingrid. "Ps [Ps]." *Bergens Tidende*, 27 May 2011, 36.
Freud, Sigmund. *Civilization and its discontents*. (1930). https://archive.org/details/in.ernet.dli.2015.221667/page/n7.
Friedan, Betty. *The feminine mystique*. London: Penguin, 2010.
Fromm, Erich. *Escape from freedom*. New York: Farrar & Rinehart, 1941.
———. *The sane society*. New York: Holt, Rinehart & Winston, 1976.
Frosh, Stephen. "Psychososial studies and psychology: is a critical approach emerging?". *Human Relations* 56, nr. 1545–1567 (2003).
Frøyland, Lars Roar, and Tilmann von Soest. "Trends in the perpetration of physical aggression among Norwegian adolescents 2007–2015." *Journal of Youth and Adolescence* (2017): 1–14.
———. "Ungdomsvold halvert på åtte år. Mindre alkohol og mer skjermbruk kan være forklaringer [Youth violence halved in eight years]." *Aftenposten* (2018, 12 February). https://www.aftenposten.no/viten/i/8wQA8W/Ungdomsvold-halvert-pa-atte-ar-Mindre-alkohol-og-mer-skjermbruk-kan-vare-forklaringer.
Fugelli, Per. *Rød resept: essays om perfeksjon, prestasjon og helse* [Red prescription]. Oslo: Universitetsforlaget, 1999.
Furedi, Frank. *Therapy culture: cultivating vulnerability in an uncertain age*. London: Routledge, 2004.
Galdas, Paul M., Francine Cheater, and Paul Marshall. "Men and health help-seeking behaviour: literature review." *Journal of Advanced Nursing* 49, nr. 6 (2005): 616–23.
Generasjon Prestasjon. *Våkn opp – En reklamefilm for Generasjon Prestasjon* [Wake up]. 2016 https://www.youtube.com/watch?v=Eg-0KPfLkrA&t=2s.

Geulayov, Galit, Navneet Kapur, Pauline Turnbull, Caroline Clements, Keith Waters, Jennifer Ness, Ellen Townsend, and Keith Hawton. "Epidemiology and trends in non-fatal self-harm in three centres in England, 2000–2012: Findings from the Multicentre Study of Self-harm in England." *BMJ Open* 6, nr. 4 (2016).

Giddens, Anthony. *The third way: the renewal of social democracy*. London: Polity Press, 1998.

Gilbert, Elisabeth. *Eat, pray, love*. Riverhead Books: New York, 2006.

Gill, Rosalind. *Gender and the media*. London: Polity Press, 2007.

Goethe, Johann Wolfgang Von. *The sorrows of young Werther*. London: Penguin, 1989.

Goodhart, David. *The road to somewhere*. London: Hurst, 2017.

Gran, Sissel. "På innsiden [On the inside]." *Aftenposten*, 19 August 1995, 38.

Grinde, Eva. "Ja til flinke piker! [Yes to good girls]" *Dagens Næringsliv*, 16 May 2011, 22.

Guneriussen, Willy. *Å forstå det moderne: framskrittstro, rasjonalitet, ambivalens og irrasjonalitet i diskursen om modernitet* [Understanding modernity]. Oslo: Tano Aschehoug, 1999.

Habermas, Jürgen. *The philosophical discourse of modernity: twelve lectures*. Cambridge: Polity Press, 2007.

Hacking, Ian. "Deres Kongelige Høyhet Kronprinsesse Mette-Marit, statsråd, Deres Eksellense, Ludvig Holbergs minnefond og gjester [Your Royal Highness Crown Princess, cabinet minister, Your Excellency, Ludvig Holberg's Prize and guests]." In *Prisseremoni Holbergs internasjonale minnepris og Nils Klim-prisen 25. november* 2009, edited by Holbergprisen, 7–8, 2009.

———. "The looping effects of human kinds." In *Causal cognition: a multi-disciplinary debate*, edited by D. Sperber, D. Premack and A. J. Premack, 351–83. New York: Oxford University Press, 1995.

———. *Mad travelers: reflections on the reality of transient mental illnesses*. Cambridge, MA: Harvard University Press, 1998.

———. "Making up people." *London Review of Books* 28, nr. 16 (2006): 23–26.

———. "Pathological withdrawal of refugee children seeking asylum in Sweden." *Studies in History and Philosophy of Biological and Biomedical Sciences* 41, nr. 309–317 (2010).

———. *Rewriting the soul: multiple personality and the sciences of memory*. Princeton, NJ: Princeton University Press, 1995.

———. *The social construction of what?* Cambridge, MA: Harvard University Press, 1999.

Hafstad, Anne. "Drikker for å finne seg selv [Drinking to find oneself]." *Aftenposten*, 26 October 1999, 2.

Hageberg, Arne Olav. "Ein generasjon av stressa jenter [One generation of stressed girls]." *Tidsskrift for Norsk psykologforening* 51, nr. 11 (2014): 961–63.

Hallström, Lasse. *Mitt liv som hund* [My life as a dog]. Stockholm: AB Svensk Filmindustri, 1985.

Hamar Dagblad. "Starter angstgruppe [Starting anxiety groups]." *Hamar Dagblad*, 26 September 2003, n. p.

Hamsun, Knut. *Børn av tiden* [Children of the present]. Kristiania: Gyldendalske forlag, 1913.

———. *Hunger*. Edinburgh: Canongate, 2016.

Han, Buyung-Chul. *The burnout society.* Stanford, CA: Stanford University Press, 2015.

Haneke, Michael. *Benny's Video*. Austria/Switzerland: Bernard Lang, 1992.

Hans Majestet Kong Harald V of Norway. "Nyttårstalen 2016 [New Year's Speech 2016]." *The Royal House of Norway* (2016, 31 December). http://www.kongehuset.no/nyhet.html?tid=139780&sek=26939.

Hansen, Bue Rübner. "Danmark-koden [The Denmark Code]." *Manifest tidsskrift* (2016, 17 April). http://www.manifesttidsskrift.no/danmark-koden-13/.

Hansen, Frode, and Asbjørn Svarstad. "Kvinnene krever bedre sex – Og bidrar til at Norge er i Viagra-toppen [Women demand better sex]." *Dagbladet*, 7 October 1999, 8.

Hansen, Vilde Bratland. "Jakten på den uoppnåelige sikkerhet [The search for unobtainable safety]." *Oppland Arbeiderblad*, 19 January 2016, 14.

Harvey, David. *A brief history of neoliberalism*. Oxford: Oxford University Press, 2005.

Harvey, Samuel B, Mark Deady, Min-Jung Wang, Arnstein Mykletun, Peter Butterworth, Helen Christensen, and Philip B Mitchell. "Is the prevalence of mental illness increasing in Australia? Evidence from national health surveys and administrative data, 2001–2014." *The Medical Journal of Australia* 206, nr. 11 (2017): 490–493.

Haugsbø, Frank. "Eksperter roser Trondheim kommunes selvmordsalarm [Experts praise Trondheim municipality's suicide alarm]." (2017, 12 May). http://www.vg.no/nyheter/innenriks/psykisk-helse/eksperter-roser-trondheim-kommunes-selvmordsalarm/a/23995106/.

Hay, Louise. *You can heal your life*. Carlsbad, CA: Hay House, 1984.

Heelas, Paul. "Reforming the self. Enterprise and the characters of thatcherism." In *Enterprise culture*, edited by Russell Keat and Nicholas Abercrombie, 72–92. London: Routledge, 1991.

Hegge, Per Egil. "Kaci Kullmann Five: Pen, flink pike fra Bærum [Kaci Kullmann Five: Pretty, good girl from Bærum]." *Aftenposten*, 23 January 1988, 7.

Hegna, Kristinn, Guro Ødegård, and Åse Strandbu. "En 'sykt seriøs' ungdomsgenerasjon? [A 'sickly serious' youth generation?". *Tidsskrift for Norsk psykologforening* 50, nr. 4 (2013): 374–77.

Heian, Hilde. "-Stadig flere unge sliter med angstsymptomer [-An increasingly number of young people struggle with anxiety symptoms]." *Bergens Tidende*, 28 June 2017, 10–11.

Helliwell, John F., Richard Layard, and Jeffrey D. Sachs. *World happiness report 2018*. New York: Sustainable Development Solutions Network, 2018.

HelpLink Psykologsenter. "Spørsmål og svar om flink pike-syndrom [Q&A on the good girl syndrome]." (2015, 5 February). http://helplink.no/flink-pike-syndrom/.

Helsedirektoratet. "Veiledende materiell for kommunene om forebygging av selvskading og selvmord [Advisory material for municipalities on prevention of self-harm and suicide]." (2017). https://helsedirektoratet.no/folkehelse/psykisk-helse-og-rus/selvmord-og-selvskading/veiledende-materiell-for-kommunene-om-forebygging-av-selvskading-og-selvmord#om-selvskading.

Hernes, Gudmund. "Det mediavridde samfunn [The media's distortion of society]." In *Forhandlingsøkonomi og blandingsadministrasjon*, edited by Gudmund Hernes, 181–95. Oslo: Universitetsforlaget, 1978.

Hertz, Kine B. "Spiser på kommando [Eats on command]." *Dagbladet*, 27 July 2002, 14.

Hewitt, John P. *The myth of self-esteem*. New York: St. Martin's Press, 1998.

Hobbes, Michael. "Generation screwed." (2017, 15 December). https://highline.huffingtonpost.com/articles/en/poor-millennials/.

Hofgaard, Tor Levin. "Psykologi må bli pensum! [Psychology must become compulsory reading]" *NRK Ytring* (2015, 17 August). http://www.nrk.no/ytring/psykologi-ma-bli-pensum_-1.12499881.

Holberg, Ludvig. *Epistler* [Episteles]. Copenhagen: Ludvig Holberg, 1748–1754.

Holden, Stephen. "Antonioni's nothingness and beauty." *New York Times* (2006, 4 June). https://www.nytimes.com/2006/06/04/movies/04hold.html.

Holmlund, Jan Thomas. "Elin Tvedt er tatt av skjermen [Elin Tvedt removed from the screen]." *Dagbladet* (2013, 13 February). http://www.dagbladet.no/kjendis/elin-tvedt-er-tatt-av-skjermen/66756059.

Holst, Inga Ragnhild. "Hurra for flinke piker! [Hurrah for good girls!]" *KK*, 10 June 2016, 14–17.

Holstad, Grete. "Forsker anbefaler kjønnsdeling [Researcher recommends gender distribution]." Adresseavisen, 21 January 2016, 8.

Holtan, Kai. "La-la land [La-la land]." *Moss Avis*, 25 March 2017, 31.

Honneth, Axel. "Organized self-realization: some paradoxes of individualization." *European Journal of Social Theory* 7, nr. 4 (2004): 463–78.

Hvattum, Torstein. "'Sykt perfekt' på TV 2: Modige jenter viser vei ['Sickly perfect' on TV2]." *Aftenposten* (2016, 12 January). https://www.aftenposten.no/kultur/i/63L3/Sykt-perfekt-pa-TV-2-Modige-jenter-viser-vei.

Hverven, Tom Egil. "Megalomani og selvutslettelse [Megalomania and self-effacement]." *Samtiden* 120, nr. 4 (2011): 78–90.

Hvidsten, Ingrid. "Bryter tabuet og forteller [Breaks the taboo and tells]." *Dagsavisen*, 4 August 2012, 12.

Høgskolen i Oslo and Akershus. "Ikke de mest ambisiøse jentene som sliter mest [Not the most ambitious girls that struggles the most]." (2015, 16 August). https://www.ntbinfo.no/pressemelding/ikke-de-mest-ambisiose-jentene-som-sliter-mest?publisherId=15678779&releaseId=15768335.

Høstmælingen, Andreas. "Et forsvar for sykeliggjøring [A defence of pathologisation]." *Tidsskrift for Norsk psykologforening* 54, nr. 6 (2017): 570–71.

Høye, Elisabet, and Ida Louise Rostad. "*Paracetamol-misbruket [The paracetamol misuse]. NRK.*" (2016, 17 February). https://www.nrk.no/livsstil/xl/paracetamol-misbruket-1.12755817.

Illouz, Eva. *Saving the modern soul: therapy, emotions, and the culture of self-help*. Berkeley, CA: University of California Press, 2008.

Jakobsen, Jonas. "Å lide av ubestemthet. Axel Honneths hegelianske samtidsdiagnose [To suffer from indeterminacy]." *Agora – Journal for metafysisk spekulasjon* 27, nr. 4 (2009): 5–22.

Jensen, Henrik. *Det faderløse samfund* [The fatherless society]. Copenhagen: People's Press, 2006.

Jetter, Michael. "The effect of media attention on terrorism." *Journal of Public Economics* 153 (2017): 32–48.

Joakimsen, Trygve Strand. "Ber foreldre være på vakt etter selvmord i Trondheim [Ask parents to be on the watch for suicide in Trondheim]." (2017, 10 May). https://www.nrk.no/trondelag/ber-foreldre-vaere-pa-vakt-etter-selvmord-i-trondheim-1.13509097.

Johannisson, Karin. "Om begreppet kultursjukdom [On the concept of culture diseases]." *Läkartidningen* 105, nr. 44 (2008): 3129–32.

Johansen, Glenn Slydal. "Forskere uenige om venstrevridde journalister [Researchers disagree about left-wing journalists]." (2015, 22 May). https://journalisten.no/2015/05/forskere-delt-om-venstrevridde-journalister.

Johansen, Marianne. "Høyre-veteran ber Erna gå av [Conservative party veteran ask Erna to retire]." *Dagbladet*, 4 April 2006, 10.

Kant, Immanuel. "Svar på spørsmålet: Hva er opplysning?" [Answer to the question: What is enlightenment?]. In *Store pedagoger i egne skrifter. III. Opplysningstiden*, edited by Reidar Myhre, 14–15. Oslo: Fabritius & Sønners forlag, 1969.

Kardefelt-Winther, Daniel. *How does the time children spend using digital technology impact their mental well-being, social relationships and physical activity? An evidence-focused literature review. Innocenti Discussion Paper 2017–02*. Florence: UNICEF Office of Research – Innocenti, 2017.

Karlsvik, Line. "Verdensdagen for psykisk helse [World day for mental health]." *Tidens Krav*, 21 October 2016, 8–9.

Kaspersen, Line. Altfor få tør å følge drømmene sine [Too few dare to follow their dream]." *Dagens Næringsliv* (2016, 7 February). https://www.dn.no/jobbledelse/2016/02/07/1201/Karriere/-altfor-f-tr%2D%2Dflge-drmmene-sine.

Kierkegaard, Søren. *Begrepet angst* [The concept of anxiety]. Oslo: Oktober, 2001.

Kingsrød-Olsen, Marie Moen, and Kaja Storrøsten. "Slik tok Therese og Jannicke kontroll over panikkangsten [This is how Therese and Jannicke took control over panic disorder]." *VG+* (2018, 15 January). http://pluss.vg.no/2018/01/15/3027/3027_24232719.

Kitzinger, Jenny. "Media templates: patterns of association and the (re)construction of meaning over time." *Media, Culture & Society* 22, nr. 1 (2000): 61–84.

Kjærstad, Jan. *Menneskets vidde* [Humankind's breadth]. Oslo: Aschehoug, 2013.

Kleive, Johanna Holt. "Forbanna på følelses-tv [Furious with emotional TV]." *Dagens Næringsliv* (2016, 20 April). http://www.dn.no/etterBors/2016/04/20/1130/Psykisk-helse/forbanna-p-flelsestv.

Klinger, Don A., John G. Freeman, Ludwig Bilz, Krystine Liiv, Daniela Ramelow, Stefanie S. Sebok, Oddrun Samdal, Wolfgang Dür, and Mette Rasmussen. "Cross-national trends in perceived school pressure by gender and age from 1994 to 2010." *European Journal of Public Health* 25, nr. suppl_2 (2015): 51–56.

Klyve, Arne. "Samtidsdiagnose [Diagnosis of the present]." *Tidsskrift for Psykisk Helsearbeid* 14, nr. 1 (2017): 73–79.

Knapstad, Miriam Lund. "På videregående var de slitne, stressa og 'sykt flinke' [During upper secondary school they were tired, stressed and 'sickly good']." *Aftenposten*, 22 October 2016, 34–37.

———. "Sykt flinke [Sickly good]." *Aftenposten*, 17 August 2013, 22–25.

Knudsen, Ann Kristin, and Arnstein Mykletun. "Det du trenger å vite om forekomsten av psykiske lidelser i Norge [What you need to know about the prevalence of mental illnesses in Norway]." *Tidsskrift for Norsk psykologforening* 47, nr. 4 (2010): 342–43.

Knutsen, Tove Karoline. "Vi snakker forbi hverandre [We talk at cross purposes]." *Klassekampen*, 21 July 2015, 22.

Kongsnes, Ellen. "Blir syk av 'flink pike'-stempel [Become ill from the good girl mark]." *Stavanger Aftenblad*, 22 September 2005, 38.

Korsbrekke, Marte. "Sjekk om du lider av flink pike-syndromet." *ABC Nyheter* (2014, 14 January). https://www.abcnyheter.no/livet/2014/01/14/191162/er-du-flink-pike.

Korsvold, Kaja. "Profilen: Flink pike [The profile: Good girl]." *Aftenposten*, 14 June 1988, 9.

Kreutz-Hansen, Hanne, Kari Mette Hole, and Christine Rian Johannessen. "Generasjon prestasjon [Generation achievement]." *VG+* (2014, 13 September). http://pluss.vg.no/2013/09/13/1359/1759_23293421?order_id=101848081&code=42f41cbdabd17a52fa3a85c20246e851d15be3f4.

Kvaal, Julie Nybakk. "Ny behandling reduserer selvskading hos ungdom [New treatment reduces self-harm among youth]." *Suicidologi*, nr. 1 (2017): 28–29.

Kvale, Steinar, and Svend Brinkmann. *Interviews: learning the craft of qualitative research interviewing (2nd edition)*. Los Angeles, CA: Sage.

LaMothe, Ryan. "The travails and tragedies of a market civilization: a psychology of faith perspective." *Pastoral Psychology* 67, nr. 2 (2017): 155–73.

Landsvik, Solveig Oterhals. "–Ikke la samfunnspress og en hashtag ta styringen [Don't let societal pressure and a hashtag take control]." *Romsdal Budstikke* (2014, 15 June). http://www.rbnett.no/nyheter/article9808306.ece.

Larssen, Lars Døvle. "Ber deg ta ansvar [Asks you to take responsibility]." *Tønsbergs Blad*, 15 March 2011, 11.

Laustsen, Eliese. "Stresstest deg selv [Stress test yourself]." *VG*, 22 May 2013, 24–25.

Lemke, Thomas. "The birth of bio-politics: Michel Foucault's lecture at the Collège de France on neo-liberal governmentality." *Economy and Society* 30, nr. 2 (2001): 190–207.

Lillehammer Tilskuer. "Lørdagskroken [The Saturday corner]." *Lillehammer Tilskuer*, 31 July 1948, 6.

Luhrmann, Tanya M. *When God talks back*. New York: Vintage Books, 2012.

Lunde, Charlotte. "Generasjon prestasjon [Generation achievement]." *Morgenbladet*, 16 December 2011, 12–13.

Lunde, Trine. "Flinke jenter møter veggen [Good girls hit the wall." *Stavanger Aftenblad*, 17 September 2005, 68.

Lundeby, Maria Celine. "Ferdig prestert [Achievement all set]." *Dagen*, 1 November 2014, 37.

Lystrup, Marianne. "Knus koppen, ta vare på kroppen [Break the cup, take care of the body]." *Vårt Land*, 10 October 2004, n. p.

Løkke, Per Are. "Diagnoser skjuler jenters raseri [Diagnosis conceals girls rage]." *Aftenposten*, 14 September 2014, 14–15.

———. "Jenters stumme raseri – i diagnosenes tidsalder [Girls silent rage – in the age of diagnosis]." *Tidsskrift for Norsk psykologforening* 51 (2014): 767–72.

———. "Å gå seg vill i åpenheten [To loose oneself in the openness]." *Morgenbladet* (2017, 10 October). https://morgenbladet.no/ideer/2017/10/gar-seg-vill-i-apenheten?utm_content=buffer2c9f1&utm_medium=social&utm_source=facebook.com&utm_campaign=buffer.

———. "Å hakke seg ut av egget [To hatch out of the egg]." *Tidsskrift for Norsk psykologforening* 53, nr. 3 (2016): 200–06.

MacLuhan, Marshall. *The medium is the massage*. London: Penguin, 1971.

Madsen, Ole Jacob. *The therapeutic turn: how psychology altered Western culture*. London: Routledge, 2014.

———. *Optimizing the self: social representations of self-help*. London: Routledge.

———. "Helsestasjonismen [Public health centrism]." *Morgenbladet*, 29 July 2016, 30–31.

———. "Hinsides sant eller falskt: En undersøkelse av Ian Hackings teori om mentale lidelsers sosiale dynamikk [Beyond truth and false]." *Tidsskrift for Norsk psykologforening* 51, nr. 9 (2014): 745–52.

———. "'Hva gjør det med oss?' ['What does it do to us?']." *Tidsskrift for Norsk psykologforening* 51, nr. 11 (2014): 936–40.

———. "Hvordan har dere det egentlig? Som man spør får man svar [How are you doing really?]." *Samtiden* 125, nr. 3 (2017): 40–45.

———. "Modernity." In *Encyclopedia of critical psychology*, edited by Thomas Teo, 1199–203. New York: Springer, 2014.

———. "Nyliberalismens sosialpsykologi – Dany-Robert Dufours kritikk av nyliberalismen [The social psychology of neoliberalism]." *Agora. Journal for metafysisk spekulasjon*, nr. 1 (2011): 94–117.

———. "Psykologiens innflytelse i velferdsstaten [The influence of psychology in the welfare state]." In *Forvaltning av makt og moral i velferdsstaten: Fra sosialt arbeid til "arbeid med deg selv"?*, edited by Randi Kroken and Ole Jacob Madsen, 86–111. Oslo: Gyldendal Akademisk, 2016.

Malt, Ulrik F., Nils Retterstøl, and Alv A. Dahl. *Lærebok i psykiatri (2nd edition)*. Oslo: Gyldendal Akademisk, 2009.

Martín-Baró, Ignacio. "The role of the psychologist." In *Writings for a liberation psychology*, edited by Ignacio Martín-Baró, Adrianne Aron and Shawn Corne, 33–46. Boston: Harvard University Press, 1995.

Martin, Jack, and Ann-Marie McLellan. *The education of selves: how psychology transformed students*. New York: Oxford University Press, 2013.

Marx, Karl, og Friedrich Engels. *Økonomisk-filosofiske manuskripter og andre ungdomsverker* [Economic-philosophic manuscripts and other youth works]. Oslo: Falken, 1991.

Masvie, Susanne. "Sunn og usunn skam [Healthy and unhealthy shame]." *Vårt Land*, 6 October 2016, 20–21.

Mathiesen, Jan Schjelderup. "'Satte meg på to skift på Rådhusstrøket' ['Put me on two shifts around the city hall district']." *VG*, 26 September 1969, 8.

Mathiesen, Pål. "Livet som filosofi [Life as a philosopher]." *Dagbladet*, 24 January 1999, 4.

Meisingset, Kristian. "–Vi risikerer en profesjonalisering av demokratiet [-We run the riks to professionalise democracy]." *Minervas* (2017, 20 December). https://www.minervanett.no/vi-risikerer-en-profesjonaliseringav-demokratiet/.

Melkeraaen, Solveig. *Flink pike. En feelgood film om depresjon* [Good girl]. Norge: Tour de Force, 2014.

Melsom, Kaja. *Den fordømte friheten [The damned freedom]*. Oslo: Gyldendal, 2016.

Mercado, Melissa C., Kristin Holland, Ruth W. Leemis, Deborah M. Stone, and Jing Wang. "Trends in emergency department visits for nonfatal self-inflicted injuries among youth aged 10 to 24 years in the United States, 2001–2015." *JAMA* 318, nr. 19 (2017): 1931–33.

Merkesvik, Viktoria. "Skolen – en besettelse [The school – an obsession]." *Bergens Tidende*, 30 January 2016, 56.

Merton, Robert K. "The self-fulfilling prophecy." *The Antioch Review* 8, nr. 2 (1948): 193–210.

———. "Social structure and anomie." *American Sociological Review* 3, nr. 5 (1938): 672–82.

Midttun, Silje. "Raskt til topps [Quickly to the top]." *Cosmopolitan*, 7 August 2006, i. s.

Mitscherlich, Alexander. *Society without the father: a contribution to social psychology*. New York: Harper Perennial, 1993.

Moe, Hallvard, and Hilde Sakariassen. "Bruksmønstre for digitale nyheter [Utility patent for digital news]." Bergen: University of Bergen, 2018.

Morgan, Catharine, Roger T Webb, Matthew J Carr, Evangelos Kontopantelis, Jonathan Green, Carolyn A Chew-Graham, Nav Kapur, and Darren M Ashcroft. "Incidence, clinical management, and mortality risk following self harm among children and adolescents: Cohort study in primary care." *BMJ* 359 (2017).

Moscovici, Serge. "The phenomenon of social representations." In *Social representations: explorations in social psychology*, edited by Gerard Duveen, 18–77. Cambridge: Polity Press, 2000.

Myhre, Aslak Sira. "Ikke følg drømmen din [Don't follow your dream]." *Dagsavisen* (2016, 2 September). http://www.dagsavisen.no/nyemeninger/ikke-f%C3 %B8lg-dr%C3 %B8mmen-din-1.773216.

Myhre, Linnea. "Åpenhet for alle [Openness for all]." (2017, 3 November). https://morgenbladet.no/ideer/2017/11/myhre-apenhet-alle.

Myhre, Reidar. *Innføring i pedagogikk* [Introduction to pedagogy]. Oslo: Fabritius & Sønners Forlag, 1969.

Mæland, Eivor. Slutt å bruk begrepet flink pike [Stop using the phrase good girl]." *forskning.no* (2016, 21 February). https://forskning.no/kjonn-og-samfunn/2016/02/hvorfor-er-vi-sa-besatt-av-flinke-piker.

Naterstad, Svanhild. "Møter slagene [Meeting the blows]." *Adresseavisen*, 31 December 2011, 25–27.

National Centre for Suicide Research and Prevention. "Självmord i Sverige [Suicide in Sweden]." (2020, 8 August). https://ki.se/nasp/sjalvmord-i-sverige.

Nehring, Daniel, Emmanuel Alvarado, Eric C. Hendriks, and Dylan Kerrigan. *Transnational popular psychology and the global self-help industry*. London: Palgrave, 2016.

Nielsen, Torben Hviid. "De 'frisatte'. Om individualisering og identitet i nyere samtidsdiagnoser [The liberated.]" In *Klassebilder: Ulikheter og sosial mobilitet i Norge*, edited by Kenneth Dahlgren and Jørn Ljunggren, 169–81. Oslo: Universitetsforlaget, 2010.

Nietzsche, Friedrich. *Twilight of the idols/The anti-Christ*. London: Penguin, 1990.

———. *Thus spoke Zarathustra*. London: Penguin, 1969.

Nilsen, Lisbeth. "Færre unge tok sitt eget liv [Fewer took their own lives]." *Dagens Medisin* (2016, 11 February). https://www.dagensmedisin.no/artikler/2016/11/02/farre-unge-tok-sitt-eget-liv/.

Nordengen, Per Anders. "Pjusk eller syk? [Bedraggled or sick?]". *Tidsskriftet Den Norske Legeforeningen* 137, nr. 1 (2017): 80.

Nordtug, Birgit, and Gunn Engelsrud. "Fra forskning til politikk [From research to politics]." *Klassekampen*, 24 July 2015, 18.

Nordtug, Birgit. "Utvendig og innvendig forståelse [External and internal understanding]." *Klassekampen*, 17 July 2015, 18.

Norheim, Marta. *Oppdateringar frå lykkelandet. Røff guide til samtidslitteraturen* [Updates from the happy nation]. Oslo: Samlaget, 2017.

NOU. "NOU 2015: 8 Fremtidens skole: Fornyelse av fag og kompetanser [NOU 2015: 8 The future school]." Oslo: Kunnskapsdepartementet, 2015.

Norwegian Institute of Public Health. "Fakta om selvmord og selvmordsforsøk [Facts about suicide and attempted suicide]." (2017, 20 June). https://www.fhi.no/fp/psykiskhelse/selvmord/selvmord-og-selvmordsforsok%2D%2D-fakta/.

———. "Forekomsten av psykiske plager og lidelser i befolkningen – stabil eller i endring? [Prevalence of mental health complaints and illnesses in the population]" (2015). https://www.fhi.no/globalassets/dokumenterfiler/moba/pdf/forekomsten-av-psykiske-plager-og-lidelser-i-befolkningen%2D%2D-stabil-eller-i-endring-pdf.pdf.

———. "Forventet levealder i Norge [Life expectancy in Norway]." (2017, 7 February). https://www.fhi.no/nettpub/hin/befolkning/levealder/.

———. "Psykisk helse i Norge [Mental health in Norway]." Oslo: Folkehelseinstituttet, 2018.

———. "Selvmordsrisikoen redusert med en firedel på én generasjon [Suicide risk reduced with a quarter in one generation]." (2017, 13 December). https://www.fhi.no/nyheter/2017/selvmordsrisikoen-redusert-med-en-firedel-pa-en-generasjon/.

Norwegian Media Authority. "Dataspill: Fortsatt store kjønnsforskjeller [Computer games]." (2018, 13 February). http://www.medietilsynet.no/om/aktuelt/dataspill-og-kjonnsforskjeller/.

Norwegian Psychological Association, Pupil's Organization, Mental Health Youth, Norwegian Lector Team, Norwegian Psychiatric Organization, and Council for Mental Health. "Boken som mangler [The book that is missing]." 2015 https://www.psykologforeningen.no/foreningen/nyheter-og-kommentarer/aktuelt/krever-psykologi-i-skolen#opprop.

NRK P1. *Deprimert og ulykkelig i lykkelandet* [Depressed and unhappy in the happy nation] Podcast audio 2016. http://podtail.com/podcast/nrk-psykologen/deprimert-og-ulykkelig-i-lykkelandet/.

NRK P2. *Selvrealiseringens tyranni* [The tyranny of self-realisation]. Debatt i P2. 2018 https://radio.nrk.no/serie/debatt/KMTE82010518/09-04-2018.

NRK Presse. "Finalistene i MGPjr 2017 er klare [The finalists in MGPjr 2017 are ready]." (2017, 28 April). https://www.nrk.no/presse/finalistene-i-mgpjr-2017-er-klare-1.13492215.

NRK TV Brennpunkt. *Arnar og Mia* [Arnar and Mia]. Oslo: NRK, 2017 https://tv.nrk.no/serie/brennpunkt/MDDP11001117/19-09-2017.

NTB. "Unge voksne sliter mer med søvnen [Young people struggles with sleep]." *Aftenposten* (2016, 12 October). https://www.aftenposten.no/norge/i/PAnOR/Unge-voksne-sliter-mer-med-sovnen.

Næs, Simon Thorsell. "En katalysator for økte forskjeller [A catalyst for increased inequality]." *Morgenbladet* (2017, 3 November). https://morgenbladet.no/ideer/2017/11/en-katalysator-okte-forskjeller.

Odinsen, Hege Lyngved. "Åpen om sønnens psykiske problemer [Open about the son's mental health problems]." *VG+* (2016, 7 August). http://pluss.vg.no/2016/08/06/2495/2396_23673654.

OECD. "CO4.4: Teenage suicides (15–19 years old)." (2017, 17 October). https://www.oecd.org/els/family/CO_4_4_Teenage-Suicide.pdf.

———. "Investing in Youth Norway." Paris: OECD Publishing, 2018.

Office for National Statistics, "Suicides in England and Wales: 2019 registrations " (2020), https://www.ons.gov.uk/peoplepopulationandcommunity/birthsdeathsandmarriages/deaths/bulletins/suicidesintheunitedkingdom/2019registrations.

Orben, Amy. "Social media and suicide: a critical appraisal." *Medium* (2017, 14 November). https://medium.com/@OrbenAmy/social-media-and-suicide-a-critical-appraisal-f95e0bbd4660.

Ordnett.no. "Flink [Good]." (2018). https://www.ordnett.no/search?language=no&phrase=flink.

———. "Kjekk [Nice]." (2018). https://www.ordnett.no/search?language=no&phrase=kjekk.

———. "Symptom [Symptom]." (2018). https://www.ordnett.no/search?language=no&phrase=syndrom.

Otnes, Per. "Innledning [Introduction]." *Sosiologisk Årbok*, nr. 2 (2001): iii-vi.

P4. *Kvinner syke av egne krav* [Women ill from own demands]. P42005. Radio.

Pallesen, Ståle, Børge Sivertsen, Inger Hilde Nordhus, and Bjørn Bjorvatn. "A 10-year trend of insomnia prevalence in the adult Norwegian population." *Sleep Medicine* 15, nr. 2 (2014): 173–79.

Pascal, Blaise. "Veddemålet [The wager]." In *Pascal*, edited by Francois Mauriac, 90–99. Oslo: Gyldendal, 1954.

Paulsen, Roland. *Arbetssamhället. Hur arbetet överlevde teknologin* [The working society]. Stockholm: Atlas, 2017.

Pedersen, Ole Petter. "Kommunebarometeret [The municipality barometer]." *Kommunal Rapport*, 14 April 2011, 10–12.

Pedersen, Willy. *Ungdom er bare et ord* [Youth is just a word]. Oslo: Universitetsforlaget, 1994.

Petersen, Anders. *Præstationssamfundet* [The achievement society]. Copenhagen: Hanz Reitzel, 2016.

Petersen, Anders, and Ole Jacob Madsen. "Depression: Diagnosis and suffering as process." *Nordic Psychology* 69, nr. 1 (2017): 19–32.

Peterson, Jordan B. *12 rules for life: an antidote to chaos*. London: Allen Lane 2018.

Phoenix, Ann. "Analysing narrative contexts." In *Doing narrative research*, edited by M. Andrews, C. Squire og M. Tamboukou, 64–77 London: Sage, 2008.

Pinker, Steven. "The media exaggerates negative news. This distortion has consequences." (2018, 18 February). https://www.theguardian.com/commentisfree/2018/feb/17/steven-pinker-media-negative-news.

Psycritic. "About that Jean Twenge smartphone article." *Psycritic* (2017, 5 October). http://www.psycritic.com/2017/10/about-that-jean-twenge-smartphone-article.html.

Psykologisk Salong. *Psykologisk Salong* [Psychological saloon]. Podcast audio. Blir vi bare psykere og psykere? 2018. https://podtail.com/no/podcast/psykologisk-salong/psykologisk-salong-2-blir-vi-bare-psykere-og-psyke/.

Public Health Agency of Sweden. "Varför har den psykiska ohälsan ökat bland barn och unga i Sverige?" [Why is mental health complaints increasing among youths in Sweden?], edited by Public Health Agency of Sweden. Stockholm, 2018.

Raftery, Adrian E., Alec Zimmer, Dargan M. W. Frierson, Richard Startz, and Peiran Liu. "Less than 2 °C warming by 2100 unlikely." *Nature Climate Change* 7 (2017): 637.

Raknes, Solfrid. *Psykologisk førstehjelp barn* [Psychological first aid children]. Oslo: Gyldendal Akademisk, 2010.

———. *Psykologisk førstehjelp ungdom* [Psychological first aid adolescents]. Oslo: Gyldendal Akademisk, 2010.

Ramberg, Eirik. "'Grillet' av førstegangsvelgere ['Grilled' by first-time voters]." *Aftenposten*, 17 April 1993, 4.

Rekaa, Karoline K. "Det er ok ikke å være best i alt [It is Ok to not be best at everything]." *Aftenposten*, 24 September 2014, 11.

Ridar, Therese R. "Skal få P4 til å sprudle [Aims to get P4 to shine]." *VG*, 20 May 2001, 33–34.

Rieff, Philip. *Freud, the mind of the moralist (3rd edition.)*. Chicago: University of Chicago Press, 1979.

Riessman, Catherine Kohler. *Narrative analysis*. Newbury Park, CA: SAGE, 1993.

Ringheim, Gunnar. "Vår tåleevne er svekket [Our tolerance is watered]." *Dagbladet*, 21 November 2009, 16–17.

Rogalands Avis. "Flinke jenter sliter [Good girls struggle]." *Rogalands Avis*, 4 October 2004, n. p.

Romerikes Blad. "Ros for åpenhet [Praise for openness]." *Romerikes Blad*, 27 September 2014, 2.

Rosa, Hartmut. *Alienation and acceleration. Towards a critical theory of late-modern temporality*. New York: Columbia University Press, 2015.

Rose, Nikolas. *Governing the soul: the shaping of the private self (2nd edition.)*. London: Free Association Books, 1999.

———. *Inventing our selves: psychology, power and personhood*. Cambridge: Cambridge University Press, 1996.

Rosenthal, Robert, and Lenore Jacobson. "Pygmalion in the classroom." *The Urban Review* 3, nr. 1 (1968): 16–20.

Rothschild, David, and Neil Malhotra. "Are public opinion polls self-fulfilling prophecies?". *Research & Politics* 1, nr. 2 (2014): 1–10.

Roy, Olivier. *Globalized Islam: the search for a new Ummah*. New York: Columbia University Press, 2004.

Royal Society for Public Health. *"#Status of mind. Social media and young people's mental health and wellbeing."* 2017.

Ruud, Solveig. "Hvordan har du det? Det vil fire partier på Stortinget nå ha svar på [How are you doing?]." *Aftenposten* (2018, 11 February). https://www.

aftenposten.no/norge/politikk/i/RxrpEO/Hvordan-har-du-det-Det-vil-fire-partier-pa-Stortinget-na-ha-svar-pa.

Ryan, Richard M., and Edward L. Deci. "Self-determination theory and the facilitation of intrinsic motivation, social development, and well-being." *American Psychologist* 55, nr. 1 (2000): 68–78.

Røed, Runa. "Bekymring etter flere selvmord og selvmordsforsøk på Lillehammer [Worried after several suicides and suicide attempts in Lillehammer]." *VG* (2017, 26 May). http://www.vg.no/nyheter/innenriks/psykisk-helse/bekymring-etter-flere-selvmord-og-selvmordsforsoek-paa-lillehammer/a/24007585/.

Salmenniemi, Suvi, and Laura Kemppainen. "Masculine performers and good girls"". In *The Routledge international handbook of global therapeutic cultures*, edited by Daniel Nehring, Ole Jacob Madsen, Edgar Cabanas, China Mills, and Dylan Kerrigan, 278–292. London: Routledge, 2020.

Salvesen, Geir. "Verdikommisjonen liv laga? [Is there a future for the value commission?]" *Aftenposten*, 13 March 1999, 35.

Sanden, Monica. "Ja, eg er flink! Eg har ikkje eit syndrom [Yes, I am good!]." *Bergens Tidende*, 9 April 2016, 68–69.

Sauar, Arne. "Verken ja eller nei til kommunereformen [Neither yes or no to the municipality reform]." *Agderposten*, 29 February 2017, 19.

Schille-Rognmo, Marthe. "Ungdata, mental health and gender differences." Tromsø: University of Tromsø, 2017.

Schopenhauer, Arthur. *Verden som vilje og forestilling* [The world as will and representation]. Oslo: Solum, 2000.

Schott, Robin May, and Dorte Marie Søndergaard, ed. *School bullying: new theories in context*. Cambridge: Cambridge University Press, 2014.

Scott-Heron, Gil. "The revolution will not be televised." In *Small talk at 125th and Lenox*, 1970.

Seale, Clive. "Health and media: an overview." *Sociology of Health & Illness* 25, nr. 6 (2003): 513–31.

Seierstad, Dag. "Sosialismen og utdanningssamfunnet." In *Ny radikalisme i Norge. 34 skribenter i samfunnsdebatten*, edited by Torild Skard, 172–81. Oslo: Gyldendal, 1967.

Seligman, Martin E. P., and Steven F. Maier. "Failure to escape traumatic shock." Journal of Experimental Psychology 74 (1967): 1–9.

Selmer-Anderssen, Per Christian. "Generasjon Depresjon speiler seg selv [Generation Depression mirrors itself]." *Aftenposten*, 2 April 2017, 5.

Shafir, Eldar. "Opposites can't both be right." In *This idea must idea*, edited by John Brockman, 406–08. New York: Harper Perennial, 2015.

Simmel, Georg. "The metropolis and mental life." In *Simmel: on individuality and social forms*, edited by Donald Levine, 324–39. Chicago: Chicago University Press, 1971.

Skagestad, Linn Julie. "Man blir så redd for å gå glipp av seg selv. En narrativ analyse av depresjon hos unge voksne i lys av et samfunnspsykologisk perspektiv [I get so afraid of missing out on myself – A thematic analysis of depression among young adults]." Oslo: University of Oslo, 2014.

Skagestad, Linn Julie, and Ole Jacob Madsen. "'Man blir så redd for å gå glipp av seg selv' – En tematisk analyse av depresjon hos unge voksne [I get so afraid of missing out on myself – A thematic analysis of depression among young adults]." *Tidsskrift for Norsk psykologforening* 52, nr. 9 (2015): 750–61.

Skard, Torild. "Norge – på vei mot prestasjonssamfunnet? [Norway – on the way to the achievement society?]". In *Intelligensen som overklasse*, edited by Michael Young, 142–59. Oslo: Pax, 1966.

Skartveit, Hanne. "Det tause opprøret [The silent rebellion]." *VG*, 20 September 2014, 2–3.

Skjeldal, Eskil. "-Det ville nok vore lurt å gje meg aktiv dødshjelp [-It would be a good idea to admit me euthanasia." *Syn og Segn* 124, nr. 2 (2018): 10–22.

Skjeseth, Eli. "Digitale misjonærer [Digital missionaries]." *Aftenposten*, 21 September 2014, 2.

Skogstrøm, Lene. "TV-psykologen gråt da han tok avskjed med de åtte: – Jeg ble så glad i alle sammen [TV-psychologist cried when saying goodbye]." *Aftenposten* (2016, 20 April). https://www.aftenposten.no/osloby/i/ddRyo/TV-psykologen-grat-da-han-tok-avskjed-med-de-atte%2D%2D-Jeg-ble-sa-glad-i-alle-sammen.

Skårderud, Jo Røed. "Jentene stresser seg syke [Girls stress themselves sick]." *Klassekampen*, 22 August 2017, 6–7.

Sletten, Mira Aaboen. "Psykiske plager blant ungdom – og hva ungdom selv tror er årsaken [Mental health among youth] [PPT-presentasjon]." 2015.

———. "Psykiske plager blant ungdom: sosiale forskjeller og historien om de flinke pikene [Mental health complaints among youth]." *Oppvekstrapporten 2017* (2017): 124–47.

Sletten, Mira Aaboen, og Anders Bakken. "Psykiske helseplager blant ungdom – tidstrender og samfunnsmessige forklaringer. Notat nr 4/16 [Mental health complains among youth]." Oslo: NOVA, 2016.

Smedsland, Stine, and Thea Ågedal Mjåland. "17. mai i Grindheim 2014 [17th of May in Grindheim 2014]." In *Avis frå Byremoelevar*, edited by Janne Åvesland, Ingrid Stulien og Elise Hobbesland, 63–66, 2014.

Smith, Roger. *Being human: historical knowledge and the creation of human nature*. New York: Columbia University Press, 2007.

Smith, Steven B. *Modernity and its discontents: making and unmaking the bourgeois from Machiavelli to Bellow*. New Haven: Yale University Press, 2016.

Solberg, Per Olav. "Mener Ungdata gir et nyansert bilde [Thinks Ungdata gives a nuanced picture]." *Tidsskrift for Norsk psykologforening* 55, nr. 2 (2018): 89.

Sowell, Thomas. "Mascots of the anointed." In *The Thomas Sowell reader*, edited by Thomas Sowell, 57–59. New York: Basic Books, 2011.

Språkrådet. "Identitet [Identity]." (2009). http://www.sprakradet.no/Vi-og-vart/hva-skjer/Aktuelt-ord/Identitet/.

Stafne, Anne Lise. "Frekk dans på Black Box [Kinky dance on Black Box]." *Aftenposten*, 3 May 1993, 15.

———. "Oss i mellom: Må vi alltid lykkes? [Between the two of us: Do we always have to succeed?]" *Aftenposten*, 29 August 1987, 25.

Statistics Norway. "Døde, etter region, alder, kjønn, statistikkvariabel og år [Deceased, after region, age, gender, statistics variable and years]." *SSB* (2018). https://www.ssb.no/statbank/table/08426/tableViewLayout1/?rxid=ed401dfe-2d0d-4b38–8c37–6dd8f1d0ee88.

———. "Levekårsundersøkelsen om helse 2015 [Living conditions in health 2015]." Oslo: Statistics Norway, 2017.

———. "Tidene skifter: Tidsbruk 1971–2010 [Times are changing]." Oslo: Statistics Norway, 2012.

Stavanger Aftenblad. "Når sunnhetsiveren tar overhånd [When eagerness for fitness takes over]." *Stavanger Aftenblad*, 2 December 2011, 30–31.

Steers, Mai-Ly N., Robert E. Wickham, and Linda K. Acitelli. "Seeing everyone else's highlight reels: How Facebook usage is linked to depressive symptoms." *Journal of Social and Clinical Psychology* 33, nr. 8 (2014): 701–31.

Stigum, Hein, Sven O. Samuelsen, and Bente Traeen. "Analysis of first coitus." *Arch Sex Behav* 39, nr. 4 (2010): 907–14.

Stoknes, Per Espen. "Feil medisin! [Wrong medicine!]" *Klassekampen*, 24 August 2017, 23.

Store norske leksikon. "Selvoppfyllende profeti [Self-fulfilling prophecy]." *Store norske leksikon* (2017). https://snl.no/selvoppfyllende_profeti.

Stortingsmelding. "Meld. St. 28. Fag – Fordypning – Forståelse. En fornyelse av Kunnskapsløftet [Deposit report St. 28]." Oslo: Kunnskapsdepartementet, 2016.

Storvik, Knut. "Her er Marte Sklet Johansens tale til kongeparet [Here is Marte Sklet Johansens talk to the royal couple]." *Gudbrandsdølen Dagningen* (2017, 13 June). https://www.gd.no/kongehus/maihaugen/tale/her-er-marte-sklet-johansens-tale-til-kongeparet/s/5-18-463522.

Stridsberg, Sara. "Et åpent ansikt [An open face]." *Klassekampen*, 11 February 2017, 4–6.

August Strindberg, *The dream play* (1902), https://www.gutenberg.org/files/45375/45375-h/45375-h.htm.

Strømman, Trude W. "Fugelli vil ha politikk mot hodepine [Fugelli want politics for headaches]." *Dagbladet*, 4 November 1999, 6.

Strømmen, Kjersti. "Norge kåret til verdens lykkeligste land [Norway ranked world's happiest country]." *NRK* (2017, 20 March). https://www.nrk.no/norge/norge-karet-til-verdens-lykkeligste-land-1.13435868.

Strømø, Camilla Klovning. "'Generasjon prestasjon' med psykiske konsekvenser ['Generation achievement' with mental implications]." *Haugesunds Avis*, 3 October 2014, 13.

Stänicke, Line Indrevoll, Hanne Haavind, and Siri Erika Gullestad. "How do young people understand their own self-harm? A meta-synthesis of adolescents' subjective experience of self-harm." *Adolescent Research Review* 3, nr. 2 (2018): 173–91.

Sundbye, Bodil. "Kunsten å tenke seg glad [The art of positive thinking]." *VG*, 20 March 2018, 25–27.

Susegg, Monica Irén Solberg. "'Galskap å si at det der er en tjukk jente' ['Crazy to say that she is an overweight girl]." *Trønder Avisa*, 20 June 2014, 10.

Svenaeus, Fredrik. *Homo patologicus: medicinska diagnoser i vår tid.* Hägersten: TankeKraft, 2013.

Sweeting, Helen, Patrick West, Robert Young, and Geoff Der. "Can we explain increases in young people's psychological distress over time?". *Social Science & Medicine* 71, nr. 10 (Nov 2010): 1819–30.

Syvertsen, Bjørn Olaf. "'Flink pike'-syndromet [The good girl syndrome]." *Universitas*, 30 March 2006, n. p.

Taylor, Charles. *The ethics of authenticity.* Cambridge, MA: Harvard University Press, 1991.

Tekin, Serife. "The missing self in Hacking's looping effects." In *Mental kinds and natural kinds*, edited by H. Kincaid and J. Sullivan. Cambridge, MA: MIT Press, 2014.

Thombs, Brett D., Linda Kwakkenbos, Alexander W. Levis, and Andrea Benedetti. "Addressing overestimation of the prevalence of depression based on self-report screening questionnaires." *Canadian Medical Association Journal* 190, nr. 2 (2018): E44–E49.

Thompson, John B. *Ideology and modern culture*. London: Polity Press, 1990.

Tiller, Per Olav. "Verdiorienteringer hos tre grupper av norske skolebarn [Value orientations among three groups of Norwegian pupils]." In *Sosialpsykologi I. Familie, ungdom og kjønnsroller*, edited by Lars Hem and Harriet Holter, 86–101. Oslo: Universitetsforlaget 1978.

Trier, Joachim. *Oslo, August 31st*. Oslo: Motlys, 2011.

Troms Folkeblad. "Kom, vær med [Come, join us]." *Troms Folkeblad*, 3 October 2012, 2.

Trondhjems Adresseavis. "[Annonse] [Advertisement]." *Trondhjems Adresseavis*, 16 March 1903, 4.

Træen, Bente, Sven Ove Samuelsen, and Katrina Roen. "Sexual debut ages in heterosexual, lesbian, gay, and bisexual young adults in Norway." *Sexuality & Culture* 20, nr. 3 (2016): 699–716.

Trønderavisen. "Rekordsøkning til Sund [Record search to Sund]." *Trønderavisen*, 13 February 2016, 33.

Tuft, Anne-Berit. "Flink pike! Så god at du ikke har godt av det [Good girl! So good that it is not good for you] [personal communication]." 2018, 8 March.

TV2. "Sykt perfekt trailer [Sickly perfect trailer]." (2016). https://www.tv2skole.no/ung/artikkel/67541.

Tveit, Andreas Kokkvoll. "–Fjernt fra grasrota [-Far from the grass root]." *Klassekampen*, 21 September 2007, 5.

Twenge, Jean M. *Generation me – why today's young Americans are more confident, assertive, entitled – and more miserable than ever before*. New York: Free Press, 2006.

———. "Have smartphones destroyed a generation?" *The Atlantic*, nr. September (2017). https://www.theatlantic.com/magazine/archive/2017/09/has-the-smartphone-destroyed-a-generation/534198/.

———. *iGen: why today's super-connected kids are growing up less rebellious, more tolerant, less happy--and completely unprepared for adulthood--and what that means for the rest of us*. New York: Atria Books, 2017.

Twenge, Jean M., and W. Keith Campbell. *The narcissism epidemic: living in the age of entitlement.* New York: Free Press, 2009.

Twenge, Jean M., Thomas E. Joiner, Megan L. Rogers, and Gabrielle N. Martin. "Increases in depressive symptoms, suicide-related outcomes, and suicide rates among U.S. adolescents after 2010 and links to increased new media screen time." *Clinical Psychological Science* 6, nr. 1 (2018): 3–17.

Twenge, Jean M., and Heejung Park. "The decline in adult activities among U.S. adolescents, 1976–2016." *Child Development* (2017): 1–17.

Tybring-Gjedde, Mathilde. "Mobiltelefonen er ungdommens nye rusmiddel [Smartphone is adolescents new drug]." *Aftenposten*, 24 February 2018, 30–31.

Tørmoen, Anita Johanna. "Self-harm among adolescents: from identification to tailored treatment." Oslo: University of Oslo, 2017.

Ukeavisen Ledelse. "Egenmeldingen [Self-report]." *Ukeavisen Ledelse*, 15 January 2016, 38.

Undset, Sigrid. *Jenny*. Kristiania: Aschehoug, 1911.

Utaker, Arild. "Michel Foucault om liberalisme og nyliberalisme [Michel Foucault on liberalism and neoliberalism]." *Sosiologi i dag* 35, nr. 2 (2005): 9–31.

Valdimarsson, Emil. "Kig op, drop selviscenesættelsen, og forpligt dig til noget større [Look up, drop the performance and commit yourself to something bigger]." *Politiken*, 21 July 2018.

Vetlesen, Arne Johan. "Det døgnåpne mennesket [The open 24/7 human being]." *Morgenbladet*, 4 September 2014, 26–27.

Vetlesen, Arne Johan, and Rasmus Willig. *Hvad skal vi svare?* [What should we answer?] Copenhagen: Hans Reitzel, 2017.

Vettestad, Mia Olea. "Generasjon prestasjon [Generation achievement]." *Aftenposten*, 26 September 2014, 15.

VG. "Anmeldelse: Mot stupet [Review: Legacy]." *VG*, 2 October 1978, 40.

———. "Cappy og den nye kokken [Cappy and the new cook]." *VG*, 19 August 1952, 7.

———. "Sint veps ville stikke Anne Marie [Angry wasp wanted to sting Anne Marie]." *VG*, 5 August 1959, 5.

Vidal, Fernando. "Brainhood, anthropological figure of modernity." *History of the Human Sciences* 22, nr. 1 (2009): 5–36.

Villa, Mariann. "Materialistisk ungdom? Verdiorienteringar hos by- og bygdeungdom [Materialistic youth?]." *Tidsskrift for Ungdomsforskning* 2, nr. 1 (2002): 51–74.

von Soest, Tilmann. "Tidstrender for depressive symptomer blant norske ungdommer fra 1992 til 2010 [Time trends for depressive symptoms among Norwegian youths from 1992 to 2010]." *Tidsskrift for Ungdomsforskning* 12, nr. 2 (2012): 3–20.

von Soest, Tilmann, and Lars Wichstrøm. "Secular trends in depressive symptoms among Norwegian adolescents from 1992 to 2010." *Journal of Abnormal Child Psychology* 42, nr. 3 (2014): 403–15.

Vårt Land. "La oss oppmuntre hverandre til gode gjerninger! [Let us encourage each other to good deeds!]" *Vårt Land*, 24 November 1999, n. p.

Weber, Max. *The protestant ethic and the spirit of capitalism* (1920), https://pages.uoregon.edu/kimball/Wbr%20Protestant.Eth.ch5.htm.

Weissmann, Myrna M. "The changing rate of major depression." *Journal of the American Medical Association* 268 (1992): 3098–105.

Welzel, Christian. *Freedom rising: human empowerment and the quest for emancipation*. Cambridge: Cambridge University Press, 2013.

West, Patrick, and Helen Sweeting. "Fifteen, female and stressed: changing patterns of psychological distress over time." *Journal of Child Psychology and Psychiatry* 44, nr. 3 (2003): 399–411.

WHO. "Suicide rates, age-standardized." (2017, 4 April). http://apps.who.int/gho/data/node.main.MHSUICIDEASDR?lang=en.

Wiig, Terje. "Naturen styrker kropp og sjel [Nature strengthens body and soul]." *Aftenposten*, 22 August 1999, 20.

Wolfe, Tom. "The 'me' decade and the third great awakening." *New York Magazine*, 23 August 1976.

Wæraas, Gerd Søvli. "Fybriomyalgi/flink-pike-syndrom [Fibromyalgia/good girl syndrome]." *Adresseavisen*, 22 November 2011, 14.

Yalom, Irvin David. *Existential psychotherapy*. New York: Basic Books, 1980.

Young, Michael. "Down with meritocracy." *The Guardian* (2001, 29 June). https://www.theguardian.com/politics/2001/jun/29/comment.

———. *Intelligensen som overklasse* [The rise of the meritocracy]. Oslo: Pax, 1966.

Young, Neil. "On the beach." In *On the beach*. New York: Reprise, 1974.

Zahrnt, Heinz. *Hvorfor jeg tror* [Why I believe]. Oslo: Gyldendal, 1977.

Ziehe, Thomas. *Pubertät und narzissmus: Sind jugendliche entpolitisiert?* [Puberty and narcissism.] Hamburg: Europäische Verlagsanstalt, 1984.

———. "Ungdom och modernitet." In *Kulturanalyser. Ungdom, utbilding, modernitet* [Cultural analysis], edited by Johan Fornäs and Joachim Retzlaff, 50–61. Stockholm: Brutus Östlings Bokförlag Symposion, 1994.

Øia, Tormod, and Viggo Vestel. "Generasjonskløfta som forsvant [The generation gap that disappeared]." *Tidsskrift for Ungdomsforskning* 14, nr. 1 (2014): 99–133.

Øimoen, Marit. "Generasjon prestasjon [Generation achievement]." *Dagsavisen*, 17 September 2014, 6–7.

Index[1]

A

Addiction, 55, 175, 198
Alcohol, 115, 116, 137, 142, 235, 239, 244, 255
Anomie, 24–25, 171
Anthropological mutation, 50–52, 61, 68
Antidepressants, 9, 11, 72, 84, 111, 112, 114, 127, 155
Anywheres, 61, 91, 240

B

Body image, 107, 187
Bullying, 3, 73, 75, 80, 81, 88, 89, 93, 117, 244
Burn-out, 60, 157, 250

C

Cannabis, 115, 116, 127
Codependency, 174, 175
Collective representations, 129, 130
Community, 21, 27, 28, 34, 46, 51, 58, 62, 70, 75, 82–83, 88, 91, 93, 105, 135, 214, 215, 217, 218, 239
Competition state, 14, 132
Consciousness-raising, 252
Critique of modernity, 64, 67, 71
CV Generation, 256

D

Desymbolization, 53, 54, 67
Diagnoses of the contemporary era, 14
Disenchantment, 30, 171

[1] Note: Page numbers followed by 'n' refer to notes.

O. J. Madsen, *Deconstructing Scandinavia's "Achievement Generation"*,
https://doi.org/10.1007/978-3-030-72555-6

E

Economy of desire, 50, 52, 54, 60
Existentialism, 249–251

F

False self, 253
The Fatherless Society, 36, 37
Feminism, 241
First world problems, 6, 216
Flexibility, 50, 63, 78, 87

G

Generation Me, 123
Generation Perfection, 256
Generation snowflake, 241, 242
Generation X, 123, 124
Generation Y, 2, 123
Guilt, 10, 27, 30, 36, 54–56, 85

H

Happiest country, 9, 10, 58, 264
Happiness, 11, 12, 15, 21, 22, 27, 28, 32, 34, 37, 38, 45, 58, 59, 64, 135, 245, 250
Hash, 72, 77, 116
Healthism, 22
Homo oeconomicus, 69

I

Identity crisis, 34–35, 73
Identity politics, 52, 242
Ideological work, 220, 223
IGeneration, 123
Illness prestige, 235
Illness template, 237
Indecision, 7
Individualization, 43–45, 50, 57, 62, 71, 80–81, 87, 90–93, 109, 185, 219, 248, 252
Individuation, 20, 21, 253
Interactive kinds, 195
Iron cage, 25–27, 65

L

Last man, 21, 22
Late capitalism, 14, 48–50, 62–63, 68, 69
Late modernity, 14, 16, 17, 19, 35, 36, 41–65, 67, 71, 88, 89, 93, 171, 227, 263
Life mastery, 221, 224, 247, 248
Liquid modernity, 45–46
Loneliness, 72, 88, 101, 106, 107, 118, 121, 147, 159, 240, 253

M

Makeover self, 63
Marijuana, 116
Meaninglessness, 33, 249
Media templates, 232–233, 236
Medicalization, 140, 194
Meritocracy, 177–181
Millennials, 123, 240, 241
Modernity, 6, 11, 12, 17, 19–39, 41, 43–47, 56, 64, 65, 71, 227

N

Narcissism, 43, 123–125
Neoliberalism, 14, 48–51, 53, 56, 63, 67, 68, 219
New individualism, 14, 57, 58, 244

New openness, 162, 195
1968 generation, 123, 238

O

The obedience generation, 143, 144
The open 24/7 human being, 5

P

Paradox of health, 15, 18, 193–224, 228
Perfectionism, 100, 101, 132, 161
Performance anxiety, 152, 154, 156, 216, 237, 246
Plasticity, 43, 63
Postmodernity, 6, 45, 55, 85
Psychologizing, 155

R

Recognition, 47, 56, 82, 83, 86, 88, 107, 165, 166
Reflexivity, 43, 172, 218–222

S

The Schooled Society, 126, 127
School stress, 3, 108, 188, 218
Self-development, 58
Self-discipline, 109
Self-esteem, 100, 123, 125, 198, 199, 215, 216, 246
Self-fulfilling prophecies, 17, 169–191, 206, 210, 223, 228
Self-harm, 18, 72, 112–114, 113n63, 114n64, 140, 147
Self-help, 14, 50, 57, 59, 63, 134, 145, 156, 162, 173, 198, 221, 251, 264
Self-regulation, 247, 248
Sexual debut, 114, 115, 227
Shame, 9, 54–56, 59, 62, 121, 146, 168, 190, 240
Sleep, 5, 86
Smartphone, 120
Social acceleration, 46–47
Social media, 4, 15, 96, 105, 107, 108, 118–121, 142, 156, 167, 176, 183, 184, 187, 207, 226, 229, 239, 255, 264, 265
Social pathologies, 69, 70
Social representations, 17, 18, 129–168, 228
Somewheres, 6, 16, 86, 90–92, 240, 255
Stagnation generation, 239–241
Stress and pressure, 4, 14, 106, 112, 118, 187, 218, 221, 222, 229, 247, 252
Stressism, 220
Stress mastery, 221, 222, 224, 246, 252
Subjectivation, 14, 17, 21, 56, 61

T

Therapeutic culture, 17, 57, 199, 251
Therapeutic turn, 33–34, 59, 256
The thin self, 264, 265
Time pressure, 47, 176
Tobacco, 115
To talk about it, 190, 191, 234, 246–248, 259
Tragedy, 47, 252

U

Übermensch, 21, 22
Unemployment, 44, 49, 50, 100, 133, 226
Ungdata, 2, 3, 15, 105–107, 109, 112, 115, 116, 140, 183, 188, 195, 209, 211–214, 217, 228, 235, 236, 244, 256

V

Vandalism, 116
Violence, 62, 68, 117, 136

W

Work of culture, 51, 54

The manufacturer's authorised representative in the EU is Springer Nature Customer Service Centre GmbH, Europaplatz 3, 69115 Heidelberg, Germany. If you have any concerns regarding our products, please contact ProductSafety@springernature.com

Printed and bound by CPI Group (UK) Ltd, Croydon, CR0 4YY
22/09/2026
02221066-0009